INTUITIVE
EATING

INTUITIVE EATING

A Revolutionary Program That Works

EVELYN TRIBOLE, M.S., R.D., and
ELYSE RESCH, M.S., R.D., F.A.D.A.,
C.E.D.R.D.

St. Martin's Griffin
New York

In the writing of this book, we have changed the names and occupations of all of our personal clients so that their true identities will not, in any way, be revealed, in order to maintain their anonymity. In addition, we use the pronouns *we* and *us* when referring to our work with individual clients, rather than specifying each time which of us has worked with a particular client. It should be noted, however, that each of us has a private clientele; we do not see clients together as a team. When referring to an event in the private life of either of us, we do differentiate between us by putting in parenthesis the initials of the one involved—hence, (ET) refers to Evelyn Tribole and (ER) refers to Elyse Resch.

INTUITIVE EATING. Copyright © 1995, 2003, 2012 by Evelyn Tribole, M.S., R.D., and Elyse Resch, M.S., R.D., F.A.D.A., C.E.D.R.D. All rights reserved. Printed in the United States of America. For information, address St. Martin's Press, 175 Fifth Avenue, New York, N.Y. 10010.

www.stmartins.com

ISBN 978-1-250-00404-8 (trade paperback)
ISBN 978-1-250-01418-4 (e-book)

10 9 8 7 6

To all of our clients and patients,
who have taught us so much

Contents

Contents

Acknowledgments

There are many people whom we would like to thank, without whose help, encouragement, and inspiration this book would not have been possible.

David Hale Smith, Inkwell Management, LLC, our agent, who was instrumental in generating overwhelming interest in this concept.

Jennifer Weis, our editor, for her enthusiasm and support of Intuitive Eating and for her practical vision and input.

Mollie Traver, editorial assistant, for her clear and prompt communication, inspired ideas, and boundless encouragement in bringing the third edition of *Intuitive Eating* to fruition; Robin Carter, assistant editor, who good-naturedly helped expedite the publication of the second edition of *Intuitive Eating*; and Tina Lee, editorial assistant, who cheerfully kept us on the straight and narrow with details in the first edition.

Desy Safan Gerard, Ph.D., for her psychological support.

Marc Weigensberg, M.D., who contributed spiritual guidance for the second and third editions.

Sue Luke, R.D.; Elaine Roberts; Diane Keddy, M.S., R.D.; and Kristin Loberg, B.A., member of the Authors Guild, for their review and comments.

Arthur Resnikoff, Ph.D., for his feedback on the psychological principles used in this book.

Andrea Volz, secretarial assistant, for her endless hours in the library.

And lastly, our families and friends, whose unselfish understanding gave us the freedom to complete this book.

Foreword

This [the brain's] integrative function illuminates how reasoning,
once thought to be a "purely logical" mode of thinking, is in fact,
dependent on the nonrational processing of our bodies.
—Daniel Siegel, M.D., *Mindsight,* 2010

Intuitive Eating was originally published in 1995. Over the years, thousands of people have read this book. While reading it, they have had a sense, at a gut level, of "getting it." We've gotten many letters and e-mails saying, "you're writing about me," or "how did you know I felt this way," or "finally someone gets it." Just as so many have "gotten it"—there are others who have asked what Intuitive Eating really means. Are we just driven by instinct? Do we just "know" what and how much and when to eat? In introducing this third edition, we'd like to take this opportunity to be as clear as we can in answering the question of what Intuitive Eating really is.

Knowing a bit about the human brain can help to understand why we're born with all the wisdom we need to be Intuitive Eaters. It can also help us to see how we're able to live an Intuitive Eating life, even while being bombarded by the unending choices of natural and refined foods available to us every day—and the relentless diet messages that abound.

Humans are privileged to experience a dynamic interplay of instinct, emotion, and thought, which work together to orchestrate life, and are mediated by the brain. Psychiatrist and mindfulness expert, Daniel Siegel, M.D., calls this process "Mindsight." There are three regions of the brain responsible for this powerful integration.

The first region is called the reptilian brain, because when the early reptiles roamed the earth, they acted and responded exclusively by instinct.

They didn't rationalize or feel—they simply just went for it. As life evolved, another level of brain function developed, called the limbic brain, which mammals also possess. Emotions and social behaviors originate here. In the limbic brain, feelings are layered upon the instincts of the reptilian brain. The instincts originating from the reptilian brain are sent to the limbic brain, which serve to expand the awareness (Levine 1997). Eventually, the third key region of the brain evolved, called the rational brain, or the neocortex. The rational brain integrates instincts and feelings from the other two brain regions. The rational brain does not control instincts—instead, it perceives the instinctual and feeling parts of our beings and reflects upon them. The rational brain creates thoughts and language.

Intuitive Eating embraces all three parts of the human brain. In infancy and toddlerhood, eating is mostly instinctual. As we grow older, thoughts and feelings often play a part in our decisions about eating. As we often tell our clients, our bodies are not just composed of the tongue and the stomach, but also the mind. We have often heard someone say, "I thought that as an Intuitive Eater, I could eat whatever I wanted. So, now I eat whatever I want and as much as I want, whenever I feel like it!" This comment actually distorts the premise of Intuitive Eating. Yes, make peace with food, and eat what pleases your palate. Yes, give yourself the freedom to eat unconditionally, and eat as much as you need to satisfy your body. But, eating whenever you feel like it, without regard to hunger and fullness, might not be a very satisfying experience and might also cause physical discomfort. Attunement with your body's satiety cues is an important part of this process.

As an Intuitive Eater, you will be honoring your brain, because it is part of your body. As you go through the principles of Intuitive Eating, you will be storing information in the memory "files" that you create and house in your brain. When you feel hungry, you will need to pull up several of these files, while deciding what to eat. You will evaluate how hungry you feel and then think about what foods might satisfy your hunger and your taste buds. You might even go through a series of sensual imaginings of the taste and texture and temperature of different foods. You also may open the file to reflect on past eating experiences. You might ask yourself whether your present eating choice has worked out for you when you've eaten it in the past. Did it sustain you long enough? Did it make your blood sugar crash? Did you end up with indigestion? Or did you thoroughly enjoy the food and want to have it again? Your emotions may also come into play when you have the desire to eat. Might you be upset and are craving food to comfort and soothe yourself? Or are you bored and thinking about eating as a distraction? Considering these possibilities might inform your decision of what to eat, or even whether to eat at all.

In the beginning of your journey to reclaim your Intuitive Eater, you will probably be hyperconscious of hunger, fullness, satisfaction, thoughts, and emotions. Your brain will need to be highly in tune with your tongue and your stomach. As you become more adept at recognizing your inner signals, you may find that your instincts and intuitive wisdom take more of a prominent role in your eating experience. So, Intuitive Eating is truly about trusting that you will be able to access all of the information you need to have, by using all of the aspects of your brain—your reptilian instincts, your limbic connection with your emotions, and your rational thoughts.

Getting back to the roots of this book, it is hard for us to believe that it has been seventeen years since *Intuitive Eating* was originally published. Although the time has flown by rapidly, the years have been packed with profound experiences. We have received an innumerable number of phone calls, e-mails, and letters from people in all parts of the country and around the world. These communications have brought us into the lives of people we could never have known without this book. We have heard stories about how *Intuitive Eating* has changed lives and healed relationships with food and body. We have talked with people who are in the beginning of their journey and are reaching out to us for more individualized intensive work—whether in person or by telephone. We have also received thanks from those who have used the book as a springboard for their own personal healing and have easily succeeded in the process on their own.

We have been asked to refer people to nutrition therapists in other locales who are familiar with Intuitive Eating. We have given talks at professional meetings, as well as to students and to the lay public, and have made television appearances and been interviewed on the radio. We have been quoted in articles in newspapers, magazines, and on the Internet. *Intuitive Eating* is being used throughout the country in numerous eating disorder treatment programs. In addition, professional colleagues have asked our permission to use *Intuitive Eating* as the basis of college lectures, workshops, and seminars of their own.

The impact of all of these experiences has been deeply meaningful for us. It has given us the opportunity to broaden the work that we had previously done in our offices or by telephone, working with individuals one-on-one. We have been able to extend the philosophy of *Intuitive Eating* to those whom we would have never been able to reach, if not for the book.

It has touched our souls to be able to hear how *Intuitive Eating* has changed the lives of so many. One of the most frequent comments that we have heard from people concerns the despair that was felt after years and years of failed dieting experiences and the new hope that blossomed after finding and reading *Intuitive Eating*. We have heard how some have cleared their minds of punitive and obsessive thoughts about their eating and body perception. This clearing has made room for positive thinking and determination to make serious life changes. Self-esteem has cata-pulted, as people have reported the empowerment they have felt by work-ing with a process that honors the validity of one's inner voice. Through Intuitive Eating, they have learned to trust the wisdom that has always been within, but has been blunted by years of self-doubt. Doubting their innate eating signals had extended to doubting their beliefs about many other aspects of their lives.

We have heard stories about people who have left abusive relationships, made peace with estranged loved ones, and have made significant career changes, once their struggle with food and body has been resolved. We have also heard about new romances that, for some, could not have been possi-ble while they were occupied with body concerns and focused on the latest doomed diet attempt. Intuitive Eating has freed all of these people to go on with their lives, while leaving behind self-doubt and despair.

Intuitive Eating has also changed the lives of many of our professional colleagues. At every conference we attend, we hear comments from nutri-tion therapists and psychotherapists about how grateful they are to have this book to give to their patients. They tell us how it makes their lives easier, having it for use as a guidebook in their private practices, for classes they teach, and for seminars they give. We have also found, in our own profes-sional lives, that having a book available, which we have written, allows our patients to take something home with them to use as a reference. We've been told that it helps some people feel that they can carry a part of us with them for support when they need it!

In this third edition, there are some new additions that we hope will reach a broader base of readers and will offer some new tools for everyone. Firstly, we have added a chapter that looks at how Intuitive Eating works with kids and adolescents. Our goal is to help parents protect their children's inner wisdom about eating, with which they were born. We also want to give advice to parents about repairing a fractured relationship that they may have with their children around the eating experience. How wonderful it would be if all children were able to retain their inborn Intuitive Eating throughout their lives!

Secondly, we have included a chapter on the research validating the benefits of Intuitive Eating. When we originally cultivated the premise of Intuitive Eating, we reviewed evidence from hundreds of studies, which, in addition to our clinical experience, ultimately formed the basis behind the ten Intuitive Eating principles. Although our original concept is evidence-based (or more accurately said, evidence-inspired)—it's really not the same thing as saying, "studies show that Intuitive Eating works." Until recently, that is.

When we first wrote *Intuitive Eating,* we had no idea that our concept would generate many studies, which we find absolutely exciting! To date, there are over twenty-five studies on Intuitive Eating, with several that are currently underway.

We have also updated the chapter on eating disorders, to present our current thinking about when and how to apply Intuitive Eating principles in the treatment of eating disorders. We have also shifted our focus to finding satisfaction and have come to see it as a driving force in the Intuitive Eating process. You will see how finding satisfaction in your eating will be profoundly affected by all of the other principles in the book. Updates have also been made throughout. Over the years, we have especially become sensitive to the impact that any mention of numbers has on our readers. Whether the numbers refer to weight, height, or serving sizes and recommendations, these numbers can trigger comparison and negative feelings. So, wherever possible, numbers have been removed.

In addition, be sure to check out our new Intuitive Eating resources section, which provides information on resources (including our new Intuitive Eating Online Community)—to give you the tools and information to further support your Intuitive Eating journey.

We have also felt that it was very important to keep the appendix, entitled "Step-by-Step Guidelines" in this version of the book. This readily accessible outline will be a boon to old and new readers as you go through this journey. If it's your first time around with the book, you can choose to read the book in its entirety and then use the outline to remind you of the whole process. Or, you might decide to read about one principle at a time and then use the part of the outline that refers to that principle to fortify your focus on each step. Readers already familiar with the Intuitive Eating process can use this section as a way to review the entire concept and as a handy shorthand method of checking to see if they're on track. Whatever you choose, we hope that "Step-by-Step Guidelines" will provide a helpful tool for you in your Intuitive Eating work.

Finally, we would like to express our gratitude to the many people with whom we have had the honor to meet and work with over the years. You have been our teachers, even as we have counseled you on your healing path. You have inspired us to continue this work and bring out this third edition of *Intuitive Eating*. Thank you!

Introduction

If you could cash in every diet like a frequent flyer program, most of us would have earned a trip to the moon and back. The nearly $60 billion a year weight-loss industry could finance the trip for generations to come (Bacon and Aphramor 2011). Ironically, we seem to have more respect for our cars than for ourselves. If you took your car to an auto mechanic for regular tune-ups, and after time and money spent the car didn't work, you wouldn't blame yourself. Yet, in spite of the fact that 90 to 95 percent of all diets fail—you tend to blame yourself, not the diet! Isn't it ironic that with a massive failure rate for dieting—we don't blame the *process* of dieting?

Initially, when we ventured into the world of private practice we did not know each other. Yet, separately, each of us had remarkably similar counseling experiences that caused us to rethink how we work. This led to a considerable change in how we practice and years later was the impetus for this book.

Although we practiced independently of each other, unknowingly each of us got started by making a vow to avoid the trap of working with weight control. We didn't want to deal with an issue that was only set up to fail. But while we tried to avoid weight-loss counseling, physicians kept referring their patients to us. Typically, their blood pressure or cholesterol was high. Whatever their medical problems, weight loss was thought to be the key to treatment. Because we wanted to help these patients, we embarked on the weight-loss issue with a commitment to do it differently: Our patients would succeed. They would be among that small 5 to 10 percent success group.

We created beautiful meal plans according to our patients' likes and dislikes, lifestyles, and specific needs. These plans were based on the widely accepted "exchange system" commonly used for diabetic meal planning and weight control. We told them that this was not a diet, for even back then we knew diets didn't work. We rationalized that these meal plans were not diets, because patients could choose among chicken, turkey, fish, or lean meat. They could have a bagel, a muffin, or toast. If they really wanted a cookie, they could have one (not five!). They could fill up with "free foods" galore, so that they never had to feel hungry. We told them that if they had a craving for a particular food, they could go ahead and eat it without guilt. But we also reinforced gently, yet firmly, that sticking to their personalized plans would help them achieve their goals. As the weeks went by, our clients were eager to please us and followed their meal plans. We weighed them each week, and finally, their weight goals were met.

Unfortunately, however, some time later we started getting calls from some of these same people telling us how much they needed us again. Somehow, the weight had come back on. Their calls were very apologetic. For some reason, they couldn't stick to the plan anymore. Maybe they needed someone to monitor them. Maybe they didn't have enough self-control. Maybe they just weren't any good at this, and definitely, they felt guilty and demoralized.

In spite of the "failure," our patients put all the blame on themselves. After all, they trusted us—we were the "great nutritionists" who had helped them lose weight. Therefore, *they* had done something wrong, not us. As time went on, it became clear that something was very wrong with this approach. All of our good intentions were only reinforcing some very negative, self-effacing notions that our patients had about themselves—that they didn't have self-control, they couldn't do it, therefore they were bad or wrong. This led to guilt, guilt, guilt.

By this time, we had both reached a turning point in the way we counseled. How could we ethically go on teaching people things that seemed logical and nutritionally sound, yet triggered such emotional upheaval? Yet, on the other hand, how could we neglect an area of treatment that could have such a profound effect on a patient's future health?

As we struggled with these issues we began to explore some of the popular literature that suggested a 180-degree departure from dieting. It proposed a way of eating that allowed for any and all food choices, without regard for nutrition. Our initial reactions were highly skeptical, if not downright rejecting. We reacted with self-righteous indignation. How could we, as nutritionists (registered dietitians), trained to look at the connections between nutrition and health, sanction a way of eating that seemed to reject the very foundation of our knowledge and philosophy?

The struggle continued. The healthy meal plans were not helping people maintain permanent weight control, yet the "throw-out nutrition approach" was a dangerous option. The suggestion to ignore nutrition and disregard how the body feels in response to eating "whatever you want" discounts the respect for one's body that comes along with the gift of life.

Eventually, we resolved the conflict by developing the Intuitive Eating process. This book is a bridge between the growing anti-diet movement and the health community. While the anti-dieting movement shuns dieting and hails body acceptance (thankfully), it often fails to address health risks. How do you reconcile forbidden food issues and still eat healthfully, while not dieting? We will tell you how in this book.

If you are like most of our clients, you are weary of dieting and yet terrified of eating. Most of our clients are uncomfortable in their bodies—but don't know how to change. *Intuitive Eating* provides a new way of eating that is ultimately struggle-free and healthy for your mind and body. It is a process that unleashes the shackles of dieting (which can only lead to deprivation, rebellion, and rebound weight gain). It means getting back to your roots—trusting your body and its signals. *Intuitive Eating* will not only change your relationship with food; it may change your life.

We hope you find that *Intuitive Eating* will make a difference in your life—it has for our clients. In fact, when our clients learned that we were writing this book, they wanted to share some specific turning points with you:

- "Be sure to tell them that if they have a binge, it can actually turn out to be a great experience, because they'll learn so much about their thoughts and feelings, as a result of the binge."
- "Tell them that taking a time-out to see if they're hungry doesn't mean that they can't eat if they find they're not hungry. It's just a time-out to make sure that they're not eating on autopilot. If they want to eat anyway, they can!"
- "When I come to a session, I feel as if I'm going to the priest for confession. That comes from all the times I used to go to the diet doctor, and I would have to tell him how I had sinned after he had weighed me. This isn't coming from you, but the inner Food Police."
- "I feel like I'm out of prison. I'm free and not thinking about food all the time anymore."
- "Sometimes I get angry, because food has lost its magic. Nothing tastes

quite as good as it did when it was forbidden. I kept looking for the old thrill that food used to give me until I realized that my excitement in life wasn't going to come from my eating anymore."

- "With permission, comes choice. And making choices based on what I want and not on what somebody else is telling me, feels so empowering."

- "After giving up bingeing, I ended up feeling pretty low some of the time and even rageful at other times. I realized that the food was covering up my bad feelings. But it was also covering up my good feelings. I'd rather feel good and bad rather than not feeling at all!"

- "When I saw how much I was using dieting and eating to cope with life, I realized that I had to change some of the stress in my life if I ever wanted to let go of food as a coping mechanism."

- "Sometimes I have hungry days, and sometimes I have full days. It's so nice to eat more sometimes and not feel guilty that I'm going against some plan."

- "I get so exhilarated when I see a food I used to restrict. Now I think—it's free, it's there, and it's mine!"

- "I'm so glad you're writing this book; it will help me explain what I'm doing. All I know is that it works!"

- "When I'm in the diet mentality, I can't think about the real problems in my life."

- "This is the best I've ever taken care of myself in my life."

MINDFUL EATING VERSUS INTUITIVE EATING—IS THERE A DIFFERENCE?

When the first edition of *Intuitive Eating* was published in 1995, the term "mindful eating" was not in the public vernacular. Consequently, we used the term "conscious eating" to describe the process of being aware while eating. Four years later, in 1999, the first mindful eating study was published (Kristeller and Hallett 1999). We actually now often use the term "mindful eating," because it has become commonly used and practiced.

The Center for Mindful Eating states that mindfulness in eating includes:

- Allowing yourself to become aware of the positive and nurturing opportunities that are available through food preparation and consumption, by respecting your own inner wisdom.

cont.

Continued

- Choosing to eat food that is both pleasing to you and nourishing to your body, by using all your senses to explore, savor, and taste.
- Acknowledging responses to food (likes, neutral, or dislikes), without judgment.
- Learning to be aware of physical hunger and satiety cues to guide your decision to begin eating and to stop eating.

While *Intuitive Eating* includes the principles of mindful eating, it also encompasses a broader philosophy, addressing the issues of cognitive distortions and emotional eating. It includes seeing satisfaction as a focal point in eating, physical activity/movement for the sake of feeling good, rejecting the dieting mentality, using nutrition information without judgment, and respecting your body, regardless of how you feel about its shape.

Intuitive Eating is a dynamic process—integrating attunement of mind, body, and food. For those who struggle with eating issues, both mindful eating and Intuitive Eating can help facilitate normal eating.

Chapter 1

Hitting Diet Bottom

I just can't go on another diet, you're my last resort." Sandra had been diet-ing all her life and knew she could no longer endure a single diet. She'd been on them all, Atkins, Dukan, The Zone, South Beach, grapefruit diet . . . diets too numerous to itemize. Sandra was a dieting pro. At first dieting was fun, even exhilarating. "I always thought, this diet would be different, *this time*." And so the cycle would recharge with each new diet, each and every summer. But the weight lost would eventually rebound like an unwanted tax bill.

Sandra had hit diet bottom. By now, however, she was more obsessed about food and her body than ever. She felt silly. "I should have had this dealt with and controlled long ago." What she didn't realize was that it was the *process* of dieting that had done this to her. *Dieting* had made her more preoccupied with food. *Dieting* had made food the enemy. *Dieting* had made her feel guilty when she wasn't eating diet-types of foods (even when she wasn't officially dieting). *Dieting* had slowed her metabolism.

It took years for Sandra to truly know dieting doesn't work (yes, she was familiar with the emerging concept that dieting doesn't work, but she always thought she would be different). While most experts and consumers accept the premise that fad diets don't work—it's tough for a nation of people ob-sessed with their bodies to believe that even "sensible dieting" is futile. Sandra had been hooked into modern-age social mythology, the "big diet hope," for most of her life since her first diet at the age of fourteen.

By the age of thirty, Sandra felt stuck—she still wanted to lose weight and was uncomfortable in her body. While Sandra couldn't bear the thought of another diet, she didn't realize that most of her food issues were actually *caused* by her dieting. Sandra was also frustrated and angry—"I know everything about diets." Indeed, she could recite calories and fat grams like a walking nutritional database. That's the big caveat—losing weight and keeping it off is not usually a knowledge issue. If all we needed to be normal weight was knowledge about food and nutrition, most Americans wouldn't have weight problems. The information is readily available. (Pick up any women's magazine, and you'll find diets and food comparisons galore.)

Also, the harder you try to diet, the harder you fall (it really hurts not to succeed if you did everything right). The best description for this effect is given by John Foreyt, Ph.D., a noted expert in dieting psychology. He likened it to a Chinese finger puzzle (the hollow cylindrical straw puzzle, into which you insert an index finger on each end). The harder you try to get out, the more pressure you exert, the more difficult it is to get out of the puzzle. Instead you find yourself locked in tighter . . . trapped . . . frustrated.

SYMPTOMS OF DIET BACKLASH

Diet backlash is the cumulative side effect of dieting—it can be short term or chronic, depending how long a person has been dieting. It may be just one side effect or several.

By the time Sandra came to the office, she had the classic symptoms of diet backlash. Not only diet weary, she was eating less food, yet had trouble losing weight during her more recent diet attempts. Other symptoms included:

- *The mere contemplation of going on a diet brings on urges and cravings* for "sinful" foods and "fatty favorites," such as ice cream, chocolate, cookies, and so forth.
- *Upon ending a diet, going on a food binge and feeling guilty.* One study indicated that post-dieting binges occur in 49 percent of all people who end a diet.
- *Having little trust in self with food.* Understandably, every diet has taught you not to trust your body or the food you put in it. Even though it is the process of dieting that fails you, the failure continues to undermine your relationship with food.
- *Feeling that you don't deserve to eat,* because you're overweight.
- *Shortened dieting duration.* The life span of a diet gets shorter and shorter. (Is it no wonder that Ultra Slim-Fast's sales pitch is, "Give us a week . . . and we'll . . ."

- *The Last Supper.* Every diet is preceded by consuming foods you presume you won't eat again. Food consumption often goes up during this time. It may occur over one meal or over a couple of days. The Last Supper seems to be the final step before "dietary cleansing"—almost a farewell-to-food party. For one client, Marilyn, *every* meal felt as if it were her last. She would eat each meal until she was uncomfortably stuffed, as she was terrified she would never eat again. For good reason! She had been dieting since the sixth grade—over two-thirds of her life! She had attempted periods of fasting and a series of low calorie diets. As far as her body was concerned, a diet was only around the corner—so better eat while you can. Each meal for Marilyn was famine relief.

- *Social withdrawal.* Since it's hard to stay on a diet and go to a party or out to dinner, it just becomes easier to turn down social invitations. At first, social food avoidance may seem like the wise thing to do for the good of the diet, but it escalates into a bigger problem. There's often a fear of being able to stay in control. It's not uncommon for this experience to be reinforced by "saving up the calories or fat grams for the party," which usually means eating very little. But by the time the dieter arrives at the party, ravenous hunger dominates and eating feels very out of control.

- *Sluggish metabolism.* Each diet teaches the body to adapt better for the next self-imposed famine (another diet). Metabolism slows as the body efficiently utilizes each calorie, as if it's the last. The more drastic the diet, the more it pushes the body into the calorie-pinching survival mode. Fueling metabolism is like stoking a fire. Remove the wood, and the fire diminishes. Similarly, to fuel metabolism, we must eat a sufficient amount of calories, or our bodies will compensate and slow down.

- *Using caffeine to survive the day.* Coffee and diet drinks are often abused as management tools to feel energetic, while being underfed.

- *Eating disorders.* Finally, for some, repeated dieting is often the stepping-stone to an eating disorder (ranging from anorexia nervosa or bulimia, to compulsive overeating).

Although Sandra felt she could never diet again, she still engaged in the Last Supper phenomenon. (We regularly encounter this when we see someone for the first time.) She literally ate higher quantities of food than usual, and ate plenty of her favorite foods (she thought she would never see these foods again). It's as if she were getting ready for a long trip and was packing extra clothes. Just the thought of working on her food issues put her into the pre-diet mentality, a common occurrence.

While Sandra was just beginning to understand the futility of dieting, her desire to be thin had not changed—clearly a dilemma. She held on to the allure of the noble American dream.

THE DIETING PARADOX

In our society, the pursuit of thinness (whether for health or physique)— has become the battle cry of seemingly every American. Eating a single morsel of any high fat or non-nutritionally redeeming food is punishable by a life sentence of "guilt" by association. You may be paroled, however, for "good behavior." Good behavior, in our society, means starting a new diet, or having good intentions to diet. And so begins the deprivation cycle of dieting—the battle of the bulge and the indulge. Rice cakes one week, Häagen-Dazs the next.

"I feel guilty just letting the grocery clerk see what I buy," lamented another client, who happened to have her cart stocked with fruits, vegetables, whole grains, pasta, and a small pint of *real* ice cream. It's as if we live in a Food Police state run by the food mafia. And there always seems to be a dieting offer you can't refuse. Exaggeration? No. There's a good reason for this perception. A study published in 1993 in *Eating Disorders—The Journal of Treatment and Prevention* found that between 1973 and 1991, commercials for dieting aids (diet food, reducing aids, and diet program foods) increased nearly linearly.

The researchers also noted that there is a parallel trend in the occurrence of eating disorders. They speculate that the media pressure to diet (via commercials) is a major influence in the eating disorder trend.

The pressure to diet is fueled beyond television commercials. Magazine articles and movies contribute to the pressure to be slim. Even subtle cigarette billboards aim for the female Achilles' heel—weight—with names such as Ultra Slim 100, Virginia Slims, and so on. A Kent cigarette, "Slim Lights," especially characterizes this tug on women's body issues. Their ad reads more like a commercial for a weight loss center than for a cigarette, by highlighting slender descriptions: "long," "lean," "light." Of course the models in cigarette ads are especially slender. It is no surprise that the

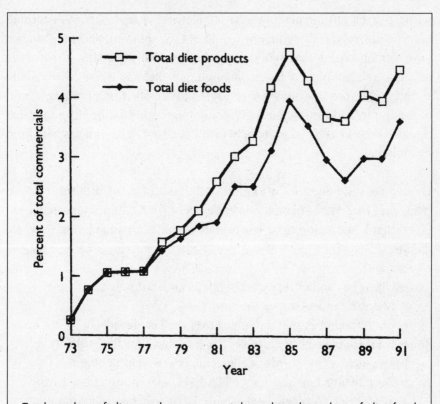

Total number of diet product commercials and total number of diet food commercials as a percent of total commercials, 1973–1991.

Reprinted with permission from: Wiseman, Claire et al. Increasing pressure to be thin: 19 years of diet products in television commercials. Eating Disorders: The Journal of Treatment & Prevention. 1(1):55, 1993.

Center for Disease Control (CDC) attributed an increase in smoking by women to their desire to be thinner. Sadly, we have heard women contemplate in our offices that they too have considered taking up smoking again as a weight loss aid.

But weight loss is not just a women's issue (although clearly there's added pressure on women). The proliferation of light-beer commercials has planted the seed of body consciousness in men's minds, as well—a lean belly is better than a beer belly. It's no coincidence we've seen the launch of magazines aimed at men, such as *Men's Fitness* and *Men's Health*.

While the pursuit of leanness has crossed over the gender barrier, sadly, we have given birth to the first generation of weight watchers. A disturbing new dieting trend is affecting the health of U.S. children. Shocking studies have demonstrated that school-age children are obsessing about their weight—a reflection of a nation obsessed with diet and weight. Around the country, children as young as six years old are shedding pounds, afraid of being fat, and are increasingly being treated for eating disorders that threaten their health and growth. Societal pressure to be thin has backfired on children.

Dieting not only does not work, it is at the root of many problems. While many may diet as an attempt to lose weight or for health reasons, the paradox is that it may cause more harm. Here's what our nation has to show for dieting:

- Obesity is higher than ever in adults and children.
- Eating disorders are on the rise.
- Childhood obesity has doubled over the last decade.
- Even though there are more fat-free and diet foods than ever before, nearly two-thirds of adults are overweight or obese.
- Over twelve hundred tons of fat have been liposuctioned from 1982 to 1992. (A recent study showed that only one year after having a liposuction procedure the fat returned, but to a different part of the body.)
- Dieting increases your chance of gaining even more weight than you lost! (See "Dieting Increases Your Risk for Gaining More Weight!" on page 7.)

DIETING CAN'T FIGHT BIOLOGY

Dieting is a form of short-term starvation. Consequently, when you are given the first opportunity to *really* eat, eating is often experienced at such intensity that it feels uncontrollable, a desperate act. In the moment of biological hunger, all intentions to diet and the desire to be thin are fleeting and paradoxically irrelevant. In those moments, we become like the insatiable man-eating plant in the movie *Little Shop of Horrors,* demanding to eat—"Feed me, feed me."

While intense eating may feel out of control, and unnatural, it is a normal response to starving and *dieting.* Yet so often, post-diet eating is viewed as having "no willpower," or a character defect. But when you interpret post-diet eating as such, it slowly erodes trust in yourself with food, diet after diet. Every diet violation, every eating situation that feels out of control lays the foundation for the "diet mentality," brick by brick and diet by diet. The seemingly brave solution—try harder next time—becomes as bewildering as the Chinese finger puzzle. You can't fight biology. When the body is starving, it needs to be nourished.

Yet so often a dieter laments, "If only I had the willpower." Clearly, this is not an issue of willpower. (Although glowing testimonials from weight loss clinics foster this misplaced blame on willpower.) When underfed, you will obsess about food—whether from a self-imposed diet or starvation.

Maybe you don't diet but eat vigilantly in the name of health and fitness. This seems to be the politically correct term for "dieting" in the nineties. But for many, it's the same food issue—with the same symptoms. Avoiding fat or carbohydrates, at all costs, and subsisting virtually on fat-free or carbohydrate-free foods is essentially dieting, and often results in being underfed. There are many forms of dieting and many types of dieters. We will explore your dieting personality and meet the Intuitive Eater in the next chapter.

DIETING INCREASES YOUR RISK FOR GAINING MORE WEIGHT!

If dieting programs had to stand up to the same scrutiny as medications, they would never be allowed for public consumption. Imagine, for example, taking an asthma medication, which improves your breathing for a few weeks, but in the long run, causes your lungs and breathing to worsen. Would you really embark on a diet (even a so-called "sensible diet"), if you knew that it could cause you to gain more weight?

Here are some sobering studies indicating that dieting promotes weight gain:

- A team of UCLA researchers reviewed thirty-one long-term studies on dieting and concluded that dieting is a consistent predictor of weight gain—up to two-thirds of the people regained more weight than they lost (Mann, et al, 2007).
- Research on nearly seventeen thousand kids ages nine to fourteen years old concluded, ". . . in the long term, dieting to control weight is not only ineffective, it may actually promote weight gain" (Field et al. 2003).

cont.

Continued

- Teenage dieters had twice the risk of becoming overweight, compared to non-dieting teens, according to a five-year study (Neumark-Sztainer et al. 2006). Notably, at baseline, the dieters did not weigh more than their non-dieting peers. This is an important detail, because if the dieters weighed more it would be a confounding factor (which would implicate other factors, rather than dieting, such as genetics).

A novel study on over 2,000 sets of twins from Finland, aged 16 to 25 years old showed that dieting itself, independent of genetics, is significantly associated with accelerated weight gain *and* increased risk of becoming overweight (Pietilaineet et al. 2011). Dieting twins, who embarked on just one intentional weight loss episode, were nearly two to three times more likely to become overweight, compared to their non-dieting twin counterpart. Furthermore, the risk of becoming overweight increased in a dose-dependent manner, with each dieting episode.

Studies aside—what have your own dieting experiences shown you? Many of our patients and workshop participants say their first diet was easy—the pounds just melted off. But that first dieting experience is the seduction trap, which launches the futile pursuit of weight loss via dieting. We say futile—because our bodies are very smart and wired for survival.

Biologically, your body experiences the dieting process as a form of starvation. Your cells don't know you are voluntarily restricting your food intake. Your body shifts into primal survival mode—metabolism slows down and food cravings escalate. And with each diet, the body learns and adapts, resulting in rebound weight gain. Consequently, many of our patients feel like they are a failure—but it is dieting that has failed them.

Chapter 2

What Kind of Eater Are You?

Perhaps you are still dieting and don't know it! There are many types of eating styles that are actually unconscious forms of dieting. Many of our patients have said they were *not* on a diet—but upon closer inspection of what and how they eat, they were still dieting!

Here's a good example. Ted came because he wanted to lose weight. He said that in his fifty years of living, he had been on only four serious diets. When perusing the book titles in the office (compulsive overeating texts, eating disorder books, and so forth) he stated, "You work with a lot of serious dieting problems . . . well I'm not one of those." Ted clearly did not see himself as a dieter, merely a careful eater. Yet it turned out that he was an unconscious dieter. Although Ted was not actively dieting, he was *undereating* to a level where he was nearly passing out in the afternoon. The reason—he had always been unhappy with his weight! In the mornings he would go for an intense hilly bike ride for one hour, come home, and eat a small breakfast. Lunch was usually salad with iced tea (while this sounds healthy, it's too low in carbohydrates). By suppertime, his body would be screaming for food. Ted was not only in a severe calorie deficit, but also carbohydrate-deprived. Evenings turned into a food fest! Ted had thought he had a "food volume" problem with a strong sweet tooth. In reality, he had an unconscious diet mentality that biologically triggered his night eating and sweet tooth.

Alicia also was not a conscious dieter. She came in not to lose weight, but because she wanted to increase her energy level. During the initial session, it became clear that she had complicated issues with food. So she was asked if she had been dieting a lot. She looked astonished. "How did you know that I've been on zillions of diets?" While Alicia claimed to be okay with her current weight, she was still at war with food; she didn't trust herself with food. As it turns out, Alicia had been dieting since she was a child. Although she was not officially dieting, she retained (and expanded) a set of food rules with each diet that nearly paralyzed her ability to eat normally. We see this all the time, the hangover from dieting: avoiding certain foods at all costs, feeling out of control the moment a "sinful" food is eaten, feeling guilty when self-imposed food rules are broken (such as "Thou shalt not eat past 6 P.M."), and so on.

Unconscious dieting usually occurs in the form of meticulous eating habits. There can be a fine line between eating for health and dieting. Notice how even the frozen diet foods such as Lean Cuisine and Weight Watchers are putting their emphasis on health rather than diet. As long as you are engaged in some form of dieting, you won't be free from food and body worries. Whether you are a conscious or an unconscious dieter, the side effects are similar—the diet backlash effect. This is characterized by periods of careful eating, "blowing-it," and paying penance with more dieting or extra-careful eating.

In this chapter, we will explore the various dieting/eating styles to help see where you are now. Later, you will meet the Intuitive Eater and the Intuitive Eating style, the solution to living without diets.

THE EATING PERSONALITIES

To help you clarify your eating style (or dieting) style, we have identified the following key categories of eaters that exhibit characteristic eating patterns: the Careful Eater, the Professional Dieter, and the Unconscious Eater. These eating personalities are exhibited even when not officially dieting. It's possible to have more than one eating personality, although we find that there tends to be a dominant trait. Events in your life can also influence or shift your eating personality. For example, one client, a tax attorney, was normally a Careful Eater, but during tax season he became the Chaotic Unconscious Eater.

You may find yourself occasionally possessing the eating characteristics described under the three core eating personalities. Take note of this, and if your eating exists in one of these domains most of the time, it can be a problem.

Read through each eating personality and see which one best reflects your eating style. By understanding where you are now, it will become easier to learn how to become an Intuitive Eater. For example, you may find you have been engaged in a form of dieting and not even have been aware of it. Or you may discover traits that unknowingly work against you.

The Careful Eater

Careful eaters are those who tend to be vigilant about what foods they put into their bodies. Ted was an example of a Careful Eater (by day). On the surface Careful Eaters appear to be "perfect" eaters. They are highly nutrition conscious. Outwardly, they seem health- and fitness-oriented (noble traits admired and reinforced in our society).

Eating Style. There is a range of food behaviors that the Careful Eater exhibits. At one extreme, the Careful Eater may anguish over each morsel of food allowed into the body. Grocery shopping trips are spent scrutinizing food labels. Eating out often means interrogating the waiter—what's in the food, how is the food prepared—and getting assurances that the food is prepared specifically to the Careful Eater's liking (usually not one speck of oil or other fat used). What's wrong with this? Aren't label reading and assertive restaurant ordering in the health interests of some people? Of course! *The difference, however, is the intensity of the vigilance and the ability to let go of any guilt in regard to your eating choice*. Careful Eaters tend to under eat and monitor the quantity of food eaten.

The Careful Eater can spend most of his or her waking hours planning out the next meal or snack, often worrying about what to eat. While the Careful Eater is not officially on a diet, his or her mind is—chastising every "unhealthy," fatty, or sugary food eaten. The Careful Eater can run the fine line between being genuinely interested in health, and eating carefully for the sake of body image.

Sometimes the Careful Eater is guided by time or events. For example, some Careful Eaters are meticulous during the weekdays, so that they earn their "eating right" to "splurge" on the weekends or for an upcoming party. But weekends occur 104 days of the year—the splurges can backfire with unwanted weight gain. Consequently, it's not unusual for a Careful Eater to contemplate going on a diet.

The Problem. There's nothing wrong with being interested in the well-being of your body. The problem occurs however, when diligent eating (almost bordering on militant) affects a healthy relationship with food—and negatively impacts your body. Careful Eaters, upon closer inspection, resemble a subtle dieter style. They may not diet, but they scrutinize every food situation.

The Professional Dieter

Professional dieters are easier to identify; they are perpetually dieting. They have usually tried the latest commercial diet, diet book, or new weight loss gimmick. Sometimes dieting takes place in the form of fasting, or "cutting back." Professional Dieters know a lot about portions of foods, calories, and "dieting tricks," yet the reason they are always on another diet is that the original one never worked. Today, the Professional Dieter is also well versed in counting carbohydrate grams.

Eating Style. Professional dieters also have careful eating traits. The difference, however, is that chronic dieters guide every eating choice for the sake of losing weight, not necessarily health. When the dieter is not officially on a diet, he or she is usually thinking about the next diet that can be started. She often wakes up hoping this will be a good day—the new beginning.

While Professional Dieters have a lot of dieting knowledge, it doesn't serve them well. It's not unusual for them to binge or engage in Last Supper eating the moment a forbidden food is eaten. That's because chronic dieters truly believe they will not eat this food again; for tomorrow they diet, tomorrow they start over with a clean slate. Better eat now; it's the last chance. Not surprisingly the Professional Dieter gets frustrated at the futility of the vicious cycle. Diet, lose weight, gain weight, intermittent binges, and back to dieting.

The Problem. It's hard to live this way. Yo-yo dieting makes it increasingly difficult to lose weight, let alone eat healthfully. Chronic under eating usually results in overeating or periodic binges.

For some Professional Dieters, the frustration of losing weight becomes so intensified that they may try laxatives, diuretics, and diet pills. And because these "diet aids" do not work, they may try extreme methods such as chronic restricting, in the form of anorexia nervosa, or purging (such as throwing up after a binge), in the form of bulimia. While anorexia and bulimia are multifactorial and rooted in psychological issues, a growing body of research has demonstrated that chronic dieting is a common stepping-stone into an eating disorder. One study in particular found that by the time dieters reach the age of fifteen years, they are eight times as likely to suffer from an eating disorder as non-dieters.

The Unconscious Eater

The Unconscious Eater is often engaged in paired eating—which is eating and doing another activity at the same time, such as watching television and eating, or reading and eating. Because of the subtleties and lack of awareness, it can be difficult for a person to identify this eating personality. There are many subtypes of unconscious eaters.

The Chaotic Unconscious Eater often lives an over-scheduled life, too busy, too many things to do. The chaotic eating style is haphazard; whatever's available will be grabbed—vending machine fare, fast food, it'll all do. Nutrition and diet are often important to this person—just not in the *critical moment* of the chaos. Chaotic Eaters are often so busy putting out fires that they have difficulty identifying biological hunger until it's fiercely ravenous. Not surprisingly, the chaotic eater goes long periods of time without eating.

The Refuse-Not Unconscious Eater is vulnerable to the mere presence of food regardless if hungry or full. Candy jars, food lying around at meetings, food sitting on a kitchen counter—none will usually be passed up by the Refuse-Not Eater. Most of the time, however, Refuse-Not Eaters are not aware that they *are* eating, or how much they are eating. For example, the Refuse-Not Eater may pluck up a couple of candies on the way to the restroom without being aware of it. Social outings that revolve around food such as cocktail parties and holiday buffets are especially tough for the Refuse-Not Eater.

The Waste-Not Unconscious Eater values the food dollar. His or her eating drive is often influenced by getting as much as they can for the money. The Waste-Not Eater is especially inclined to clean the plate (and others' as well). It's not unusual for a Waste-Not Eater to eat the leftovers from children or spouse.

The Emotional Unconscious Eater uses food to cope with emotions, especially uncomfortable emotions such as stress, anger, and loneliness. While Emotional Eaters view their eating as the problem, it's often a symptom of a deeper issue. Eating behaviors of the Emotional Eater can range from grabbing a candy bar in stressful times to chronic compulsive binges of vast quantities of food.

The Problem. Unconscious eating in its various forms is a problem if it results in chronic overeating (which can easily occur when you are eating and not quite aware of it).

Keep in mind that somewhere *between* the first and last bite of food is where the lapse of consciousness takes place. As in, "Oh, it's all gone!" For example, have you ever bought a large box of candy at the movies and begun to eat it only to discover your fingers *suddenly* scraping the bottom of the empty box? That's a simple form of unconscious eating. But unconscious eating can also exist at an intense level, in a somewhat altered state of eating. In this case, the person is not aware of what is being eaten, why he started eating, or even how the food tastes. This is zoning out with food.

WHEN YOUR EATING PERSONALITY WORKS AGAINST YOU

Eventually, the eating styles of the Careful Eater, the Professional Dieter, and the Unconscious Eater become an ineffective way of eating, even when on the surface they appear okay. The solution for the frustrated eater: Try harder with a new diet! At first the new diet seems exhilarating and hopeful, but eventually the familiar pounds return. Dieting gets more difficult, and even when you resume your baseline eating personality it may feel more uncomfortable than before. This is because with each diet the inner food rules get stronger. These food rules often perpetuate feelings of guilt about eating even when you are not officially dieting. Also, the biological effects of dieting (as detailed in chapter 5) make it increasingly difficult to have a normal relationship with food.

The Intuitive Eater personality, however, is the exception. It is the one eating style that doesn't work against you and can help you end chronic dieting and yo-yo weight fluctuations.

INTRODUCING THE INTUITIVE EATER

Intuitive Eaters march to their inner hunger signals, and eat whatever they choose without experiencing guilt or an ethical dilemma. The Intuitive Eater is an unaffected eater. Yet it is increasingly difficult to be an unaffected eater in today's health-conscious society when you consider the bombardment of nutrition, food, and weight messages from commercials, media, and health professionals.

When we've described the basic eating traits of the Intuitive Eater to our clients, it's amazing how often we'll hear the response, "That's how my wife eats." or "That's how my boyfriend eats." When we ask how that person's weight and relationship to food are, the response is, "No problem!"

Consider toddlers. They are the natural Intuitive Eaters—virtually free from societal messages about food and body image. Toddlers have an innate wisdom of food, if you don't interfere with it. They don't eat based on dieting rules or health, yet study after study shows that if you let a toddler eat spontaneously, he will eat what he needs when given free access to food. (This is probably the toughest thing for a concerned parent to do—to let go and trust that kids have an innate ability to eat!) (See Chapter 15 for more information on raising Intuitive Eaters.)

A landmark study, led by Leann Birch, Ph.D. and published in the *New England Journal of Medicine* confirmed that preschool-age children have an innate ability to regulate their eating according to what their bodies need for growth. This holds true, even when, meal by meal, the little tykes' eating appears to be a parent's nightmare. Researchers found that at a given meal, caloric intake was highly variable, but it balanced out over time. Yet, many parents assume that their young children cannot adequately regulate their food intake. Consequently, parents often adopt coercive strategies in an attempt to ensure that the child consumes a nutritionally adequate diet. But previous research by Birch and her colleagues indicates that such *control* strategies are counterproductive.

Furthermore, Birch notes that "parents' attempts to control their child's eating were reported more often by obese adults than by adults of normal weight." Similarly, Duke University psychologist, Philip Costanzo, Ph.D., found that excess weight in school-age children was highly associated with the degree to which parents tried to restrain their children's eating. Even well-meaning parents interfere with Intuitive Eating. When a parent tries to overrule a child's natural eating cues, the problem gets worse, not better.

A parent who feeds a child whenever a hunger signal is heard and who stops feeding when the baby shows that he's had enough, can play a powerful role in the initial development of Intuitive Eating.

In fact, groundbreaking work by therapist and dietitian Ellyn Satter has shown that if you get the parents of overweight kids to back off and let them eat without parental pressure, the kids will eventually eat *less*. Why? The child begins to hear and understand his own inner signals of hunger and satiety. The child also knows that he or she will have access to food.

According to Satter, "Children deprived of food in an attempt to be thin become preoccupied with food, afraid they won't get enough to eat, and are prone to overeat when they get the chance." We have found this to be true for adult dieters as well. Only for adults, the Intuitive Eating process has been buried for a long time, often years and years. Instead of having a parent loosen up the pressure, this loosening of pressure has to come from within and against society's myth of dieting and distorted body worship.

Fortunately, *we all possess the natural Intuitive Eating ability*; it's just been suppressed, especially by dieting. This book is devoted to showing you how to awaken the Intuitive Eater within.

HOW YOUR INTUITIVE EATER GETS BURIED

As toddlers get a little older, the mixed messages begin to creep in—from the early influences of the Saturday morning food commercial, to the well-meaning parent who coaxes his child to "Clean your plate." The assault does not stop when you are a child. There are several external forces that influence our eating, which can further bury Intuitive Eating.

Dieting. You have already seen the damage that chronic dieting plays, including but not limited to:

- Increased binge eating
- Decreased metabolic rate
- Increased preoccupation with food
- Increased feelings of deprivation
- Increased sense of failure
- Decreased sense of willpower

This only serves to erode your trust with food and urges you to rely on *external* sources to guide your eating (a food plan, a diet, the time of day, food rules, and so forth). The more you go to external sources to "judge" if your eating is in check, the *further* removed you become from Intuitive Eating. Intuitive Eating relies on *your* internal cues and signals.

Eat Healthy-or-Die Messages. Messages about eating healthfully are everywhere, from nonprofit health organizations to food companies touting the health benefits of their particular product. The inherent message? What you eat can improve your health. Conversely, take one wrong move (bite) and you're one step closer to the grave. Is this an exaggeration? No. For example, a 1994 press release issued by the Harvard School of Public Health stated that eating trans-fatty acids (found in margarine) may cause thirty thousand deaths each year in the U.S. from heart disease. That kind of message can easily leave you feeling guilty for eating the "wrong" kind of food and feeling confused about what you should eat.

Magazines and newspapers have also greatly increased their coverage of food and health. One food editor, Joe Crea, of a major metropolitan newspaper, the *Orange County Register* (California), noted that in a six-year period (1987–1993) his stories on nutrition increased fivefold. Of nearly eight hundred food stories, two hundred were on health-related issues. While there is no doubt that what you eat can have an impact on your health, the exponential media coverage has served as a conduit to building food paranoia in the consumer, especially the dieter. Joe Crea agrees, "You open the paper, see a beautiful lead story about cheesecake, and simultaneously another piece on how overeating will make you fat. It puts the reader in conflict."

Are we saying that you should ignore the virtues of healthful eating? Of course not. However, when you have a dieting mind-set, the barrage of "healthy eating" messages can make you feel guiltier about the food you choose to eat. *Obesity and Health* reported a survey on 2,075 adults in Florida that revealed that 45 percent of adults felt *guilty* after eating foods they like. (Keep in mind that this survey was conducted to reflect typical American demographics. These "guilt-by-eating" numbers would most likely be much higher if performed on dieters.)

Women may be especially guilt-ridden. An American Dietetic Association Gallup poll showed that women feel guiltier than men about the food they eat (44 percent versus 28 percent). Could this be because women diet more frequently than men? Or because women are usually the target of health messages and food ads (consider the number of women's magazines). Women are the key decision makers for the family's health care, and are usually the gatekeepers of food and nutrition issues, as well; they serve as a prime target.

We have found that establishing nutrition or healthy eating as an *initial* priority in the Intuitive Eating process is counterproductive. In the beginning we *ignore* nutrition, because it interferes with the process of relearning how to become an Intuitive Eater. Nutrition heresy? No. It's possible to respect and honor nutrition. It just can't be the first priority when you've been dieting all your life. Or look at it this way, if you have focused all your attention on nutrition, has it helped? The most nutritious eating plan (absolute) can become embraced as another form of a diet.

To get an idea of whether you are already an Intuitive Eater, or where you might need some further work, see "Are You an Intuitive Eater?" on page 19. It is adapted from research, which defines Intuitive Eating characteristics.

You can recapture Intuitive Eating, but first you have to get rid of the diet mentality rules that keep the Intuitive Eater buried. In the next chapter, we will briefly introduce you to the core principles of Intuitive Eating. The remainder of the book will show you step-by-step how to become an Intuitive Eater.

SUMMARY OF EATING STYLES

Eating Style	Trigger	Characteristic
Careful Eater	Fitness and health	Appears to be the perfect eater. Yet anguishes over each food morsel and its effect on the body. On the surface, this person seems health- and fitness-oriented.
Unconscious Eater	Eating while doing something else at the same time	This person is often unaware that she/he is eating, or how much is being eaten. To sit down and simply eat is often viewed as a waste of time. Eating is usually paired with another activity to be productive. There are many subtypes.
Chaotic Unconscious Eater	Overscheduled life	This person's eating style is haphazard—gulp 'n' go when the food is available. Seems to thrive on tension.

SUMMARY OF EATING STYLES

Eating Style	Trigger	Characteristic
Refuse-Not Unconscious Eater	Presence of food	This person is especially vulnerable to candy jars, or food present in meetings or sitting openly on the kitchen counter.
Waste-Not Unconscious Eater	Free food	This person's eating drive is often influenced by the value of the food dollar and is susceptible to all-you-can-eat buffets and free food.
Emotional Unconscious Eater	Uncomfortable emotions *unhealthiest* *binge/restrict*	Stress or uncomfortable feelings trigger eating—especially when alone.
Professional Dieter	Feeling fat *biggest drive*	This person is perpetually dieting, often trying the latest commercial diet or diet book.
Intuitive Eater	Biological hunger *paired w/ health*	This person makes food choices without experiencing guilt or an ethical dilemma. Honors hunger, respects fullness, enjoys the pleasure of eating.

ARE YOU AN INTUITIVE EATER?

This quiz is adapted from Tracy Tylka's research on Intuitive Eaters (2006). It will give you an indication of whether you are an Intuitive Eater, or perhaps where you might need some further work.

Directions: The following statements are grouped into Tylka's three core characteristics of Intuitive Eaters. Answer "yes" or "no" for each statement. If you are unsure of how to respond, consider if the description usually applies to you—is it mostly "yes" or "no"?

cont.

Continued

UNCONDITIONAL PERMISSION TO EAT

Yes No

☒ ☐ 1. I try to avoid certain foods high in fat, carbs, or kcal.

☐ ☒ 2. If I am craving a certain food, I don't allow myself to have it.

☒ ☐ 3. I follow eating rules of diet plans that dictate what, when, and/or how to eat.

☒ ☐ 4. I get mad at myself for eating something unhealthy.

☒ ☐ 5. I have forbidden foods that I don't allow myself to eat.

EATING FOR EMOTIONAL RATHER THAN PHYSICAL REASONS

☐ ☒ 1. I find myself eating when I'm feeling emotional (anxious, sad, depressed), even when I'm not physically hungry.

☐ ☒ 2. I find myself eating when I am bored, even when I'm not physically hungry.

☒ ☐ 3. I cannot stop eating when I feel full (not overstuffed).

☒ ☐ 4. I find myself eating when I am lonely, even when I'm not physically hungry.

☒ ☐ 5. I use food to help me soothe my negative emotions.

☐ ☒ 6. I find myself eating when I am stressed, even when I'm not physically hungry.

RELIANCE ON INTERNAL HUNGER/SATIETY CUES

☐ ☒ 1. I cannot tell when I'm slightly full.

☐ ☒ 2. I cannot tell when I'm slightly hungry.

☒ ☐ 3. I do not trust my body to tell me *when* to eat.

☒ ☐ 4. I do not trust my body to tell me *what* to eat.

☒ ☐ 5. I do not trust my body to tell me *how much* to eat.

☐ ☒ 6. When I'm eating, I cannot tell when I am getting full.

Scoring: Each "yes" statement indicates an area that likely needs some work. The section with the greatest amount of "yes" responses indicates the area that needs the most attention.

this ↙
is ↙
wrong
(handwritten margin note)

Chapter 3

Principles of Intuitive Eating: Overview

Only when you vow to discard dieting and replace it with a commitment to Intuitive Eating will you be released from the prison of yo-yo weight fluctuations and food obsessions. In this chapter, you will be introduced to the core principles of Intuitive Eating—a snapshot of each concept, with a case study or two. The most significant achievement of each client mentioned was gaining a healthy relationship with food and their bodies. By following the ten principles of Intuitive Eating, you will normalize your relationship with food. A focus on weight loss must be put on the back burner. If your current weight has resulted from being out of touch with your internal wisdom about eating, and as a result of tuning back in to this wisdom, weight loss occurs, so be it. If, however, you are already maintaining your set point weight through a process of restricting, overeating, restricting, and so forth, then it is especially important to put weight loss on the back burner.

Later in the book, each principle will be discussed in greater detail. You may find it useful to return to this chapter for a quick reference.

PRINCIPLE 1:

REJECT THE DIET MENTALITY

Throw out the diet books and magazine articles that offer you the false hope of losing weight quickly, easily, and permanently. Get angry at the lies that have led you to feel as if you were a failure every time a new diet stopped working and you gained back all of the weight. If you allow even one small hope to linger that a new and better diet might be lurking around the corner, it will prevent you from being free to rediscover Intuitive Eating.

James dieted most of his life, starting with the little diets his mother put him on and ending with a liquid protein fast, which gave him his most recent short-lived "success." By the time he came to the office, James weighed more than he ever had in his life. He knew he was incapable of ever going on another diet but felt guilty because he thought he "should." *Rejecting the diet mentality* was a key milestone for James. He discovered that he was not a failure, but that the system of dieting itself created the setup for failure.

Today, James is a committed ex-dieter who found his way back through Intuitive Eating. He no longer feels that he "should" be on a diet. He is pleased and amazed that his weight has normalized, while eating everything he likes. Ironically, James sadly watches his boss go from diet to diet, while truly knowing that dieting is the quickest short-circuit to a healthy relationship with food.

PRINCIPLE 2:

✖ HONOR YOUR HUNGER

Keep your body biologically fed with adequate energy and carbohydrates. Otherwise you can trigger a primal drive to overeat. Once you reach the moment of excessive hunger, all intentions of moderate, conscious eating are fleeting and irrelevant. Learning to honor this first biological signal sets the stage for rebuilding trust with yourself and food.

A critical step to becoming an Intuitive Eater for Tim, a busy physician, was learning to honor his hunger. Tim dieted all through medical school while trying to keep up with a frenetic schedule, working over eighty hours a week. He felt hungry most of the time but ignored these signals, because he was "watching his weight." By midafternoon, his eating was out of control, with snack attacks at the vending machine. His weight fluctuated with each dieting attempt (and failure). Not surprisingly, he felt low in energy most of the time.

Today, Tim has learned to pay attention to his biological signals of hunger and to honor them by taking the time to feed himself. He knows now, that if he doesn't listen to his growling stomach and eat breakfast before he leaves for work, he can't concentrate on what his patients are saying during their morning appointments. Tim has learned to *honor his hunger.*

As a result of becoming an Intuitive Eater, Tim feels full of energy throughout the day. He has ended the cycles of restriction and overeating that plagued him for twenty years and feels confident that this futile cycle is gone forever.

PRINCIPLE 3:

✱ MAKE PEACE WITH FOOD

Call a truce; stop the food fight! Give yourself unconditional permission to eat. If you tell yourself that you can't or shouldn't have a particular food, it can lead to intense feelings of deprivation that build into uncontrollable cravings and, often, bingeing. When you finally "give in" to your forbidden foods, eating will be experienced with such intensity, it usually results in Last Supper overeating and overwhelming guilt.

Nancy is a waitress, whose battleground was the gourmet restaurant where she worked. This restaurant offered an array of delicious, rich foods. Before becoming an Intuitive Eater, Nancy would valiantly refrain from all of the tempting foods available at the restaurant. She would leave each night, physically tired and with haunting visions of the foods she thought she shouldn't have. Her restraint was consistent, until making her first appointment. Suddenly in the week prior to coming in, all she wanted to do was eat. And eat, she did!

Nancy experienced the Last Supper effect that accompanies intense food deprivation. She had an eating backlash from not allowing herself to touch her favorite foods. Nancy believed any nutritionist would confirm that she had to give up these foods for good *and* follow a rigid meal plan. She acknowledged feeling scared and angry about her future food loss and automatically went into a phase of overeating, especially of foods that she perceived would be forever forbidden.

Now that Nancy is an Intuitive Eater, she eats whatever appeals to her at the restaurant (and elsewhere). She no longer restricts the foods she likes, nor does she overeat and feel guilty. She discovered that some of the foods that looked wonderful didn't even taste good! Nancy has made *peace with food* and loves the freedom that comes with it.

PRINCIPLE 4:

CHALLENGE THE FOOD POLICE

Scream a loud "no" to thoughts in your head that declare you're "good" for eating under a thousand calories or "bad" because you ate a piece of chocolate cake. The Food Police monitor the unreasonable rules that dieting has created. The police station is housed deep in your psyche, and its loudspeaker shouts negative barbs, hopeless phrases, and guilt-provoking indictments. Chasing the Food Police away is a critical step in returning to Intuitive Eating.

As an adolescent, Linda had been a competitive track sprinter and went on to qualify for the Olympic trials. Linda's coach had been a strong influence in her life, and to this day, her coach's voice reverberates, "To be competitive, you must diet to get rid of body fat." She can also hear her mother's voice chiming in about which foods are "good" and "bad."

Years of weight fluctuations resulted from obeying the monotonous dieting tapes droning in her head. These inner tapes originated from her well-meaning coach and numerous diets, only to be reinforced with negative messages that her mother doled out. Linda's Food Police strengthened with each diet, each coachly admonishment, and motherly chastisement.

Linda's breakthrough came when she discovered how to *Challenge the Food Police*. Linda learned to talk back to the inner critical voices that tried to restrict her food choices. She learned to give herself nurturing messages and make nonjudgmental decisions about her eating.

The voice of the Intuitive Eater was allowed to reemerge once the Food Police were silenced. Linda is guilt-free about her eating, and her weight has stabilized at its natural level without dieting.

PRINCIPLE 5:

FEEL YOUR FULLNESS

Listen for the body signals that tell you that you are no longer hungry. Observe the signs that show that you're comfortably full. Pause in the middle of a meal or snack and ask yourself how the food tastes, and what your current fullness level is.

Jackie was a party girl. She loved to go out to eat with her friends every night after work and felt that weekends were not complete without a party. Jackie loved life and loved to eat. But she also didn't know how to stop eating when she began to feel full. (Rather she often did not recognize feeling full until she was uncomfortably satiated, stuffed.) The morning after each social event she made the same vow, "I never want to eat again. I feel sick and stuffed and bloated, and I hate this roll around my middle."

Learning to *feel fullness* was a key element in Jackie's journey to Intuitive Eating. She began to pay attention to the transition from an empty stomach to a slightly full stomach. She soon learned to sense the signals of fullness that started to emerge in the midst of her meals.

It was easier for Jackie to honor her body's satiety signals when she truly knew she could eat again if hungry (even within the hour) and eat her favorite foods. (What starving person would stop at comfortable fullness if he thought he was never going to eat again, or have access to a particular food?) Jackie made an interesting observation while feeding alley cats during one of her out-of-town parties: The starving alley cat will eat until the bowl is licked clean, unlike finicky cats—they know they will be fed again, so can easily turn up their tails and leave food in their dish. Finicky cats can honor fullness because they know they will eat again.

Jackie also discovered that by honoring satiety signals and pushing her plate away (when *she* was ready), she felt that she was showing more respect for herself. After becoming an Intuitive Eater, Jackie felt that she had it all. She could still go out with her friends whenever she liked, and she could wake up the next morning feeling great!

PRINCIPLE 6:

DISCOVER THE SATISFACTION FACTOR

The Japanese have the wisdom to keep pleasure as one of their goals of healthy living. In our fury to be thin and healthy, we often overlook one of the most basic gifts of existence—the pleasure and satisfaction that can be found in the eating experience. When you eat what you really want, in an environment that is inviting, the pleasure you derive will be a powerful force in helping you feel satisfied and content. By providing this experience for yourself, you will find that it takes much less food to decide you've had "enough."

---

ok, great, but what if nothing satisfies?

Denise is a production assistant who was surrounded by a variety of "forbidden" foods each day when she went to the set. Instead of giving herself permission to eat what she really wanted, she would ignore her preference signals. If she wanted French fries, she would nobly substitute an austere baked potato, unadorned. If cookies beckoned, she'd settle for fruit. Rather than stopping at her substitute food choice, however, she'd continue to seek out food after food, trying to find satisfaction in unsatisfying foods.

Once Denise realized that all of these alternate food choices were only fillers, that none of them led her to feel satisfied, she decided to experiment and eat what she was craving. She was delighted to find that not only did she get true pleasure from the food, but also she stopped eating as soon as she finished the portion—sometimes even leaving some behind! She was satisfied, content—not needing to seek out yet another replacement for her "phantom food." Denise *discovered the satisfaction factor* in eating. She eats far less than ever before, and has experienced the benefits of our motto, "If you don't love it, don't eat it, and if you love it, savor it."

PRINCIPLE 7:

COPE WITH YOUR EMOTIONS WITHOUT USING FOOD

Find ways to comfort, nurture, distract, and resolve your emotional issues without using food. Anxiety, loneliness, boredom, and anger are emotions we all experience throughout life. Each has its own trigger, and each has its own appeasement. Food won't fix any of these feelings. It may comfort for the short term, distract from the pain, or even numb you into a food hangover. But food won't solve the problem. If anything, eating for an emotional hunger will only make you feel worse in the long run. You'll ultimately have to deal with the source of the emotion, as well as the discomfort of overeating.

Marsha was a writer who did most of her work at home. She loved her work, but sometimes found that she would have mini periods of writer's block. To relieve her tension about finding the right word to put on the computer, she would visit the kitchen many times during the day to get a snack. Marsha was *using* food to help her get her work done.

Lisa was a fourteen-year-old who would come home after school and plop herself down in front of the TV with a bag of potato chips. Lisa was *using* food to procrastinate doing her homework.

Cynthia's children were grown; she had an illness that depleted her energy, not allowing her to go to work, and her husband didn't pay much attention to her. Cynthia found food to keep her occupied when she was bored and to soothe her lonely soul.

Using food to cope with emotions comes in degrees of intensity. For some, food is simply a means of distraction from boring activities or a filler for empty times. For others, it can be the *only* comfort they have to get through a painful life.

Before becoming Intuitive Eaters, Marsha, Lisa, and Cynthia were coping with the problems of their lives by using food as a distracter, comforter, and calmer. But they soon learned to savor the foods they had chosen, eat in an inviting environment, and honor their biological hungers. Increased gratifying eating experiences allowed each to let go of using food as a coping mechanism. These experiences also offered clarity—it was easier to distinguish an eating urge from an emotional urge.

These women discovered that food never tasted as good or was as satisfying when they weren't really hungry, or hadn't figured out what they really wanted to eat, or bolted food down without respecting fullness. Marsha, Lisa, and Cynthia learned to *cope without using food* and to find appropriate outlets for their emotions. Now they save their eating for the times it gives them true satisfaction and eat far smaller quantities of food.

PRINCIPLE 8:

✗ RESPECT YOUR BODY *My biggest issue*

Accept your genetic blueprint. Just as a person with a shoe size of eight would not expect realistically to squeeze into a size six, it is equally futile (and uncomfortable) to have a similar expectation about body size. Respect your body, so you can feel better about who you are. It's hard to reject the diet mentality if you are unrealistic and overly critical of your body shape.

One of the most important goals that Andrea made while working toward becoming an Intuitive Eater was to *respect her body*. She was fifty years old, had given birth to four children, and was a valuable member of the community. Her body had gotten her through childbirth, traveling, working, and exercise. It was a body to respect rather than belittle. Yet, Andrea spent many of her waking hours criticizing her body and missing the days when she was younger and thinner. The more she made negative comments to herself, the more despair she felt. She would go to food when she wasn't hungry to console herself for her misery. She also found herself overeating as a way to punish herself for looking so "bad."

Once Andrea stopped comparing herself to every other woman she knew and started to respect and honor her body, she began to eat less, and to take better care of herself. Andrea became an Intuitive Eater, took pride in her achievements, and stopped trying to have the "perfect" body!

Janie, a twenty-five-year-old publicist, also played the "body-check" game. Every time she was at a party, she silently compared herself to other women, only to feel that she was the heaviest woman in attendance. Ironically, Janie had a very fit build, but felt mortified every time and would vow that night to begin a diet the next day. Only when Janie began to focus on respecting her body and its inner cues, rather than external forces (what other people look like, what other people are doing) did she make a significant breakthrough.

PRINCIPLE 9:   *I've got this one down*

EXERCISE—FEEL THE DIFFERENCE

Forget militant exercise. Just get active and *feel* the difference. Shift your focus to how it feels to move your body, rather than the calorie burning effect of exercise. If you focus on how you feel from working out, such as energized, it can make the difference between rolling out of bed for a brisk morning walk or hitting the snooze alarm. If when you wake up, your only goal is to lose weight, it's usually not a motivating factor in that moment of time.

Miranda had all the accoutrements of a regular exerciser—a membership in a gym, a stationary bike at home, athletic clothes and shoes. There was just one problem—she was *not* exercising. Miranda was burned out. She had tried almost as many new exercise programs as she had diets. It was a vicious cycle—begin a diet and simultaneously begin working out, and then quit both the diet and the exercise. That was precisely the problem. Miranda never really felt the pleasure of exercise, of moving her body. Part of the problem was that when she was underfeeding her body (dieting), she had little energy, if any, to exercise—and that *does not feel good.* Consequently, exercising was always a struggle. It was only the initial enthusiasm and momentum of the diet that would carry her through a monotonous workout. But because dieting was short-lived, so too was exercise.

When Miranda began feeding her body (by *honoring her hunger),* she felt better and entertained the idea of beginning a walking program. She discovered that by reframing the purpose of exercise from a weight loss tool to *feeling* good, she began to actually enjoy walking. For the first time in her life Miranda has consistently exercised, and *enjoys* it. She also knows that she will continue to be consistent, because she enjoys the payoff, which includes feeling better about herself.

PRINCIPLE 10:

HONOR YOUR HEALTH—GENTLE NUTRITION

Make food choices that honor your health and taste buds while making you feel good. Remember that you don't have to eat a perfect diet to be healthy. You will not suddenly get a nutrient deficiency, or gain weight from one snack, one meal, or one day of eating. It's what you eat consistently over time that matters. Progress, not perfection, is what counts.

↳ but I'm a perfectionist

Louise, like so many of our clients, had dieted all her life. She had been enlightened by the anti-dieting movement and was ahead of the game with a reject-dieting mentality. But Louise had been meticulously counting fat grams like a dieter counting calories—in essence she was still dieting. She was using nutritional information militantly to keep herself in check. Her food choices were primarily fat-free foods; they were safe and healthy, she reasoned. Yet, Louise couldn't understand why she was still bingeing. When Louise realized that she was using nutrition as a dieting weapon, rather than as an ally for health, she began to change the way she chose her foods. Louise honored her taste buds and listened to her body with respect to how food made her feel. When Louise was finally able to relax her eating, to eat with less rigidity, she discovered that it was possible to honor both the pleasure of taste and her health. And by doing this, she was more satisfied with eating, and her binges ceased.

A PROCESS WITH GREAT REWARDS

All of the clients mentioned in the previous examples had been dissatisfied with their relationship with food and their bodies. Each had tried either formal or informal dieting and had felt failure and despair. By learning the principles of Intuitive Eating and putting them to work, each found a deepening of the quality of life and resolution about eating. You can too!

Chapter 4

Awakening the Intuitive Eater: Stages

The journey to Intuitive Eating is like taking a cross-county hiking trip. Before you even strap on your hiking boots, you'd want to know what to expect during your journey. While a road map is helpful, it doesn't describe what you'll need to be adequately prepared, such as trail conditions, climate, special sightseeing spots, what kind of clothes to wear, and so forth. The purpose of this chapter is to help you understand what to expect during your journey to Intuitive Eating.

Whether it's hiking or relearning a more satisfying eating style, you will go through many stages along the way. The amount of time that you need to stay in any particular stage is variable and highly individualized. For example, traversing new hiking trails depends on how physically fit you are, how you deal with fear of new trails, how much time you have to hike, and the availability of hiking trails. Similarly, your journey back to Intuitive Eating depends on how long you've been dieting, how strongly entrenched your diet thinking is, how long you've been using food to cope with life, how willing you are to trust yourself, and how willing you are to put weight loss on the back burner and learning to become an Intuitive Eater the primary goal.

Sometimes, you'll move back and forth among the stages. If you accept that this is a normal part of the process, it will help you to keep going without feeling that you are backsliding or not making progress.

Consider this scenario: You are on a hiking trail, and encounter a fork in the road that is hard to decipher with your trail map. Do you go to the right or left? You ponder for a while and decide to go left. While walking, you spot something you've never seen before, a bright green caterpillar shimmying up a purple flower. A few steps ahead, you discover an unusual bird. But a few steps beyond these glories of nature is a big boulder signaling that you chose the wrong path. You turn around, go back to the fork, and take the other path. Was this detour a waste of time? No! Similarly, on the path to Intuitive Eating, you will take many turns and experiment with new thoughts and behaviors. You may even find that after making noticeable progress, you go back to old ways that are uncomfortable and unfulfilling. But like taking the "wrong" path on the scenic hiking trail, you'll discover that excursions into old eating patterns can be used as learning experiences. (Most hikers would not chide themselves for being unsure of which path to take; instead, they'd be grateful for the discoveries of nature that a blocked path offered.) It's important to be kind to yourself and appreciate the learning that comes out of the experience. This process involves coming from a place of curiosity rather than a place of judgment, so whatever you do, don't beat yourself up mentally!

Intuitive Eating is very different from dieting. Dieters usually get frustrated when they don't follow the diet path exactly as prescribed. We have seen many a chronic dieter merely take a wrong turn at one meal, be critical for that mistake, and "blow" the diet for that day or weekend or even longer!

Keep in mind that the journey to Intuitive Eating is a *process,* complete with ups and downs, unlike dieting where the common expectation is linear progress (losing a certain amount of weight in a specific time period).

The road to Intuitive Eating is like investing in a long-term mutual fund. Over time, there will be a return on the investment, in spite of the daily fluctuations of the stock market. It is normal and expected. How ironic that we have been taught that, in economics, the day-to-day changes in the stock market are normal, and seldom is there a quick get-rich fix, yet, in the multibillion dollar a year weight loss business, "get thin fast" is the only goal for success. We are invested, instead, in helping you bring peace to your eating life and body image. On the path to this goal, keep in mind Webster's definition of *process*: "a continuing development involving many changes" and "a particular method of doing something, generally involving a number of steps or operations."

As with any process, it's important to stay focused in the present, and grow from the many experiences you will encounter. If, however, you focus on the end result (which for many people is weight or the amount of pounds lost), it can make you feel overwhelmed and discouraged, and end up sabotaging the process. Instead, if you acknowledge small changes along the way and value the learning experiences (which can sometimes be frustrating), it will help you stay on the Intuitive Eating path and move forward. Once you truly become an Intuitive Eater, you will consistently tune in to your inner wisdom, and you will feel better in mind, body, and spirit.

At this point, we feel it is important to clarify the issue of the pursuit of weight loss. For some, your body will return to its natural weight level, which may be lower than your current weight and remain there. To see if this applies to you, ask yourself the following questions: Have you routinely eaten beyond your comfortable fullness level? Do you routinely overeat when you're getting ready for your next diet (knowing that there will be a lot of foods you won't be allowed to eat on the diet)? Do you overeat as a coping mechanism in difficult times or to fill up time when you're bored? Have you also been resistant to exercise? Do you only exercise when you are dieting? Do you skip meals or wait to eat until you're ravenously hungry, only to find that you overeat when you finally do eat? Do you feel guilty, either when you overeat or when you eat what you call a "bad food," which results in more overeating? If you answered "yes" to some or all of these questions, then it's likely that your present weight may be higher than the weight your body is meant to maintain. It is also likely that you will be able to return to your natural, healthy weight, as a result of this process. But, remember, weight loss MUST be put on the back burner. If you focus on weight loss, it will interfere with your ability to make choices based on your intuitive signals.

Once you've given up on the futility of dieting forever, you'll find yourself eating far less food with a desire to experience regular movement in your life. You'll find that your body feels so much better when your stomach isn't overfilled, when your muscles are toned, and your heart is fit. You will also find that as your thoughts about your eating and body begin to change, you will experience a more peaceful feeling, rather than the chronic background anxiety that looms with every food choice. However, if you continue to focus on weight loss as the goal, you'll get tied up in the old diet-mentality thinking, which does not serve you.

Over the years, we have seen that our patients go through a five-stage progression in learning how to become an Intuitive Eater. The following section will help you get an idea of what to expect in your own personal journey.

STAGE ONE:
READINESS — HITTING DIET BOTTOM

This is where most people begin. You are painfully aware that every attempt to lose weight has ended in "failure." You are tired of valuing each day based on whether the scale is up or down a pound or two (or if you overate the day before). You think and worry about food all the time. You talk the restrictive food talk—"If only I didn't have to watch my weight, I could eat that," or "I had two cookies—I was really bad today."

At the present time, your weight might be higher than ever before, or, while not greatly overweight, you lose and gain five or ten pounds as frequently and rapidly as you wash your clothes and they get dirty once again!

You have lost touch with biological hunger and satiety signals. You have forgotten what you really like to eat and instead eat what you think you "should" eat. Your relationship with food has developed a negative tone, and you dread eating the foods you love, because you're afraid it will be hard to stop. When you give into the temptation of forbidden foods, it's not unusual to overeat them, because you feel guilty. Yet, you sincerely vow you will never eat them again.

It's not unusual to find that you eat to comfort, distract, or even numb yourself from your feelings. If that's the case, you will sense that the quality of your life has been clouded by obsessional thinking about food and by mindless eating.

Your body image is negative—you don't like the way you look and feel in your body, and self-respect is lessened. You have learned from your own experience that dieting does not work—you have hit diet bottom and feel stuck, frustrated, and discouraged.

This stage continues until you decide that you are unhappy eating and living this way—you are ready to do something about it. Your first thoughts may veer toward finding a new diet to solve your problems. But almost immediately, you realize that you just can't do that one ever again. If this is where you find yourself, then you are ready for the process that will bring you back to eating intuitively.

STAGE TWO:
EXPLORATION — CONSCIOUS LEARNING AND PURSUIT OF PLEASURE

This is a stage of exploration and discovery. You will go through a phase of *hyperconsciousness* to help reacquaint yourself with your intuitive signals: hunger, taste preferences, and satiety.

This stage is a lot like learning how to drive a car. For the novice driver, just getting the car out of the driveway requires a lot of conscious thinking, complete with a mental checklist: Put the key in the ignition, make sure the gear is in park or neutral, turn on the engine, check the rearview mirror, remove the hand break, and so forth. This hyperconsciousness is necessary to lock in all of the steps needed just to get that car into Drive! In the same sense, you will be zooming in on details of eating that have evolved without such focused thinking. (But this is necessary to reclaim the Intuitive Eater in you.)

It may seem awkward and uncomfortable, even obsessive. However, hyperconsciousness is different than obsessive thinking. Obsessive thinking is pervasive and is characterized by worry. It fills your mind during most of the day and keeps you from thinking of much else. Hyperconsciousness is more specific. It zooms in when you have a thought about food, but goes away when the eating experience is over. And just like the steps required to drive a car become autopilot for the experienced driver, Intuitive Eating will eventually be experienced without this initial awkwardness.

You may feel that you are in a hyperconscious state much of the time during this stage. This may feel uncomfortable at first and perhaps even strange. Remember, much of your previous eating was either mostly mindless or diet-directed.

sounds good but scary

In this stage, you'll begin to *make peace with food* by giving yourself unconditional permission to eat. This part may feel scary, and you may choose to move slowly (within your comfort level). You will learn to get rid of guilt-induced eating and begin to discover the importance of the satisfaction factor with food. The more satisfied you are when eating, the less you think about food when you are not hungry—you will no longer be on the prowl.

You will experiment with foods that you may not have eaten for a long time. This includes sorting out your *true* food likes and dislikes. You may even discover that you don't like the taste of some of the foods you've been dreaming of! (Keep in mind that years of dieting, or eating what you "should" only serve to disconnect you from your internal eating drive and true food preferences.)

You will learn to *honor your hunger* and recognize your body signals that indicate the many degrees of hunger. You will learn to separate these biological signals from the emotional signals that might also trigger eating.

In this stage, you may find that you are eating larger quantities of foods than your body needs. It will be difficult to *respect your fullness* at this stage, because you need time to experiment with the quantity it takes to satisfy a deprived palate. It also takes time for you to develop trust with food again and know that it's truly okay to eat. How can you honor fullness, if you are not completely sure it's okay to eat the particular food, or if you fear it won't be there tomorrow?

If you have previously been gaining weight, weight gain usually ceases or is limited to just a few pounds. If you have been using food emotionally, you may find that you will begin to *feel* your feelings and may experience discomfort, sadness, or even depression at times.

The bulk of your eating may be foods that are heavier in fat and sugar than you've been accustomed to—although you may have been eating large quantities of these foods secretly or with guilt. *The way you eat during this stage will not be the pattern that you will establish or want for a lifetime.* You will notice that your nutritional balance is off kilter and you may not feel physically on top of things during this time. This is all normal and expected. You must let yourself go through this stage for as long as you need. Remember, you are making up for years of deprivation, negative self-talk, and guilt. You are rebuilding positive food experiences, like a strand of pearls. Each food experience, like each pearl, may seem insignificant, but collectively they make a difference.

OK I'm officially terrified of this stage

STAGE THREE:
CRYSTALLIZATION

In this stage, you will experience the first awakenings of the Intuitive Eating style that has always been a part of you, but was buried under the debris of dieting. When you enter this stage, much of the exploration work from the previous stage begins to crystallize and feels like solid behavior change. Your thoughts about food are no longer obsessive. You hardly need to maintain the hyperconsciousness about eating that was originally needed. Consequently, your eating decisions don't require quite as much directed thought. Instead, you find that your food choices and responses to biological signals are mainly intuitive.

You have a greater sense of trust—both in your right to choose what you really want to eat and in the fact that your biological signals are dependable. You are more comfortable with your food choices and will start to notice increased satisfaction at your meals.

At this point, you *honor your hunger* most of the time, and it's easier to discern what you feel like eating when you are hungry. You continue to *make peace with food*.

What feels new in this stage is that it's easier to take a time-out in the midst of your meal to consciously gauge how much your stomach is filling up. You will be able to take note of your fullness and respect the presence of that signal, although you may find that you often eat beyond the fullness mark. Just like when an archer takes aim at a new target, it often requires shooting many arrows before learning how to reach the bull's-eye. You may still be choosing previously forbidden foods most of the time, but you will find that you don't need as much of them to satisfy you.

If you've been an emotionally cued eater, you'll become quite adept at separating biological hunger signals from emotional hunger. Because of this clarity, more often than not, you will be experiencing your feelings and finding ways to comfort and distract yourself without the use of food.

Remember to put weight loss on the back burner. Far more important than weight loss, is the sense of well-being and empowerment that begins to take place. You won't feel helpless and hopeless anymore. You will begin to respect your body and understand that if you're over your natural weight, it's a result of the dieting mentality, rather than lack of willpower.

STAGE FOUR:
THE INTUITIVE EATER AWAKENS

By the time you reach this stage, all of the work you have been doing culminates in a comfortable, free-flowing eating style. You consistently choose what you really want to eat when you are hungry. Because you know that you can have more food, of your choosing, whenever you are hungry, it's easy to stop eating when you feel comfortably full.

You may begin to find that you choose healthier foods, not because you think you should, but because you *feel* better physically when you eat this way. The urgent need to prove to yourself that you can have previously forbidden foods will have diminished. You truly know and trust that these foods will always be there, and if you really want to eat them, you can—so they lose their alluring quality. Chocolate starts to take on the same emotional connotation as a peach. You won't need to test yourself anymore, and your deprivation backlash with food will be gone.

When you do choose the foods you used to restrict, you will get great pleasure, and feel satisfied with a much smaller quantity than ever before, and without guilt. (When you feel guilty eating a food, it takes away much of the pleasure from eating.)

If coping with your feelings had been difficult for you, you will be less afraid to experience them, and become more adept at sitting with them. Finding healthy alternatives to distract and comfort yourself when necessary will become natural for you.

Your food talk and self talk will be positive and noncritical. Your peace pact with food is firmly established, and you will have released any conflict or leftover guilt about food choices that you have carried around.

You have stopped being angry with your body and making disrespectful comments about it. You respect it and accept that there are many different sizes and shapes in the world. At this point, and if it's meant to be, your body will be on its way to approaching its natural weight.

STAGE FIVE:
THE FINAL STAGE—TREASURE THE PLEASURE

At this point your Intuitive Eater has been reclaimed. You will trust your body's intuitive abilities—it will be easy to *honor your hunger* and *respect fullness*. Finally, you will feel no guilt about your food choices or quantities. Because you feel good about your relationship to food and treasure the pleasure that eating now gives you, you will discard unsatisfying eating situations and unappealing foods.

You will want to experience eating in the most optimal of conditions and not taint it with emotional distress. You will feel an inner conviction to give up using food to cope with emotional situations, if that has been your habit. When emotions become too overwhelming. you will find that you would much rather deal with your feelings or distract yourself occasionally from them with anything other than food.

Because your eating style has become a source of pleasure rather than an affliction, you will experience nutrition and movement in a different way. The *burden* of exercise will be removed, and exercising will begin to look enticing to you. Exercise will no longer be used as a driving force to burn more calories; rather, you become committed to exercise as a way to *feel* better, physically and mentally. Likewise, nutrition will no longer be another mechanism to make you feel bad about the way you eat; instead, it becomes a path to feeling as physically good and healthy as you can.

When you reach the final stage, your weight will settle into what is natural for you—a place that is comfortable and appropriate for your height and body frame. If your weight was already normal, you will find that you will maintain it with no effort and will be rid of the emotional ups and downs that accompany the restriction/overeating cycles.

At last, you will feel empowered and protected from outside forces telling you what and how much to eat, and how your body should look. You will feel free from the burden of dieting. And you will be an Intuitive Eater once again.

YOU CAN DO IT!

These stages and the changes that occur with your eating and thoughts may seem impossible. Or, it might seem too scary. For example, the thought of giving yourself unconditional permission to eat may seem terrifying—and you might fear that you will never stop eating or gaining weight. The remainder of the book explains in great detail how to implement each principle, why it is needed, and the rationale behind it. You will also learn how other chronic dieters became Intuitive Eaters and how it changed their lives. By the time you finish reading this book, you will know that you too can become an Intuitive Eater, and stop the madness of dieting.

Chapter 5

PRINCIPLE 1:
Reject the Diet Mentality

Throw out the diet books and magazine articles that offer you false hope of losing weight quickly, easily, and permanently. Get angry at the lies that have led you to feel as if you were a failure every time a new diet stopped working and you gained back all of the weight. If you allow even one small hope to linger that a new and better diet might be lurking around the corner, it will prevent you from being free to rediscover Intuitive Eating.

If you're like most clients we see, the idea of *not* dieting can be scary (even when you know that you can't choke down one more diet plan or drink). It's normal to feel panicky about letting go of dieting, especially when the world around you is on some diet. It has been the only tool you have known to lose weight (albeit temporarily).

Hitting diet bottom is a paralyzing feeling—damned if you diet and damned if you don't. Many of our clients feel stuck between two conflicting fears: "If I continue dieting, I'll ruin my metabolism and gain weight" and "If I stop dieting I'll gain *more* weight." Other common fears that we hear are:

FEAR: If I stop dieting, I won't stop eating.

REALITY: Dieting is often the *trigger* for overeating. Of course it's hard to stop eating when you've been undereating and restricting food. It's a normal response to starvation (you'll learn more about that in the next chapter). But once your body learns (and trusts) that you will not be starving it anymore (through dieting), the intense drive for eating will decrease.

FEAR: I don't know how to eat when I'm not dieting.

REALITY: When you banish diets and become an Intuitive Eater, you will be eating in response to inner signals, which will guide your eating. This is like learning how to swim for the first time. The feeling of being surrounded by water can be terrifying to the novice swimmer, especially when totally submerged. Similarly, being surrounded by food can be terrifying to the chronic dieter, who is learning how to eat again. But you will not learn how to swim by merely standing at the edge of the pool (even while believing that learning how to swim is a good thing). First you begin by getting your feet wet and learning how to breathe in the water. Eventually you will put your head in the water when you are ready—and you get more comfortable.

FEAR: I will be out of control.

REALITY: Control is not an issue in Intuitive Eating. Instead, you will be relying on your internal signals, rather than on external factors and authority figures (whom you're bound to defy). Nobody can be the expert of "you." Only *you* know your thoughts, feelings, and experiences. You will learn to trust your internal wisdom and will learn to listen to and honor your inner cues (both physical and emotional), all of which feels empowering.

THE DIET VOID

For many people dieting has been a way to cope with life, from filling up time, to serving as a symbol of control over your life. Think of the times in your life in which you started a diet. How often did your diets coincide with difficult times or transitions in your life? It's not unusual to begin a diet during the following life transitions: passing from childhood to adolescence, leaving home, marrying, starting a new job, or when experiencing marital difficulties. While dieting may have been futile, it offered excitement and hope—the exhilaration of quick weight loss and the excitement of watching the scale inch downward. The hope—that this diet will be it. It's similar to going to a hairstylist for a new cut, with the expectation that it will revolutionize the way you look and feel about yourself and maybe change your life. But when you say good-bye to the thrill and excitement of dieting, you'll also be letting go of the false hope and disappointments from dieting.

There's a social element to dieting that you may miss, *diet bonding*. When you decide to give up dieting, you might be surprised how often new diets and dieting are the topics of conversation at parties, with friends, at work—and now you won't be playing *that* game. It might feel like a must-see movie everyone is talking about, only you haven't seen it and have no plans to view it either. You might feel a little left out, detached.

Remember, as long as there is money to be made, there will always be a new gimmick or diet for a quick weight loss fix. At one point, the manufacturer of a product called "Sleepers Dieter" claimed to help people attain greater weight loss while sleeping. Talk about dreaming! The manufacturer was fined by the FTC for making unsubstantiated claims. But people still shelled out the money for this new gimmick.

THE ONE-LAST-DIET TRAP

The initial step to becoming an Intuitive Eater is to reject the diet mentality. Yet even when you come to terms with the futility and harm that dieting unleashes on the body (and mind), it can be a difficult first step, as described in a letter below from a client, Lisa:

> *I have been in the dieting dilemma all my life. Every diet I've ever been on has worked for me, at least what I thought of as worked. Worked in the past was losing a certain number of pounds, never considering the reality of regaining the weight, plus more, with each and every diet I went on. At age thirty-six, I came to a point in my life where I was dieted-out. I knew there had to be another way. Yet my first thought was to let myself find* one *more diet for the last time, and I would make a promise to myself to never gain the weight back through a change in lifestyle.*

Lisa's letter represents a common conflict of chronic dieters. You've hit diet bottom, you know dieting doesn't work, but you're desperate—just one more diet, just this time, "I'll be good." And so begins the familiar chronic dieter's plea: Just let me lose the weight now, and *after* I lose the weight, I'll figure it out. But as long as you cling to a small hope that a quick little diet will turn your weight around, or jump-start you into a new person, you won't be free from the tyranny of dieting. Giving into just-one-more-diet is one of the biggest traps, because it doesn't face the reality—diets do not work. So how could another diet truly be part of the solution?

Jackie, another client, had been consistently dieting since the age of twelve. By the time she came in, Jackie thought she was ready to give up dieting. Jackie made a lot of progress in three months, which for her was stabilizing weight, rather than gaining weight. For the first time, she began to have a normal relationship with food rather than constant food worry and obsession. But she wanted to take a break from our work together. Five months later, Jackie called—she desperately needed to come back. Jackie said that she "finally got it." She knew once and for all that dieting creates *more* problems. Jackie revealed that during her initial work with Intuitive Eating, she had secretly hoped that a little diet was all she needed. She thought losing some quick pounds would allow her to work on her "real food issues," without worrying about her body, and then she would have more patience. It was part of her reason for leaving.

When Jackie left, she dabbled with two serious quickie diets, which resulted in disaster. She lost ten pounds quickly (through juice fasting and intense exercise) and got excited. She was so "motivated" that she was sure if she lost another ten pounds, through a different food-combining diet, her problems would be over. Jackie couldn't have been further from the truth. She became more obsessed with food and began bingeing. Not only did she gain back every pound, she was *heavier,* more frustrated, and had less trust in herself with food.

Every diet is like a hula hoop flung onto your body. At first it's effortless to keep the hoop in motion. But eventually massive layers of hula hoops disrupt normal rhythm and become binding. You cannot rotate the hula hoop—you can't even move. To get yourself out of the last-chance diet trap, you need to come to terms with the fact that dieting doesn't work and can, in fact, be harmful. (Remember, a body of research shows that the act of dieting increases your risk of gaining even more weight. This holds true for kids, teens, and adults. We believe that if people really knew that embarking on a diet could cause your body to gain more weight, they would not go down the futile dieting path.)

Perhaps you're inclined to argue, however, that you'll *feel* better about yourself *when* you lose the weight. But studies have shown that improvements in psychological well-being associated with weight loss are just as temporary as the pounds lost and regained. The "good feelings" diminish with regained weight, and existing issues of self-worth and general psychological function return to initial levels when the weight is regained.

PSEUDO-DIETING

Many of our clients state, "I've given up dieting" but they still have trouble shaking the diet mentality. They may be physically off of a diet, but the dieting thoughts remain. The problem is that dieting thoughts usually translate into diet-like behaviors, which becomes *pseudo-dieting* or unconscious dieting. Consequently, these clients will still suffer the side effects of dieting, but it's much harder to spot (and then they really feel out of control with their eating). *Pseudo-dieting* behaviors are not usually apparent to the person engaged in them. Keep in mind that eating is so universal that it's hard to be objective. It can be difficult to find the loopholes in your own eating mentality/behavior if you don't know what you are looking for. To the surprise of our clients they often don't discover that they have been pseudo-dieting until *together* we review their Intuitive Eating journal. Here are some examples of pseudo-dieting:

• *Meticulously counting carbohydrate grams* is the modern version of counting calories. While being conscious of what you eat has its merits, the act of counting carbohydrate grams to control weight is really no different than counting calories. Many of our chronic dieters are pros at rationing their carbohydrate grams for the day—and they are stuck.

• *Eating only "safe" foods.* This usually means sticking with fat-free and/or low-calorie foods, beyond counting carbohydrate grams. For example, one client would not eat any food that listed more than one gram of fat on the food label, regardless of what her total fat and calorie intake for the day was. Remember, however, that one food, one meal, or one day will not make or break your health or your weight.

• *Eating only at certain times of the day,* whether or not you are hungry, is a common leftover habit from dieting, especially *not* eating after a certain time of night, such as after 6 P.M. Reality check: Our bodies do not punch time clocks; we do not suddenly turn off our need for energy at a certain time. This can especially be a problem for a dieter who exercises after work, comes home late around 7:30 P.M., and decides it's too late to eat for fear that the fat meter is in high gear. While it is reasonable not to want to go to bed on a full stomach because it would be uncomfortable, to deny a hungry body *any* food or energy is unreasonable.

⭐*Paying penance for eating "bad" foods* such as cookies, cheesecake, or ice cream. The penalty can include skipping the next meal, eating less, vowing to be "good" tomorrow, or doing *extra* exercise.

⭐ *Cutting back on food,* especially when feeling fat or when a special event such as a wedding or class reunion comes up. While cutting back sounds innocent enough, it's amazing how often this gets acted out in the form of unconscious *undereating*. Remember, under eating usually triggers overeating.

• *Pacifying hunger by drinking coffee or diet soda.* This is a common dieting trick to assuage hunger pangs without eating or calories.

• *Limiting carbohydrates.* We are struck by the number of clients who profess they know of the importance of consuming this form of fuel, yet eat an *inadequate* amount of carbohydrates, such as bread, pasta, rice, etc., because they are afraid they will gain weight.

• *Putting on a "false food face" in public.* You only eat what is "proper" in front of other people. One client, Alice, ate an enjoyable meal with friends. When the dessert tray came around she really wanted a piece of pie, but fought the urge, because she wanted to appear to be the healthy/weight-conscious eater. However, on her way home, the urge for the pie swelled into an uncontrollable craving. Alice stopped at the store, bought a whole pie, and ate one-fourth of it—*more* than she would have eaten had she honored her true food preference! This social dieting behavior of putting on a false food face backfired (and it often does).

• *Competing with someone else who is dieting . . .* feeling obligated to be equally virtuous (if not more). Because dieting is viewed as a virtuous trait in our society, it is not unusual that you would get sucked into appearing virtuous. This can easily occur when friends, family, or a significant other is dieting.

• *Second-guessing or judging what you deserve to eat* based on what you've eaten earlier in the day, rather than on hunger cues. One client, Sally, ate two large bowls of puffed rice cereal for breakfast after running for one hour. She thought that was too much food and later in the midmorning did not allow herself to eat, although she was ravenous. Sally thought, "How could I be hungry only two hours after I ate a big breakfast?" The reality for Sally was that while her volume of food in the morning was larger than her norm, it was still *inadequate* for the amount of exercise she did. Her body was trying to tell her, "I need more fuel." Yet Sally felt guilty for being hungry. She also felt guilty for eating a big breakfast, until she realized that in actuality she had *under eaten.* Just because a meal or snack does not fit the "standard" portion size from your dieting days, it does not mean you are overeating!

• *Becoming a vegetarian or eating a gluten-free diet only for the purpose of losing weight.* A vegetarian lifestyle can be a healthy way of eating and living, but if it is embraced with a diet mentality, it becomes merely another diet. For example, Karen began eating meatless to lose weight. But a month into her vegetarian eating, she began craving meat. Never before had she experienced meat cravings! Karen realized she never really intended to become a vegetarian. She wasn't interested in vegetarian eating for health or ethical issues, only as a vehicle to lose weight, and so her diet backfired.

THE DIETER'S DILEMMA

Whether you are engaged in bona fide dieting or pseudo-dieting, any form of dieting is bound to lead to problems. The inherit futility of dieting is explained in the Dieter's Dilemma chart created by psychologists, John P. Foreyt and G. Ken Goodrick, shown below. The Dieter's Dilemma is triggered by the desire to be thin, which leads to dieting. That's when the dilemma unfolds. Dieting increases cravings and urges for food. The dieter gives into the craving, overeats, and eventually regains any lost weight. He

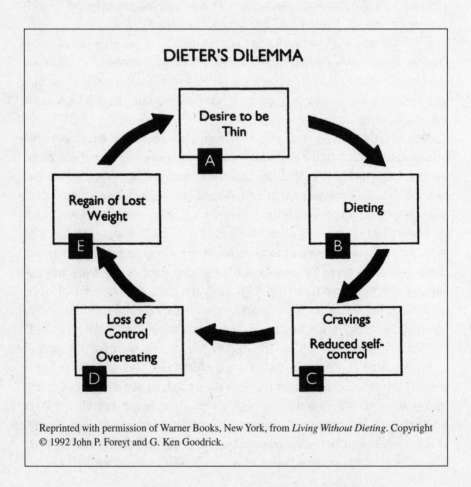

Reprinted with permission of Warner Books, New York, from *Living Without Dieting*. Copyright © 1992 John P. Foreyt and G. Ken Goodrick.

is back to where he started, with the original weight—or higher. And once again the dieter has the desire to be thin . . . and so another diet begins. The Dieter's Dilemma is perpetuated and gets worse with each turn of the cycle. The dieter is heavier and feels more out of control with eating.

How do you break the futile Dieter's Dilemma? You must simply make the decision to give up dieting. Although the anti-dieting movement is growing in popularity, there is always a new diet or program around the corner.

HOW TO REJECT THE DIET MENTALITY

To let go of the dieting myth and the dieting mentality, our minds require a new frame of reference. In the best-selling book, *The 7 Habits of Highly Effective People,* author Stephen Covey popularized the concept of paradigm shifts. A paradigm is a model or frame of reference by which we perceive and understand the world. In the world of weight management, dieting is the cultural paradigm by which we attempt to control our weight. A paradigm shift is a break with tradition, with old ways of thinking, with old paradigms. We must change our paradigm to reject dieting; only then can we build a healthy relationship with food and our bodies.

While Covey's work is aimed at the business community, he hits upon an issue that rings true for chronic dieters. He believes that people are often drawn to remedy the problem without regard to the long-term implications of this "quick fix." He feels that this approach actually exacerbates the problem rather than permanently solving it. He points to the physical body as a prized asset that often is ruined while one is on the race for rapid results and short-term benefits.

Here are the steps to begin your paradigm shift of rejecting the diet mentality.

STEP 1:
RECOGNIZE AND ACKNOWLEDGE THE DAMAGE THAT DIETING CAUSES

There is a substantial amount of research on the harm that dieting causes. Acknowledge that the harm is real, and that continued dieting will only perpetuate your problems. Some of the key side effects gleaned from major studies are described below in two categories, biological and emotional. As you read, take a personal inventory, and ask yourself which of the problems you are already experiencing. Recognizing that dieting is the problem will help you break through the cultural myth that diets work. Remember, *if dieting is the problem, how can it be part of the solution?*

Damage from Dieting: Biological and Health

In every century, famine and human starvation have existed. Sadly, this is true even today. Survival of the fittest in the past meant survival of the fattest—only those with adequate energy stores (fat) could survive a famine. Consequently, our bodies are still equipped in this modern age to combat starvation at the cellular level. As far as the body is concerned, dieting is a form of starvation (even though it's voluntary).

• *Chronic dieting teaches the body to retain more fat when you start eating again.* Low-calorie diets double the enzymes that *make* and store fat in the body. This is a form of biological compensation to help the body store more energy, or fat, after dieting.

• *Chronic dieting slows the rate of weight loss* with each successive attempt to diet. This has been shown in both rat and human studies.

• *Decrease metabolism.* Dieting triggers the body to become more efficient at utilizing calories by lowering the body's need for energy.

• *Increase binges and cravings.* Both humans and rats have been shown to overeat after chronic food restriction. Food restriction stimulates the brain to launch a cascade of cravings to eat *more.* After substantial weight loss, studies show that rats prefer eating more fat, while people have been shown to prefer foods both high in fat and sugar.

• *Increase risk of premature death and heart disease.* A thirty-two-year study of more than three thousand men and women in the Framingham Heart Study has shown that *regardless of initial weight,* people whose weight repeatedly goes up and down—known as weight cycling or yo-yo dieting—have a higher overall death rate and twice the normal risk of dying of heart disease. These results were independent of cardiovascular risk factors, and held true regardless if a person was thin or obese. The harm from yo-yo dieting may be equal to the risks of staying obese.

Similarly, results of the Harvard Alumni Health Study show that people who lose and gain at least eleven pounds within a decade or so, don't live as long as those who maintain a stable weight.

• *Cause satiety cues to atrophy.* Dieters usually stop eating due to a self-imposed limit rather than inner cues of fullness. This, combined with skipping meals, can condition you to eat meals of increasingly larger size.

• *Cause body shape to change.* Yo-yo dieters who continually regain the lost weight tend to regain weight in the abdominal area. This type of fat storage increases the risk of heart disease.

Other documented side effects include headaches, menstrual irregularities, fatigue, dry skin, and hair loss.

Damage from Dieting: Psychological and Emotional

Psychological experts reported the following adverse effects at the landmark 1992 National Institutes of Health, Weight Loss and Control Conference:

• Dieting is linked to eating disorders. (In an unrelated study, dieters were eight times as likely to suffer from an eating disorder by the age of fifteen, than non-dieters.)
• Dieting may cause stress or make the dieter more vulnerable to its effects. Independent of body weight itself, dieting is correlated with feelings of failure, lowered self-esteem, and social anxiety.
• The dieter is often vulnerable to loss of control over eating when violating "the rules" of the diet, whether there was an actual or *perceived* transgression of the diet. The mere perception of eating a forbidden food (regardless of actual calorie content) is enough to trigger overeating.

In a separate report, psychologists David Garner and Susan Wooley make a compelling case against the high cost of false hope from dieting. They conclude that:

• Dieting gradually erodes confidence and self-trust.
• Many obese individuals assume they could not have become obese unless they possessed some *fundamental character deficit.* Garner and Wooley argue that while many obese individuals may experience binge eating and depression, these psychological and behavioral symptoms are the *result of dieting.* But these overweight

individuals easily interpret these symptoms as further evidence of an underlying problem. Yet, obese people do not have inordinate psychological disturbances compared to normal-weight people.

Step 2:
Be Aware of Diet Mentality Traits and Thinking

The diet mentality surfaces in subtle forms, even when you decide to reject dieting. It's important to recognize common characteristics of the diet mentality; it will let you know if you are still playing the dieting game. Forget about willpower, being obedient, and failing. The general traits of how the dieter versus the non-dieter view eating, exercise, and progress are summarized by a chart at the end of this section.

Forget Willpower. While no doctor would expect a patient to "will" blood pressure to normal levels, physicians frequently expect their overweight patient to "will" their weight loss by restricting their food, according to Susan Z. Yanovski, M.D. This is also a prevailing attitude among our clients and many Americans—all you need is willpower and a little self-control. In a 1993 Gallup Poll, the most common obstacle cited to losing weight by women was willpower.

For example, Marilyn is a highly successful lawyer who climbed to the top of the corporate ladder. She credits her success with her determination, willpower, and self-discipline. Yet, when she tried to use these exemplary principles in her dieting attempts, she always failed. Whatever success she had achieved in her professional life was dulled by her sense of failure with her eating.

Why was Marilyn able to be so disciplined in one area of her life but not in the other? The word "discipline" derives from the word disciple. According to Stephen Covey's work, if you are a disciple to your own deep values that have an overriding purpose, it's likely that you'll have the *will* to carry them out. Marilyn believed deeply that writing exacting contracts and keeping immaculate records were requisites to building confidence with her clients and her law firm. But, somehow, hearing that bread was wrong on one diet and anything with sugar was wrong on another, did not engender the same kind of deep beliefs. Try as she might, she couldn't really believe that chocolate chip cookies were that evil!

Willpower can be defined as an attempt to counter natural desires and

replace them with proscriptive rules. It also implies the ability to do unpleasant tasks that are not essential. The desire for sweets is natural, normal, and quite pleasant! Any diet that tells you that you can't have sweets
is going against your natural desire. The diet becomes a set of rigid rules,
and these kinds of rules can only trigger rebellion.

Willpower does not belong in Intuitive Eating. As Marilyn became an
Intuitive Eater, she found that listening to her personal signals reinforced her
natural instincts, rather than countering them. She had no one else's proscriptive rules to follow or to rebel against. Marilyn has stopped fighting the
phantom willpower battle and has made peace with food and her body.

Forget Being Obedient. A well-meaning suggestion by a spouse or significant other such as: "Honey, you *should* have the broiled chicken . . ." or
"You *shouldn't* eat those fries . . ." can set off an inner food rebellion. In
this type of food combat, your only arsenal to fight back becomes a double
order of fries. Our clients call this "forget-you eating."

In physics, resistance always occurs as a reaction to force. We see this
principle in action in society—riots often erupt when the force of authority
becomes too great. Similarly, the *simple act of being told* what to do (even
if it's something you want to do), can trigger a rebellious chain reaction.
Just like "terrible two-year-olds" or teenagers who revolt to prove they are
independent, dieters can initiate rebellious eating in response to the act of
dieting, with its set of rigid rules. And so, it's not surprising to hear from
our clients that breaking the rules of a diet makes them feel just like they
did when they were defiant teens.

But take heart, rebellion is a normal act of self-preservation—protecting
your space, or personal boundaries.

Think of a personal boundary as a tall brick fence surrounding you, with
only one gate. Only you can open that gate, if you choose. Therefore, no one
is allowed inside, unless you invite the person in. Within your fence reside
private feelings, thoughts, and biological signals. People who *assume* they
know what you need and tell you what to do are picking the lock to your
gate, or invading your boundaries. Remember, nobody can be the expert of
"you." Only *you* know your thoughts, feelings, and experiences. No one
could possibly know what's inside, unless you tell him, by inviting him in.

What diet or diet counselor can possibly know when you are hungry or
how much food it will take to satisfy you? How can anyone but you know
what texture and taste sensations will be pleasing to your palate? In the world

of dieting, personal boundaries are crossed at many levels. For example, you are told what to eat, how much of it to eat, and when to eat it. These decisions should all be personal choices, with respect for individual autonomy and body signals. While food guidance may come from elsewhere, *you* should ultimately be responsible for the *when, what,* and *how much* of eating.

When a diet doctor or a diet plan invades your boundaries, it's normal to feel powerless. The longer you follow the food restrictions, the greater the assault to your autonomy. Here is where the paradox lies. When dieting, you will likely rebel by eating more—to restore your autonomy and protect your boundaries. But the act of rebelling can make you feel as out of control as a city riot. Instead, you have an inner food fight on your hands. But once the food rebellion is unleashed, its intensity reinforces feelings of lack of control and the belief that you don't possess willpower. Ultimately you begin to drown in a sea of self-doubt and shame. *What begins as a psychologically healthy behavior, ends in disaster.* Ultimately, a healthy relationship with food and your body is sabotaged, as a result of personal boundary protection. With Intuitive Eating there will be no need to rebel, because you become the one who is finally in charge!

Boundaries are also invaded when someone makes comments about your weight or how you should look. Again, you are bound to rebel by over-eating. It's a way of saying, "forget you" once again, and "you have no right to tell me what to weigh."

Rachel is an artist who had dieted all of her life. She was married to a successful lawyer who wanted to show off his beautiful *slim* wife to all of his colleagues. He would continually make subtle remarks that she wasn't as thin as she could be. He would even go so far as to give her dirty looks when she would reach for a rich dessert at a party. Rachel rebelled against her husband by sneaking foods behind his back (free from his evil eye). While going through the Intuitive Eating process, Rachel discovered that she was actually keeping extra weight on as the ultimate form of rebellion toward her husband.

But, instead of feeling strong and powerful from her rebellion, she found that she actually felt weak, out of control, and miserable. She knew that she would feel better if she ate according to her body's hunger and fullness signals, but "something" kept making her turn to the hidden extra foods. Rachel had been trapped in a game of control, boundary invasion, and rebellion all her life. Her husband and the world of dieting had been trying to control this free-spirited woman. To protect her boundaries, she would fight the diets by overeating and fight her husband's inappropriate demands by staying overweight.

Eventually Rachel stood up to her *well-meaning* husband and told him that he had no right to make comments about her food or her weight. Although initially resistant, he began to respect her boundaries. She also made a firm commitment to give up dieting. As a result, Rachel was shocked to find that her secret eating disappeared, as did her self-doubt, and she began to eat less, by listening to her intuitive signals.

Forget About Failure. All of our chronic dieters walk into our offices feeling as if they are failures. Whether they are highly placed executives, prominent celebrities, or straight-A students, they all talk about their food experiences shamefully, and they doubt whether they'll ever be able to feel successful in the area of eating. The diet mentality reinforces feelings of success or failure. You can't fail at Intuitive Eating—it's a learning process at every point along the way. What used to be thought of as a setback, will instead be seen as a growth experience. You'll get right back on track when you see this as progress, not failure.

STEP 3:
GET RID OF THE DIETER'S TOOLS

The dieter relies on external forces to regulate his eating, sticking to a regimented food plan, eating because it's time, or eating only a specified (and measured) amount, whether hungry or not. The dieter also validates progress by external forces, primarily the scale, asking, "How many pounds have I lost?" "Is my weight up or down?" It's time to throw out your dieting tools. Get rid of the meal plans and the food and bathroom scales. If all it took was a good "sensible" calorie-restricted meal plan to lose weight, we'd be a nation of thin people—free meal plans are readily available from magazines, newspapers, the Internet, and even some food companies.

The Scale as False Idol. "Please, please, let the number be . . ." This wishful number prayer is not occurring in the casinos of Las Vegas, but in private homes throughout the country. But just like a desperate gambler waiting for his lucky number to come in, so is it futile for the dieter to pay homage to the "scale god." In one sweep of the scale roulette, hopes and desperation combine to form a daily drama that will ultimately shape what mood you'll be in for the day. Ironically a "good" or "bad" scale number can *both* trigger overeating—whether it's a congratulatory eating party or a consolation party.

The scale ritual sabotages body and mind efforts; it can in one moment devalue days, weeks, and even months of progress, as illustrated with Connie.

Connie had been working very hard at Intuitive Eating and refrained from weighing herself, which in itself had been a feat since she originally weighed in daily, and sometimes even twice a day at home. But Connie felt she had made so much progress in three months that she was certain she had lost a significant amount of weight. To "confirm" her progress, Connie stepped on the scale. But the number of pounds that she lost was disappointing compared to how great she felt. The momentary brush with the scale boomeranged Connie right back to the diet mentality. That week, Connie cut back her food intake, which resulted in a large binge. Stepping on the scale was a step back into the diet mentality. It was no surprise that Connie countered her scale experience with a dieting approach. She also thought, "I must be doing something wrong." Her newfound trust began to erode—all with a single trip to the scale.

So much power is given to the almighty scale that it ultimately sabotages our efforts. But in the case of Sherry, she found the weighing process to be so humiliating that she had postponed going to the doctor for fifteen years! At the age of fifty-five, Sherry had not had a mammogram or other essential physical exams because she did not want to be weighed at the doctor's office (although she weighed in at home daily). In this case the scale was getting in the way of Sherry's health; she was at risk for breast cancer because it ran in her family. Getting the mammogram was more important than any number on the scale, but Sherry couldn't face the routine admonishments from the nursing staff. It was standard procedure—weigh the patient regardless of the reason for the appointment. Sherry did not realize that she had the right to refuse to be weighed. She finally got the courage after our work together. She made a doctor's appointment and refused to be weighed, since it was not an essential component of her medical care at the moment. Fortunately her physical exam results were healthy.

We have found that the "weigh-in" factor usually detracts from a person's progress. In the "old days" when we used to weigh all patients, we found that sessions were often spent on why the weight went up or did not move at all, and they became scale-counseling sessions. Our patients also dreaded the weighing-in part as much as we did.

When a Pound Is Not a Pound. Many factors can influence a person's weight, though *not* reflect a person's body fat. For example, two cups of water weighs one pound. If you tend to retain water or bloat, the scale can easily rise a few pounds without a change in what you have eaten. But for the oft guilt-ridden dieter, the consequences of water weight can seem severe. For example, we have had many patients feel bad about eating an extra dessert over the weekend and weigh themselves on the following Monday. The scale shoots up five pounds—and they *believe* they gained five pounds of *fat*. We explain to them that it is impossible for this one dessert to cause a true five-pound weight increase. So how do you explain the weight gain? Water weight. Anytime the scale suddenly rises or falls, it is usually because of a fluid shift in the body. Many factors can influence fluid retention— hormones, excessive sodium intake, and even the weather! Yet how easily chronic dieters believe they did something wrong—they must have single-handedly gobbled five pounds' worth of food! No! No! No! Similarly, losing two pounds immediately from an hour of aerobics is not a two-pound fat loss. Rather it's mostly water loss from sweat.

Jubilant dieters who think that they have lost ten pounds in a week might be in for an unwanted surprise. While it may be true that the scale indicated ten pounds less than when they weighed one week before, the question is, what *kind* of weight did they lose? To lose ten pounds of fat in one week requires an enormous energy deficit. The sad reality is that this person is losing a lot of water weight, usually at the expense of muscle-wasting. Muscle is made up of mainly water (70 percent). When a hungry body is not given enough calories, the body cannibalizes itself for an energy source. The prime directive of the body is that it must have energy, at any cost— it's part of the survival mechanism. The protein in muscles is converted to valuable energy for the body. When a muscle cell is destroyed, water is released and eventually excreted—there's your precious weight loss. The whittled-away muscle contributes to lowering your metabolism. Muscles are metabolically active tissue—generally the more muscle we have, the higher our metabolic rate. That's one of the reasons men burn more calories than women—they have more muscle mass.

Increased muscle mass, while metabolically more active and desirable, weighs more than fat. Muscle also takes up less space than fat. While this is certainly beneficial, a chronic dieter often gets frustrated by the rising, or unchanging, scale number. *The scale does not reflect body composition—* just like weighing a piece of steak at the butcher's does not tell you how lean the meat is.

Weighing in on the scale only serves to keep you focused on your weight; it doesn't help with the *process* of getting back in touch with Intuitive Eating. Constant weigh-ins can leave you frustrated and impede your progress. Best bet—stop weighing yourself.

STEP 4:
BE COMPASSIONATE TOWARD YOURSELF

When the world around you is dieting, and euphoric about how weight is melting away as a result of the latest diet craze—it's understandable that you can get pulled in. But this pull is more than just aesthetics.

In her book, *The Religion of Thinness,* Harvard-trained theologian and scholar, Michelle M. Lelwica makes a compelling argument about how the endless pursuit of thinness, through dieting, fulfills a spiritual hunger. The pursuit of dieting serves as an "ultimate purpose" by:

- Providing a set of myths to believe regarding the "rewards" of thinness.
- Offering rituals to organize the daily lives of women.
- Creating a moral code of which to live and eat by.
- Creating a common bond and a community for women.

When you consider these covert "benefits" of dieting, no wonder you can get seduced by the "rewards" of dieting. Don't beat yourself up for entertaining fantasies of trying one more diet or just wanting to diet. It takes a while to let go of this desire, even when you intellectually understand that the pursuit of dieting is truly futile.

Intuitive Eating Tools

The tools of the Intuitive Eater are internal cues—not outside forces telling you what, when, and how much to eat. But to acquire and understand these internal cues, you need a new set of power tools, rather *empowerment* tools, which will be discussed in the following chapters.

SUMMARY: THE DIET MENTALITY **VERSUS THE NON-DIET MENTALITY**		
Issue	Dieting Mentality	Non-Diet Mentality
Eating/Food Choices	★Do I deserve it? ★If I eat a heavy food, I try to find a way to make up for it. ★I feel guilty when I eat heavy foods. ★I usually describe a day of eating as either good or bad. • I view food as the enemy.	★Am I hungry? ★Do I want it? • Will I be deprived if I don't eat it? ★Will it be satisfying? ★Does it taste good? • I deserve to enjoy eating without guilt.
Exercise Benefits	• I focus primarily on the calories burned. ★I feel guilty if I miss a designated exercise day.	★I focus primarily on how exercise makes me feel, especially the energizing and stress-relieving factors.
Progress is viewed as:	• How many pounds did I lose? ★How do I look? ★What do other people think of my weight? ★I have good willpower.	• Rather than being concerned with my weight, I trust that my weight will normalize when I am attuned to my internal eating signals. My weight is not my primary goal or an indicator of my progress. • I have increased trust with myself and food. • I am able to let go of "eating indiscretions." • I recognize inner body cues.

A DIET IS A DIET, IS A DIET

Whether you count calories or points, even so-called sensible weight loss programs, such as Weight Watchers, use the tools of dieting. People often express surprise when they hear that counting points is a dieting behavior. That's when we will gently ask, "What do you do if you are hungry, and your points are used up?" The reply to this question is usually, "Ohhh—how did you know?"—which is followed by a deep sigh.

Deconstructing Weight Watchers. Any way you look at it, Weight Watchers is a diet in every aspect. Here are six examples:

1. The focus on points pulls one away from internal signals of hunger and fullness.
2. The points become obsessional. For years after someone gets off of Weight Watchers, the points stay embedded in the brain to haunt him or her.
3. It encourages overeating. If you can eat as much as you want of vegetables (in the old days) and fruits (now), it promotes eating to push away feelings, eating of foods that give false fullness signals, and substituting these foods for foods that might be more satisfying.
4. It promotes the concept of "good" and "bad" foods. Foods that have a low amount of points become the good foods, and vice versa.
5. If there are points left over at the end of the day, the person will be apt to eat beyond need, because she doesn't want to waste the points.
6. If a person is hungrier one day than the allowed points, she either has to "starve" or eat beyond her points. This promotes feeling guilty for going beyond, and/or the intention to make up the points the next day. If able to do this, it leads, once again, to semi-starvation, restricting, or not being able to do it, leading to more guilt.

Here are some other dieting examples, which might not be so obvious:

- Drinking a weight loss beverage for breakfast and lunch; followed by a "sensible" dinner.
- Detox fast—which usually consists of some type of liquid fast, in order to "remove toxins" from your body. Our bodies are built with an amazing inner cleansing system—the liver, kidneys, and digestive system.
- Colon cleanse, which involves a process forcing the colon to empty its contents (ultimately resulting in diarrhea). The process may be via laxatives, enemas, or colon irrigation, known as a high colonic.

Chapter 6

PRINCIPLE 2:
Honor Your Hunger

Keep your body biologically fed with adequate energy and carbohydrates. Otherwise you can trigger a primal drive to overeat. Once you reach the moment of excessive hunger, all intentions of moderate, conscious eating are fleeting and irrelevant. Learning to honor this first biological signal sets the stage for rebuilding trust with yourself and food.

A dieting body is a starving body. Drastic comparison? No. While a dieting body may not *look* like a starving person in Ethiopia or Somalia, the "symptoms" from dieting exhibit a striking resemblance to the starvation state. The body does not know that there is a McDonald's on every corner as you embark on a diet. As far as the body is concerned it is living in a famine state and adapts. Our need for food (energy) is so essential and primal that if we are not getting enough energy, our bodies naturally compensate with powerful biological and psychological mechanisms.

The power of food deprivation was keenly demonstrated in a landmark starvation study conducted by Dr. Ancel Keys during World War II, designed to help famine sufferers. The subjects of the study were thirty-two healthy men who were selected because they had superior "psychobiological stamina"—superior mental and physical health.

During the first three months of the study the men ate as they pleased, averaging 3,492 calories. The next six months was the semistarvation period. The men were required to lose 19–28 percent of their weight depending on their body composition. Calories were cut nearly in half to an average 1,570 per day. The effects of the semistarvation were startling, and strikingly mirrored the symptoms of chronic dieting:

- Metabolic rate decreased 40 percent.
- The men were obsessed with food. They had heightened food cravings and talked of food and collecting recipes.
- Eating style changed—vacillating from ravenously gulping to stalling out the eating experience. Some men played with their food and dawdled over a meal for two hours.
- The researchers noted that, "Several men failed to adhere to their diets and reported episodes of bulimia." One man was reported to have suffered a complete loss of "willpower" and ate several cookies, a sack of popcorn, and two bananas. Another subject "flagrantly broke the dietary rules" and ate several sundaes, malted milks, and even stole penny candy.
- Some men exercised deliberately to obtain increased food rations.
- Personalities changed, and in many cases there was the onset of apathy, irritability, moodiness, and depression.

During the refeeding period, when the men were once again allowed to eat at will, hunger pangs became more intense, and hunger was insatiable. The men found it difficult to stop eating. Weekend binges added up to eight thousand to ten thousand calories. It took the majority of men an average of five months to normalize their eating.

It's important to remember that during the era of this classic study, there were no celebrity trainers, the TV Food Network, or fitness and food divas. Nutrition research was just in its infancy. Yet these men experienced a primal obsession with food that was not media driven or society driven; rather it was triggered by a biological survival mechanism. Such behavior was never observed in these men prior to their food deprivation encounter! Although this is a classic starvation study, the caloric level is representative of a modern weight loss diet for men of fifteen hundred calories. These men were eating fifteen hundred calories' worth of food, and still experienced marked symptoms, both physically and psychologically. Imagine if the same study was held under today's pressures to be thin.

We have had several clients read the classic Keys study, and they are struck by their own similar experiences to the semistarved men. Mary, for example, noted that after completing her second liquid fast program, she was more obsessed with food than ever before. She bought several cookbooks and major cooking appliances—a waffle maker, a bread maker, and a food processor. The biggest paradox Mary noted was that she doesn't like to cook and did not use her new appliances or cookbooks!

Jan had dieted most of her life. But the more she dieted the more she got interested in food. She collected magazine and newspaper recipes of all kinds, from rich gourmet to spartan spa cuisine, and read them as if they were engaging novels. Yet she would never dare prepare the scrumptious recipes; instead they were her food fantasy and food escapism.

interesting

Of Mice and Men. Rats are certainly not exposed to the social pressures and nuances of eating that humans are, yet when deprived of food, rats will also overeat. In one study, rats were divided into two groups, one food-deprived and one control group. The food-deprived rats went without food for up to four days, and then were allowed to eat again until they gained their weight back. Both groups of rats were then given free access to a "palatable diet"—beyond the ordinary rat chow staples, like five-star dining in the rodent world. While both groups gained weight, those in the food-deprived group gained more weight, *in direct proportion to the length of their prior deprivation.*

PRIMAL HUNGER

The psychological terror of hunger is profound, notes Naomi Wolf in her book, *The Beauty Myth.* Even after hunger has ended, the nagging terror of it remains. She cites how hungry orphans adopted from poor countries often cannot control their compulsion to smuggle and hide food, even after living for years in a secure environment. A disproportionate number of starving concentration camp survivors are now obese.

Research historians have documented that during times of famine or food shortages, food becomes an overriding preoccupation resulting in so-cietal problems: breakdown of social behavior, abandonment of cooperative effort, loss of personal pride and sense of family ties. While this preoccu-pation with food has been observed during times of food deprivation, these actions also mirror dieting behavior at the individual level. How often have you become more socially isolated while on a diet, turning down a party invitation, for instance, because you didn't want to deal with the food, or not going out altogether until you are through with your diet?

While the hunger and food obsession from dieting may not be experi-enced as a terrifying event, it does leave a lasting mark.

Karen had been on several medically supervised fasts over her lifetime and became frightened of experiencing hunger. To her, hunger was terrifying and often resulted in out-of-control eating, which reinforced her fear of hunger. Therefore, Karen always kept herself in a "fed" state between diets, never to really experience gentle biological hunger. She only knew what *extreme* hunger felt like with all of its voracious intensity. To avoid hunger she was constantly eating, but the persistent eating caused more weight gain, so she would start a new diet or fasting program and the vicious cycle would continue—hunger from dieting, followed by overeating.

MECHANISMS THAT TRIGGER EATING

Whether or not you are a chronic dieter, powerful biological mechanisms are triggered when your body does not get the energy from food that it needs. It's no accident that food is included as one the fundamental needs in Maslow's Hierarchy of Needs—a model that ranks human needs, suggesting that certain basic needs must be met before you can go on to fulfill more complex ones. Food and energy are so essential to the survival of the human species, that if we don't eat enough we set off a biological fuse that turns on our eating drive, both physically *and* psychologically. The hunger drive is truly a mind-body connection. Eating is so important that the nerve cells of appetite are located in the hypothalamus region of the brain. A variety of biological signals triggers eating. What many people believe to be an issue of willpower, is instead a *biological drive*. The power and intensity of the biological eating drive should not be underestimated. The neurochemicals from the brain coordinate our eating behavior with our body's biological need. Through a complex system of chemical and neural feedback, the brain monitors the energy needs of all our body systems, moment to moment. And it makes very emphatic chemical directives as to what we should eat. Fasting or restricting is particularly counterproductive to appetite. It simply turns on the neurochemical switches that induce us to eat.

Many studies have shown that lowering body weight by food restriction and dieting makes no sense metabolically or to our brain chemistry. In fact, it's counterproductive. The biological chemicals that regulate appetite also directly affect moods and state of mind, our physical energy, and our sex lives.

Most researchers agree that there are both complex biological *and* psychological mechanisms that influence our eating. In this chapter, we will focus on the profound biological mechanisms that turn on our desire to eat, especially if we have been food-deprived or dieting.

Heightened Digestion

In food-deprived individuals, research has shown that the body gets biologically primed for the moment of eating, like a sprinter crouched in a ready-position for an explosive start, the moment the starting pistol is triggered.

- Salivation increases with increases of food deprivation, even when there is no food present or suggestion of eating! This has been demonstrated in studies both on dieters and normal (non-dieting) individuals.
- Increased digestive hormones have been found in dieters both before and after eating.

The Carbohydrate Craver: Neuropeptide Y

Neuropeptide Y (NPY) is a chemical produced by the brain that triggers our drive to eat carbohydrates, the body's primary and preferred source of energy. While most of what we know about NPY comes from research on rats, there is a lot of evidence that shows that this brain chemical can have a profound impact on human eating behavior as well, by increasing both the size and duration of carbohydrate-rich meals.

Food deprivation or under eating drives NPY into action, causing the body to seek more carbohydrates. When the next meal or eating opportunity rolls around, it can easily turn into a high-carbohydrate binge—not because you lack willpower or are out of control, it's your biology (rather NPY) screaming, "Feed me."

NPY is revved up after any imposed period of food deprivation, including an overnight fast from dinner to breakfast. NPY's levels are naturally the highest in the morning because of the short-term food deprivation from an overnight fast. The elevated NPY levels are part of the biological basis for eating in the morning. During an overnight fast, your body's stores of carbohydrate (in the liver) are drained and need refilling. You literally wake up on empty in the morning. But if you skip breakfast, you are likely to pay for it with increases in NPY levels which can lead to midafternoon gorging.

The brain also makes more NPY when carbohydrates are being burned as fuel and under times of stress. Eating carbohydrates turns off NPY through its effect on serotonin, another brain chemical. As we eat more carbohydrates, it helps to increase the production of serotonin, which in turn shuts off the production of NPY and puts a halt to the desire for carbohydrates.

The more you deny your true hunger and fight your natural biology, the stronger and more intense food cravings and obsessions become. Fasting or restricting especially revs up the NPY and drives the body to seek more carbohydrates. So by the time the next eating opportunity occurs, it can *easily* become a high-carbohydrate binge.

Why is there such a chemical drive for carbohydrates? Let's look briefly at the critical role carbohydrates play in the body—it will help you understand the primal hunger drive.

The Importance of Carbohydrates. Carbohydrates are the gold standard of food energy to the body. Cells function best when they receive a certain level of carbohydrates, in the form of glucose, and even small decreases can cause problems. The brain, nervous system, and red blood cells rely *exclusively* on glucose for fuel. Because of the importance of glucose, the levels of it in the blood are closely regulated by two hormones, insulin and glucagon.

There is a very limited amount of carbohydrate stored in the liver, in the form of glycogen, that helps supply more glucose to the blood when levels get too low. Yet this precious fuel reserve ordinarily lasts only three to six hours. (Except at night, when liver glycogen lasts longer because the need for energy is lower.) How does it get replaced? Eating. Eating carbohydrate-rich foods, that is.

If carbohydrates are inadequate in the diet, the body has to turn to creative fueling mechanisms to supply vital energy to the body. Protein mainly from muscle will get taken apart and converted to energy, primarily in the form of glucose. It's like taking wood from the framework structure in your house to use as fuel in your fireplace. The wood will burn and provide necessary fuel, but it does so at a high price. You begin to lose the integrity of your structure!

If you think that eating a high-protein diet will prevent this dismantling from occurring, it's not so. When you eat an inadequate amount of energy or carbohydrates, the protein from the diet will *also* be diverted to be used as energy. Therefore, this "high-protein diet" is no insurance. Instead, the protein is used as an expensive source of fuel, rather than for its intended use in the body. It's like having a building supplier provide lots of wood to rebuild your house. If you are constantly using that wood pile to make bonfires, instead of repairing your home, you are still left with a weak structure. Similarly, protein is needed to maintain and build muscles, hormones, enzymes, and cells in the body. When carbohydrates and energy are lacking, protein is shifted from its primary role to provide fuel.

Many of our clients believe that when we don't have enough energy, our bodies will finally start burning fat. It doesn't work that way. Remember, the brain and other parts of the body need carbohydrates exclusively for fuel. Only a very small component (5 percent) of the stored fat can be converted to a carbohydrate fuel. On the other hand, the body has plenty of enzymes to convert protein to glucose.

One reason people lose weight so quickly on low-carbohydrate or fasting diets is that they are devouring their own protein tissues as fuel. Since protein contains only half as many calories per pound as fat, it disappears twice as fast. Also, with each pound of body protein, three or four pounds of associated water are lost. If your body were to continue to consume itself at this rate, death would occur within about ten days. After all, the liver, heart muscle, and lung tissue—all vital tissues are being burned as fuel. Even when the heart muscle is deteriorating, it still has to keep up the same amount of work, with *less* power and at a slower heart rate. In essence the cannibalized heart muscle has to work harder with a smaller, faulty engine; pumping performance is not reduced in proportion to the amount of heart tissue lost.

Eventually, the body can convert stored fat to a usable energy form for the brain and nervous system, called ketones. This is known as ketosis. Ketosis is an adaptation to prolonged fasting or carbohydrate deprivation. But only about *half* of the brain's cells can use these compounds for energy. Therefore, when fat is being used under these deprivation conditions, the body's lean tissue (protein) continues to be lost at a rapid rate in order to supply glucose to nervous system cells that cannot use ketones as fuel. The bottom line? Adequate carbohydrates and energy are important!

The Powerhouse Cell Theory

Hunger signals are not affected by low carbohydrates alone. According to the work of cellular researchers Nicolaidis and Even, the hunger signal is generated by the overall energy need of the cell. When cellular power is low, it will produce a signal that induces hunger. While cells primarily get their energy from carbohydrates, protein and fat are factored into the cellular power equation, which could trigger hunger. For example, even if one of your household appliances runs on pure electricity, it could also get its energy from batteries, or a gasoline-powered generator. They all provide energy, but have different costs and efficiencies. All nutrients that provide energy (carbohydrates, protein, and fat) eventually get converted to one universal energy denomination used by the cell, ATP. ATP is the chemical energy that powers the cells, and thus our bodies. Nicolaidis and Even propose that the hunger signal is triggered by the overall ATP need of the cell.

To sum up—we need energy. Energy comes from food.

Second-Guessing Your Biology

In spite of the complex and elegant biological systems that help ensure that our body's get enough energy (food), all too often the chronic dieter tries to outthink biology. Rather than eating when hungry, eating is often tied into a cognitive set point, based on the dieter's set of rules (Is it time? Do I deserve it? Is it fat-free? And so forth). For example, on the days Alice exercised, early in the morning, she would get mad at herself for eating a larger (but appropriate) breakfast. She was worried that her body did not deserve the "extra" portion of food, so her solution was to skip lunch. Skipping lunch was easy, because Alice was a busy executive assistant, with never enough hours in the day to get her work done. Her busyness preoccupied any afternoon hunger that would surface. But by the time Alice arrived at home in the evening, she would be so hungry she would overeat at dinner and often late into the night. Or if she were eating out at a restaurant, she would devour the bread basket and clean her plate, feeling stuffed and guilty by the end of her meal.

Even non-dieters who go too long without eating will often overeat. (Remember, even rats overeat when food deprived.) You are also likely to buy more food impulsively when you are in a ravenous state, regardless of your health and dieting intentions.

The problem with consistently denying your hunger state is twofold. First, it usually crescendos into a period of overeating. Second, when the mind gets so used to ignoring hunger signals, they begin to fade and you don't hear them anymore. Or you can only "hear" hunger in extreme, ravenous states, which can be adverse. This further conditions you to believe that you can't be trusted with food, because ravenous hunger often triggers overeating. This is explained in part by the Boundary Model for the Regulation of Eating, developed by C. Peter Herman and Janet Polivy, psychological experts in chronic dieting. This model considers both the biology and psychology of eating.

The boundary model explains how dieters, through their cognitive set point, push their normal biological cues of hunger and satiety to the extremes. The gentle sensations of hunger are atrophied for a dieter who is constantly trying to suppress them. Instead, the dieter might only feel extreme, ravenous hunger—or be so disconnected that the feeling of hunger is difficult to identify. Similarly, for this individual, it can be increasingly difficult to know what comfortable satiety feels like. Instead the dieter hovers in a gray zone of what Herman and Polivy call "biological indifference." In the zone of biological indifference, there is no clear hunger or satiety cue. This zone is so wide for the chronic dieter that instead of eating based on internal eating cues, food thoughts and judgments prevail and tell the dieter what to do. *luckily I can still fee hunger*

PRIMAL FOOD THERAPY: HONOR YOUR HUNGER

The first step to reclaiming the world of normal eating, free of dieting and food worry is to *honor your biological hunger.* Your body needs to *know* consistently that it will have access to food—that dieting and deprivation have halted, once and for all. Otherwise, your biology will always be on call, ready to avert a self-imposed food deprivation.

Your body needs to be biologically reconditioned. Diet after diet has taught your body that personal famines are frequent, so it should stay on guard. Remember, famines and food shortages have always existed, even in our modern times. Our bodies are still biologically equipped to survive famines through lowering our energy requirements, increasing biological chemicals that trigger our eating drive, and so on.

It is much easier to stop eating when you truly know you will be able to eat again. For example, imagine you are in a room and offer a *starving* child a plate of cookies. You tell the child that she can have only one cookie. You exit the room and leave the child alone with the whole plate. What would the hungry child do? Eat *all* the cookies (and lick the crumbs), of course. But if the child knew that cookies (or any other food) were always available when hungry, the intensity to eat would be greatly diminished. The same is true for dieters.

For example, Barbara usually kept herself in a hungry state. She only allowed herself to eat when extremely ravenous. By her own definition, if she allowed herself to eat when simply hungry, *but not ravenous,* she thought she was overeating. Yet because her definition of "normal" hunger was being ravenous, her eating would vacillate from feast to famine cycles.

HUNGER SILENCE

not an issue

What if you don't feel hunger anymore, or never really knew what the gentle sensation of hunger feels like? Can you get it back? Yes. But first let's look at a couple of reasons why hunger may be silenced.

• *Numbing.* Many people have learned over the years to quell, or avert hunger pangs by turning to calorie-free beverages, such as diet sodas, coffee, and tea. The liquid in the stomach temporarily tricks the gastric mechanism into a sense of fullness.

• *Dieting.* Dieters get so used to denying their hunger that it becomes easy to tune it out. Eventually, when hunger comes knocking on their inner door and there is no response, the knocking, or rather the stomach rumbling, stops.

• *Chaos.* It's very easy to suppress hunger or ignore it, when you are busy putting out the fires in your life or job. If this is a chronic pattern, hunger may slowly fade.

• *Skipping breakfast.* Some of our clients skip eating in the morning, because they say it keeps them from feeling hungrier the rest of the day. Yet hunger is a normal, welcomed body signal that should be embraced. It's a sign that you are getting back in touch with your body's needs. But because these clients are afraid of their hunger, especially when it becomes overwhelming in the evening as a result of not eating early in the day, they respond by not eating breakfast the next morning—which repeats the vicious cycle of hunger silence.

HOW TO HONOR BIOLOGICAL HUNGER

It's too hard to hear hunger if you are never listening for it. The first step to honoring your biological hunger is to begin to listen for it. The symphony of hunger has many sounds that are varied for different people. Just as an orchestra conductor can distinguish the voices of each instrument in a symphony, you will eventually be able to key in to specific bodily sensations and what they mean. In the beginning, you may be able to recognize overt ravenous hunger, but have difficulty recognizing gentle hunger pangs. Similarly, to the nontrained musical ear, loud cymbals might be easy to identify, but it will take time and listening to pick up on the subtler voices of the bassoon or oboe.

Each time you eat, ask yourself: "Am I hungry? What's my hunger level?" If the feeling of hunger is hard to identify, ask yourself: "When was the last time I *ever* felt hungry? How did my stomach feel? How did my mouth feel?" Any combination of the following can be experienced as hunger sensations or symptoms (ranging from gentle to ravenous):

- Mild gurgling or gnawing in the stomach
- Growling noises
- Light-headedness
- Difficulty concentrating
- Uncomfortable stomach pain
- Irritability
- Feeling faint
- Headache

The ebb and flow of your hunger might not match other people's—that's okay, it's individual. Take care not to get overly hungry or ravenous. If this is difficult for you to gauge, a *general* guideline is to *go no longer than five waking hours without eating.* This is based on the biology of fueling up your carbohydrate tank in the liver, which runs out every three to six hours. We have observed that clients who go longer than five hours without eating tend to overeat at the next eating opportunity. (For some people, this can happen even after three or four hours without eating.)

To get in touch with the nuances of hunger, it helps to check the pulse of hunger at regular intervals. Check in with your body, and simply inquire, What's my hunger level? It's helpful to do this every time you eat, and between eating occurrences. Remember, although this may seem hyperconscious, it's a focused step to get you reacquainted with your body and its biology.

We have used a variety of tools to help our clients check in with their hunger, but one is particularly helpful and is a little less exacting. Monitor

THE HUNGER DISCOVERY SCALE

Time	Food	Hunger Rating										
		0	1	2	3	4	5	6	7	8	9	10
10:30	breakfast				▨							
2:45	lunch				▨							
6:30	dinner			▨								
10:00	snack					▨						

```
Empty          Set     Neutral        Full      Sick
       Ravenous     Pangs        Satisfied   Stuffed
<----+----+----+----+----+----+----+----+----+----+---->
  0    1    2    3    4    5    6    7    8    9    10
```

Use this scale (0–10) to help you identify your initial hunger when you begin to eat. This rating system is purely subjective and will help you get in touch with your body's inner signals. There is no right or wrong way to use this rating system—it's merely a rating to help increase your awareness. The more you rate your hunger, the more these numbers will have meaning to you.

The neutral point is 5, when you are neither hungry nor full. Visualize your stomach getting emptier and hungrier as you go down on the scale to 0, completely empty. At 4, you begin to feel the first awakening of hunger. Hunger pangs begin there and increase to a 3. By 3, your hunger is completely set, and you're feeling quite hungry. At 2–1, you are ravenous.

Every time you start to eat, check your hunger level. Ideally, aim for around a level of 3 to begin eating. If you are at a 5 or above, you're not biologically hungry. If you're at 2 or lower, you're likely overhungry and at risk for overeating.

your hunger levels each time you eat, before and after, using the Hunger Discovery Scale on the previous page. What pattern do you see emerging? Is there a certain time interval that you eat? Is there any relationship between how much you eat and the length of time between eating?

You may discover that your eating style leans toward nibbling or grazing. Don't be alarmed. If you eat small amounts of food such as a snack or mini-meal, you may find that you are hungry more often, such as every two, three, or four hours. Not only is this normal, it may have metabolic advantages. Nibbling studies (in which people are given multiple snacks or mini-meals) have shown that the release of insulin is lower in people fed nibbling diets compared to larger traditional meals of *identical* calories. Insulin is a fat-building hormone. The more insulin released, the easier it is for the body to make fat.

Sometimes our clients get worried when they suddenly feel more hungry than usual—as if something is wrong. However, on closer inspection, they usually find that a couple of days prior, they had an unusually light day of eating—not dieting, but just not a lot of food. The body plays catch-up on its own terms, not yours. Most of our clients have difficulty remembering what they ate one day ago, let alone two days ago. Research on children has shown that they make up for their needs in an average of time such as a week or couple of days. Why would adults be any different? In fact, new research is beginning to indicate the same is true for adults. The body may do some of its energy fine-tuning over a period of days, rather than from hour to hour. We find this is especially true if you still have a tendency to eat diet types of food, such as rice cakes or salad. You may feel full but the lack of energy catches up with you. The body wants to compensate.

Other Voices of "Hunger"

A common mistake with our newer clients is that they initially embrace the *honor your hunger* concept in the form of a diet mantra, "Thou shalt eat only when hungry." The problem here is that this rigid interpretation can leave you feeling as if you have broken a "rule" or failed, if you eat for any other reason than hunger. When you feel like you have broken a rule, you get pulled right back into the diet mentality.

• *Taste hunger.* Sometimes people may eat simply because it sounds good or because the occasion calls for it. We call this *taste hunger.* Normal eaters can accept this—they don't view it as a big diet violation. In nearly every culture, food plays important roles in rites of passage and celebratory events. Would you chastise a bride or groom for eating a piece of wedding cake when she or he was not hungry? Yet it's not unusual for dieters to feel bad about *any* perceived food transgression, and then feel like they might as well throw in the towel. And that's when *overeating* often takes place.

• *Practical "hunger"—planning ahead.* While it's important to eat primarily based on your biological hunger, it's also important to be practical and not rigid. For instance, let's say you are attending a play with friends that lasts from 7 to 10 P.M. and your opportunity to eat out is at 6 P.M. You may not be hungry then, but you certainly will be later. Do you sit there at the restaurant and *not* eat, and let hunger roll in right in the middle of the play, only to culminate in ravenous hunger by the final act? No. Eating a light meal or snack is a sensible solution.

• *Emotional hunger.* Once you are truly able to identify and distinguish biological hunger, it becomes easier to clarify *why* you want to eat. It is not unusual for a number of our clients to eat because of *emotional* hunger—to quench uncomfortable feelings (such as loneliness, boredom, and anger). Ironically, many of our patients are often amazed that what they assumed to be emotional eating, was in many instances primal hunger eating. But the out-of-control feeling of eating is nearly identical, whether it was triggered emotionally or biologically. A discussion of how to distinguish the sources of hunger is found in Chapter 11.

STUDIES SHOW—EATING IN RESPONSE TO INITIAL HUNGER IMPROVES HEALTH & WEIGHT

A promising series of studies from an Italian research team in Florence shows that training people to recognize initial hunger improves insulin sensitivity and lowers body mass index.

They were able to train people to predict when blood glucose is low, by attending to their subjective experience of hunger (Ciampolini and Bianchi 2006).

There are two unique aspects to their approach. First, the focus of the training is distinguishing *initial hunger*, from the uncomfortable symptoms that occur when hunger is prolonged. Secondly, a biofeedback technique, well

cont.

Continued

known to diabetic educators, was utilized to train people how to make this distinction via blood glucose monitoring, using glucometers. (Note, these people did not have diabetes or impaired glucose tolerance.)

Initially, people were instructed to measure their blood sugar at the earliest feelings of hunger or discomfort. Next, if glucose was under 85 mg/dL, subjects were instructed to remember their physical feelings and to proceed to eat their meal. (Note, the glucose level of 85 mg/dL was chosen based on previous studies, indicating that it represents the upper limit of homeostatic control of feeding.)

If blood sugar was higher than 85 mg/dL, subjects were instructed to delay the meal. They were then asked to wait for the spontaneous development of novel hunger feelings for at least one hour, before making further blood glucose measurements.

Two other studies using this initial hunger recognition technique demonstrated that people trained in this method had improved insulin sensitivity and weight loss, compared to the non-trained controls (Ciampolini et al. 2010; Ciampolini, Lovell-Smith, and Sifone 2010). When insulin is less effective in your body, it is called "insulin resistance," which is related to chronic health problems.

The research team concluded that restoring and validating hunger and training people to recognize initial hunger could help in the prevention and treatment of diabetes and obesity and associated disorders.

Chapter 7

PRINCIPLE 3:

Make Peace with Food

Call a truce, stop the food fight! Give yourself unconditional permission to eat. If you tell yourself that you can't or shouldn't have
a particular food, it can lead to intense feelings of deprivation
that build into uncontrollable cravings and often, bingeing. When
you finally "give in" to your forbidden foods, eating will be experienced with such intensity, it usually results in Last Supper overeating and overwhelming guilt.

When I was on the grapefruit diet, all I wanted was bananas, and when
I was on a low-carbohydrate diet all I did was dream of eating bread and
potatoes," said Laurie, an inveterate dieter. Does that sound ironic? Familiar? What may seem like irony is actually the natural reaction that is triggered by the limitation and deprivation that comes with most diets.

Cravings run rampant as soon as we're restricted from any kind of
substance—whether it is clothing, fresh air, scenery, or especially food.
Scientists living in the Biosphere 2, an airtight, glass-enclosed terrarium,
coveted something as basic as fresh air, after being deprived of an open
environment for two years. But fresh air was not the only fantasy of these
researchers—so, too, was the food they had sorely missed. After they emerged
from this self-imposed captivity, the research team had more to say about
food than science at their press conference. The scientists described cravings for food that began to occupy their thoughts and led one of them to
write a cookbook!

These scientists are not unlike the dieter who has been told certain foods
are forbidden. Even though they were not on a diet, the scientists were still
preoccupied with food cravings as a result of lack of availability. They

dreamed about desserts which were nonexistent and obsessed about dinners, which were of limited variety. As cooking chores rotated, it became vitally important not to spoil the day's meal for the others. Common foods like salmon, berries, and coffee took on a heightened allure.

THE DEPRIVATION SETUP

Why would Biosphere scientists or the healthy men in the Ancel Keys study (described in the previous chapter) exhibit behaviors so unlike their normal eating patterns? Deprivation. These people had not been tainted by the dieting trap, yet their reactions to deprivation were virtually identical to those of dieters. While you have already seen the effects of *biological* deprivation in the last chapter, you should not underestimate the *psychological* effect of deprivation. This effect is the focus of this chapter.

When you rigidly limit the amount of food you are allowed to eat, it usually sets you up to crave *larger* quantities of that very food. In fact, being restricted from anything in life sets it up to be extra special, regardless of age. (Oh, maybe not in the beginning, when you are in the initial stages of diet euphoria, but the craving builds with each "dieting day.") For example, if you put a two-year-old on the floor with several brand-new toys and tell him that he can play with any one of them except for the simple oatmeal carton, which do you think he'll choose? You guessed it—the plain oatmeal carton.

One client revealed that when he was young, he had little money and the thought of buying a new car gave him a deep thrill. Yet, now that he's successful, he can buy *any* car he wants at any time. Cars are no longer a big deal, no thrill. Food has replaced the thrill that buying a new car used to provide. Paradoxically, food is the one thing out of his reach, forbidden, when dieting. The forbidden object is elevated to an overvalued level of specialness.

Psychologist Fritz Heider stated that depriving yourself of something you want can actually heighten your desire for that very item. *The moment you banish a food, it paradoxically builds up a "craving life" of its own that gets stronger with each diet, and builds more momentum as the deprivation deepens.* Deprivation is a powerful experience both biologically and psychologically. You already saw in the last chapter how food deprivation sets off a biological drive. Psychological forces wreak havoc with your peace of mind, triggering cravings, obsessive thoughts, and even compulsive behaviors.

When a diet dictates that a particular food is forbidden or should be avoided it makes you crave that food even more! If you are someone who has experienced deprivation in areas outside of food, such as love, attention, material wants, etc., the deprivation connected to dieting may be felt even more intensely by you. Bonnie is a client who grew up in a home where her father was never home, and her mother was emotionally distant. As a young child, she learned to use food as a way to substitute for the love and attention she wasn't getting. As an adult on a diet, she found that food deprivation evoked these deep feelings of deprivation from childhood. For Bonnie, this became a double whammy, which was hard to overcome. For the chronic dieter, the combination of biological changes (from under eating), psychological reactions, and cognitive distortions create just the right mix to set off the dynamite of rebound eating.

DEPRIVATION BACKLASH—REBOUND EATING

Meet Heidi. Her experience with chocolate typifies what can happen when you deprive yourself of a particular food. Heidi had been on every known diet, each forbidding one type of food or another, and chocolate was usually on the "do not eat" list. Heidi was a self-described chocoholic. She complained that the moment chocolate crossed her lips, she couldn't stop eating it. Her way of managing her chocolate problem was simply to not allow herself to eat it. But this was a vicious cycle. It was not uncommon for Heidi to consume large bags of chocolate in spite of her attempts to eliminate it from her life. The moment a box of chocolate was opened, she couldn't resist eating it to completion. Heidi's chocolate binges were triggered by the food rule she had created—"I am not allowed to eat chocolate." This meant that each time she "succumbed" and ate it, she truly believed that it was for the last time. Each chocolate episode would become a "farewell to chocolate" with all the sadness and mourning that goes along with saying good-bye to anything special in life. Since Heidi "knew" she was never, *ever* going to eat chocolate again (despite her experience demonstrating otherwise), she would consume large amounts of it as a last hurrah, or "get it while you can." When Heidi's chocolate binges occurred, she would feel guilty and as if she did not deserve to eat any food. She would compensate for her chocolate feasts by under eating or semi-fasting, which would set her up for ravenous hunger and more out-of-control eating.

Today Heidi eats chocolate but is often satisfied with a piece or two, and can easily even pass it up! To Heidi, this is a miracle. How did she overcome her chocolate problem? Heidi's solution was to learn to make peace with food—especially with chocolate—an idea that she was terrified to try in the beginning. No wonder; her only experience with chocolate was eating it in massive quantities, then feeling out of control. For Heidi, making peace with chocolate was a brave and risky step.

| Last Supper Eating | *big problem for me*

The mere *perception* that food might become banned can trigger overeating. Just thinking about going on a diet can create a sense of panic and send you on a trail of eating every food that you think won't be allowed. As we explained in Chapter 1, this is Last Supper eating. It is triggered by the sincere belief that you will never get to eat a particular food (or foods) again. The threat of deprivation becomes so powerful that all reason is lost and you find yourself eating whatever is to be forbidden, even if you are not hungry.

Clients will often overeat right before their first session. Although we make it clear that we use a non-dieting approach, they figure that we have something up our sleeves, a diet of sorts—after all, we are both registered dietitians and nutrition therapists! For example, Paul ate in an out-of-control fashion the night before his first appointment. Why? Paul was sure that he would be advised to give up most of his favorite foods, and to start eating a diet of carrots and cottage cheese. His fear increased during the week leading up to his session, and so did his intake of french fries, hamburgers, and donuts. This experience was not new to Paul—in fact, he had engaged in Last Supper eating before *every* diet he started. Likewise, nearly all of our clients engage in this pre-dieting ritual of saying good-bye to favorite foods. In fact, some of our clients tell us that Last Supper eating is one of their favorite parts of dieting—it's almost an entitlement.

For some of our clients, however, there is such an intense sense of urgency with Last Supper eating, that a period of frantic gorging ensues. One client described it as, "Hurry and get all the food while you can, and time is short, so get it all, now!" The overeating that follows falsely gives "proof" that you need to diet, as you watch in horror your inability to "control" yourself.

Each impending diet brings with it more fear of deprivation—with the knowledge that you won't get "enough" or get what you want. Then comes more overeating, loss of self-control, and finally, erosion of self-esteem. How could you possibly feel good about yourself, if you truly believe that it's possible to eliminate certain foods, only to find yourself bingeing and failing on yet another diet?

definitely feel this @ school

Rebound Eating: Subtle Forms

Food Competition. Have you ever shared a bowl of cherries or a piece of dessert with someone who eats faster than you? Watch how quickly you dig in because you're concerned that you won't get enough. Or see what happens when you hear that your favorite brand of cereal is to be discontinued; it's not unusual to buy every last box on the shelf because of fear of deprivation. Or some parents find themselves gobbling down the cookies before the kids can get their hands on them and eat them all.

Eating in a large group of people can instill a sense of future food-deprivation worry. To prevent this from occurring, there is a tendency to eat quickly, grab it while you can, or there won't be any food left. For example, Joshua was one of nine children in a family of moderate means. As a child he was worried that he wouldn't get enough food at mealtime, although in actuality there was an adequate amount of food to go around. While not overweight as a child, the fear of food deprivation taught him to grab what he could. As an adult he continued this behavior, which evolved into an obesity problem.

Returning Home Syndrome. When they return from having been away, people often overeat because they felt deprived of familiar foods while away. Kids returning home from summer camp or from their college dorms find themselves emptying the refrigerator, gorging on home cooking, or visiting their favorite local restaurants excessively. Recently, I (ER) came home to find my stepson's friend, who had just returned from Thailand, methodically eating everything in the kitchen that he hadn't seen in three years. When he began to eat the cream cheese by the forkful (without a bagel), I knew how deprived he had been! Even fresh fruits and vegetables take on a heightened allure when one is returning from a journey in which they were not available. For example, clients have described unusual cravings for salads after a two-week camping trip or trip abroad where it's been advised *not* to eat the fresh produce.

The Empty Cupboard. If there is consistently no food in the house because grocery shopping is chaotic, eating often vacillates between feast and famine, with emphasis on the former. Food in the pantry or refrigerator takes on extra specialness.

For example, Gayle is a young woman who exhibits a tendency to eat every bite of food in a meal regardless of how stuffed she feels. Gayle's parents work many hours, seldom shop for food, and eat most of their meals out. Gayle usually comes home from school to an empty house, no food or parents. With food haphazardly available, Gayle feels greatly deprived. She feels a compulsion to finish whatever food she gets, as she doesn't know where or when her next meal will appear.

Captivity Behavior. Various accounts of released hostages have reported obsessive thinking about food and cravings while "in captivity." On a somewhat lighter level, my (ER) son described his "captivity" behavior during a survival training camp out in the wilderness in Montana. To occupy his lonely hours, he would write lists of all the foods he wasn't getting. Yet, normally he is not preoccupied with food or cravings.

Depression-Era Eating. People who went through the Great American Depression hold food in special regard; it's cherished. There is a pervasive sense that there won't be enough food, or certain foods may become unavailable. And like a precious metal, you dare not throw food away, let alone waste it. "Clean your plate" takes on special meaning, and is passed on with other family traditions and values.

Once in a Lifetime. Eating a meal in a special restaurant while on vacation can stimulate a sense of future deprivation. For example, if you are in Paris eating a superb French meal, the thought of leaving even a forkful seems an impossible feat. After all, this is likely to be the one and only time you'll ever experience these particular tastes in this particular setting! You might eat until uncomfortably full, just because you're already feeling deprived.

exacerbated in college

One Last Shot. A similar experience can occur when eating a delicious meal at the home of a friend or tasting cookies that have been sent as a gift. The notion that this is your only shot at these foods drives you to eat every last bit of the meal or food.

HOW IS DIETING POSSIBLE?

If deprivation backlash is so powerful, how do dieters actually diet at all? Aren't the biological and psychological forces too compelling? Chronic dieters adapt by changing both their mind-set and their responsiveness to inner body cues. This adaptation is known as *restrained eating*. Unfortunately, these changes work against them. In the long run, deprivation backlash still prevails.

Restrained eaters, in essence, are chronic dieters who are preoccupied with dieting and weight control. To stay in control with their food, restrained eaters set up rules that dictate how they should eat, rather than listening to their bodies. Forget *honor your hunger*; instead they calculate what to eat, choosing foods with their mental brakes on, and second-guessing the needs of their bodies. Their eating appears to be fine until one of their sacred rules is violated. When a rule is broken, so is their restraint—and, wham, overeating begins. This has been described as *the what-the-hell effect* by leading researchers in this field, Janet Polivy, Ph.D., and C. Peter Herman, Ph.D., from the University of Toronto. And it is *that* phrase, rather than the term restrained eating, that most of our clients relate to! Here's what it means in eating terms:

true

- The moment a forbidden food is eaten, overeating takes place.
- The moment a calorie level is exceeded, overeating takes place.
- The mere *perception* of breaking a food rule or eating a forbidden food triggers overeating.

Restrained Eating Studies

Studies on restrained eaters have shed a lot of psychological light on the world of dieting. They show how ineffective outlawing particular foods can be and how it sets you up for overeating. Most restraint studies follow this core procedure:

A short ten-question test, called the Restraint Scale is given to identify who the restrained eaters are. (Questions include frequency of dieting, history of weight loss and gain, weekly weight fluctuations, emotional effect of weight fluctuations, effect of "others" on eating, obsessive thinking about food, and guilt feelings about eating.) Then a "preload" is given—that is, the subjects are "loaded up" with food *before* the real experiment begins. The preload is a calculated amount of food—and it's usually some sort of setup to see how the dieters versus non-dieters respond in various eating situations. Then the "real" experiment begins.

Here are a couple of particularly significant studies on restrained eaters:

Mind Games—The Counterregulation Effect. One of the classic studies involved fifty-seven female college students at Northwestern University. The students were led to believe that the goal of the study was to evaluate the *taste* of several ice cream samples. *The actual purpose of the study was to determine how diet thinking might affect eating after drinking milkshakes.* The women were arbitrarily divided into three groups, based on the number of eight-ounce milkshakes given (none, one, and two shakes). After drinking the shakes, the subjects were asked to taste and rate three flavors of ice cream. They were allowed to eat as much ice cream as they wanted and "taste tested" in privacy to guard against self-consciousness. The researchers saw to it that ample ice cream was provided so that substantial amounts could be eaten without making an appreciable dent in the supply!

Here's what happened. The non-dieters naturally regulated their eating; they ate less ice cream in proportion to the amount of milkshakes consumed. The dieters, however, had a dramatic, *opposite* behavior. Those who drank two milkshakes ate the *most* ice cream—a "counterregulation" effect. The researchers concluded that forcing the dieters to overeat or "blow their diet" caused them to release their food inhibitions. With inhibition banished, restraint was eliminated and the dieters overate the ice cream.

Perception Affects Eating. Another similar study examined the notion of how dieters perceive calories. All subjects were given snacks of chocolate pudding with a substantial calorie difference. One group was given a high-calorie pudding, and another was given a lower calorie version. But within each of these groups, half of the subjects were told that the pudding was high in calories, and half were told that it was low. Then the subjects were given a pseudo taste test. The dieters who *thought* the pudding was high in calories ate more than the dieters who *thought* the pudding was low in calories, by 61 percent! This study illustrates how much power thoughts and perception can have on eating behavior. And once again, when the dieter "blew the diet" (whether actual or perceived), overeating ensued.

The Seesaw Syndrome: Guilt vs. Deprivation

The longer foods are prohibited, the more seductive they become. Consequently, eating these "illegal" foods brings with it a compelling sense of guilt for most dieters. And as the guilt increases, so does the quantity of food intake. The more deprived you become from dieting and from specific foods, the greater the deprivation backlash. We see this all the time—we call it *the seesaw syndrome.*

When it comes to dieting, feelings of deprivation and guilt work in an opposing manner; like two kids on a seesaw—"what goes up must come down."

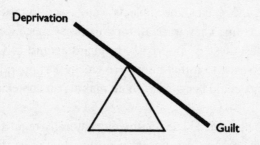

When dieting, as you restrict foods that you enjoy eating, deprivation becomes higher and higher. Meanwhile, in tandem, guilty feelings go down—because you haven't eaten any "bad" foods. But there's a limit to which the seesaw can climb. The level of deprivation rises to its highest point, where you can't bear one more meal, let alone one more day of restrictive eating. Meanwhile, guilty feelings are at their lowest, because you have not eaten any forbidden foods; you've been "good." Since you have no buildup of guilt, you're wide open to allow some forbidden foods into your life and able to tolerate the beginning feelings of guilt that these foods engender. As you eat the first forbidden food, you begin to feel guilt. That guilt triggers feelings of being "bad," which lead you to more food (the what-the-hell effect), with its accompanying guilt. Now the seesaw looks like a tug-of-war:

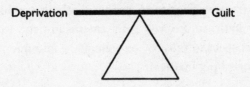

After awhile, the guilt continues to build, and in tandem, deprivation begins to recede. As the days go by, you feel worse about breaking your diet rules, and guilt rises to its highest point. Deprivation feelings are virtually nonexistent, because you've been eating all the foods that weren't allowed on the diet. Now the seesaw looks like the following diagram:

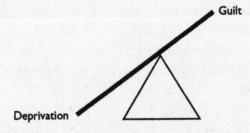

At this point the syndrome repeats itself—up and down, up and down—every time you go from diet to binge, diet to binge. The only way to get off this seesaw is to lighten up, and let go of the deprivation. And just as when one kid decides to get off the seesaw, the other is forced to stop playing, when you give yourself permission to not be deprived, you simultaneously let go of the guilt! By giving yourself permission to eat, you stop playing the futile seesaw game.

THE KEY: *UNCONDITIONAL* PERMISSION TO EAT

The key to abolishing the pattern of restraint and subsequent overeating is to give yourself unconditional permission to eat. This means:

that's really scary & hard – I'm at conditional for most foods but that's a big step

- Throwing out the preconceived notion that certain foods are "good" and others are "bad." No one food has the power to make you fat or help you to become slim.
- Eating what you *really* want. Yes, what you want.
- Eating without obligatory penance. (*"Okay, I can have the cheesecake now, but tomorrow I diet."*) These kinds of personal food deals are *not* unconditional.

When you truly free your food choices, without any hidden agenda of restricting them in the future, you eliminate the urgency to overeat. Yet it's an unsettling prospect to most of our clients, even more frightening than the initial idea of giving up diets.

The Peace Process

Making peace with food means allowing *all* foods into your eating world, so that a choice for chocolate becomes emotionally equal to a choice for a peach. It also means that your food choices do not reflect your character or morality. While for years many health professionals have agreed that there should be no forbidden foods, very few will go the distance and say, eat *whatever* you want. Eventually there is a limit imposed. And knowing there is a limit can still impart a food lust of sorts—better eat it now!

Ironically, once you truly know you can eat whatever you want, the intensity to eat greatly diminishes. The most effective way to instill this belief is to experience eating the very foods you forbid! It becomes self-evident proof that you can "handle" these foods, or better yet that they have no magic hold on you or your willpower. Ironically, once again, many of our clients discover that the very foods that they had prohibited and craved are no longer desirable once they can be eaten freely. Over and over, we hear stories of how, when they were truly allowed to eat certain foods, they discovered, to their surprise, that they really didn't like the foods to begin with! For example, Molly had relished bakery birthday cakes, but tried not to eat them. She would, however, eventually relent, especially at a party and power through two or more pieces. But when she decided to make peace with food—and come face-to-face with "official permission," she found that she did not care for most bakery birthday cakes. She had always eaten them so fast, often on the sly, that she had not truly experienced the taste and texture of the cake! With her newfound permission, Molly took the time to *taste* the cake (whether in the privacy of her home or at a party). She found more often than not that the cakes were stale or bland, and would not finish a single piece, let alone go for more pieces. Eventually, Molly would not settle for cakes that were less than superb. She now often turns down cake at parties—because she wants to, not because she is a diet martyr.

Annie had a similar "taste experience." Her commitment to making peace with food sparked an enthusiasm for taste sensations that had been buried by her restrained eating. Annie gave herself unconditional permis-

[handwritten margin note:] ok, good – I'd love some guidance on this

sion to experience forbidden foods one at a time, day after day, often in preference to all other foods. Annie went through her red licorice phase, her Pop-Tarts phase, and her mashed potato phase. While in the midst of each phase, she ate the favored food with relish and delight. For some foods, she found that it took a few weeks for the desire to peak and then slowly taper off. For other foods it took longer, and for a few she found that they didn't taste half as good as she had imagined.

To Annie's surprise (and delight), she discovered that once she completed a particular food-freeing phase, she found that *she stopped craving that food, hardly ever thought of it, and sometimes was so sick of it that she never wanted it again!* Removing deprivation from Annie's eating diminished the alluring quality of foods, and instead, put them in a reasonable, rational perspective.

Fears That Hold You Back

Even clients who come ready to give up dieting have a strong resistance to eating whatever they *really* want. They are terrified. While they feel comfortable learning to *honor their hunger,* they are ready to bolt out the door when we talk about giving unconditional permission to eat what they like.

If people are so afraid to advance to this part of the Intuitive Eating process, why do we insist that this must be explored? Legalizing food is the critical step in changing your relationship with food. It frees you to respond to inner eating signals that have been smothered by negative thoughts and guilt feelings about eating. When you don't truly believe that you can eat whatever food you like, you will continue to feel deprived, ultimately overeat, and be blocked from feeling satisfied with your eating. And when you are not satisfied, you will be on the prowl for more food! When you know the food will be there and allowed, day after day, it doesn't become so important to have it. Food loses its power.

In spite of the knowledge that deprivation leads to backlash eating, many people are apprehensive to make this peace pact with food, in part due to the following obstacles.

I Won't Stop Eating

At first you may experience an overpowering fear that you won't stop eating a favorite forbidden food. Just remember that when you know that previously forbidden foods will always be allowed, the urgency to have large quantities of them eventually dissipates. Also research shows that people will tire of eating the same kind of food—it's called habituation. *Habituation studies have shown that the more a person is exposed to a particular food the less appealing it becomes.* (See "Habituation Response Explains Why Foods Become Less Enticing with Exposure" on page 91.) In fact, you may have already witnessed this type of eating in other people. For example, observe the all-you-can-eat buffet dining that is popular in vacation spots such as Las Vegas. On the first day, people typically load up their plates and grab three or four desserts. By the last day, however, they are choosing their food selectively. The novelty has worn off, and they know there is plenty of food.

My entire family (ET) recently encountered the habituation effect when I was working on a two-hundred-recipe cookbook. Whether I was testing salads, appetizers, or casseroles, we eventually tired of eating the same kinds of food. This was especially evident while creating the dessert chapter. Not only did we tire of eating sweets, but one family member to this day cannot bear to take a bite of pineapple upside-down cake, which was once his favorite! I made that particular cake at least eight times before I decided to give up on that *particular* recipe.

The only way that *you* will come to believe that you will be able to stop eating is *to go through the food experience, to actually eat.* That's why we are fond of the word "process." This is not about knowledge of food, but rather rebuilding experiences with eating. You cannot have an experience through knowledge; rather, you need to go through it, bite by bite. Otherwise it would be like trying to learn how to play the guitar by reading a book on music theory. You may understand the components—but only when you practice and struggle with the strings personally will you truly know how to play. And the more you practice, the more confidence you will have.

Sometimes people express a fear about being addicted to food—there are many reasons, other than addiction, that can explain the reward aspect of eating. (For more information, see "Can You Really Be Addicted to Food?" on page 92.)

Pseudo-Permission: I've Tried It Before

Many of our clients will recount that when they "allowed" themselves to eat certain forbidden foods, they still overate and felt out of control. But for most people these foods were never really *unconditionally* allowed; rather, they were only given pseudo-permission. These forbidden foods were actually being eaten with a sense of temporarily breaking the rules, or with a little voice saying, "you really shouldn't eat that." The moment that food touched the tongue, feelings of guilt and remorse flooded in. And with these feelings came a conviction to limit these foods in the future and counter this indulgence by "eating right" tomorrow. Although physically eating the food, they were emotionally depriving themselves in the future. And so the cycle perpetuates. Pseudo-permission does not work—it's only an illusion. Your mouth may be chewing, but your mind is saying, "I shouldn't." Your mind is still on a diet.

Self-Fulfilling Prophecy

Sometimes just the thought that you will overeat is enough to actually make you overeat. Carolyn initially had held the strong conviction that white flour would cause her to overeat. She believed that even one bite of a bagel would trigger a binge. And it did. Carolyn had created a self-fulfilling prophecy. She "knew" these foods were fattening, she "knew" she would binge, and she "knew" she would gain weight. Every time she gave into her craving for white bread, she sincerely told herself that this would be the last time. Of course, she ended up overdoing it—the depriving thoughts and feelings, along with her sense of being bad sent her out of control.

It took a long time before Carolyn was truly able to permit herself to eat foods with white flour, but now she rarely binges on these foods. Every now and then a fleeting, archaic thought of restriction occurs and drags her back to the world of deprivation. And with that thought comes her occasional sense of loss of control. Now, though, she only has a few cookies instead of the whole bag, and this happens once every six months instead of every week. Because Carolyn has had so many positive experiences with foods containing white flour, it has become much easier for her to let go of her restrictive thinking and make peace with these foods.

I Won't Eat Healthfully

In case after case, when people are given free choice and access to all varieties of food, after going through the peace process, they end up balancing their intake to include mostly nutritious foods with a smattering of "play foods." As nutritionists, we continue to honor and respect nutrition, but at this point in the Intuitive Eating process, nutrition is not the driving force. If nutrition were the overriding priority now it would only perpetuate your restrictive thoughts. (It took us years to come to terms with this factor, and it is why nutrition issues are reserved for later in this book.) As you go further along with the process and all foods are completely allowed, your intuitive signals will give you good advice. But even right now, if you think about eating a hot fudge sundae for every meal, how soon do you think you will be craving something completely opposite, such as a salad or a piece of grilled chicken?

✦Lack of Self-Trust

A mighty obstacle to making peace with food is a strong lack of self-trust. Most clients say that they intellectually trust us and our philosophy. They truly believe that it has worked for "other" clients, but they distrust themselves and are frightened that it won't work for them.

Ironically, the process of giving yourself permission to eat is actually the stepping-stone to rebuilding your trust with food and with yourself. In the beginning, each positive food experience is like a tiny thread. They may be few and far between, and seem insignificant, but eventually the threads form a strand. The strands multiply into strong ropes and finally the ropes become the bridge to a foundation of trust in food and in yourself.

Betsy was gaining weight by the moment when she first came in. She had been on several very restricted diets and was now rebound eating in an out-of-control fashion. After a short time of giving herself permission to eat, she began to find herself eating only *one* candy bar instead of three, which was a major breakthrough. At first these experiences were sporadic and her successes were interspersed with large gaps of bingeing behavior. But Betsy was gradually able to see her successes build upon each other and watch her overeating begin to gradually disappear. Soon she began to redevelop that sense of self-trust that had been eroded by her history of dieting.

For some, the trust issue goes even deeper. Several studies have shown that the regulation of food intake has its foundation in early eating experiences. If as a child your parents took control over most of your eating without respecting your preferences or hunger levels, you easily got the message that you couldn't be trusted with food.

Sarah described this as the push-or-pull-away effect. Her mom was either pushing her to eat, while exerting pressure about Sarah's weight, or pulling food away. At dinner time, for example, Sarah's mom forced her to clean her plate, even though she was full. Sarah remembers coming home from school on several occasions feeling famished and heading for the fridge for a snack. Her mom would chastise her, "You can't be hungry," and forbid her to eat. Consequently, Sarah would sneak food when her mom wasn't looking. By that time, however, hunger was no longer mild, but intense. Sarah would overeat in response to hunger, but she felt guilty from overeating and shame from sneaking the food. And she grew to believe that her mother was right—she couldn't be trusted with food. Wrong!

Don't underestimate the profound impact self-trust can have. Psychoanalyst Erik Erikson, a noted pioneer in human development, explains how critical trust is. According to Erikson, all people must go through a series of stages throughout their lives. The first developmental stage deals with basic trust. During each stage there is a significant issue or crisis that presents itself and must be resolved. If this task is not handled well, a person will continue to struggle with it into adulthood. If food becomes a battleground during this stage, the ability to trust yourself with food becomes tarnished. The you-can't-be-trusted-around-food message becomes compounded if you were put on diets by your parents or your doctor. As an adult, try as you may, you still don't trust yourself. That child can still reside within you, making you fearful to give yourself permission to eat unconditionally.

Fortunately, Erikson had an optimistic belief that childhood crises can be resolved at any time later in life. If you take back ownership of your eating signals by making peace with food, you can heal one of the most basic trust issues and go on to a healthier relationship with food.

Five Steps to Make Peace with Food

Keep in mind as you read through these steps that it's okay to proceed at a pace with which *you* are comfortable. There is no need to feel overwhelmed by going to the grocery store and buying every single forbidden food—we find that is too big of a step and not necessary. It takes time to build up trust in yourself. Before you proceed, please be sure that you are consistently *honoring your hunger.* A ravenous person is bound to overeat regardless of his or her intention.

1. Pay attention to the foods that are appealing to you and make a list of them.
2. Put a check by the foods you actually do eat, then circle remaining foods that you've been restricting.
3. Give yourself permission to eat one forbidden food from your list, then go to the market and buy this food, or order it at a restaurant.
4. Check in with yourself to see if the food tastes as good as you imagined. If you find that you really like it, continue to give yourself permission to buy or order it.
5. Make sure that you keep enough of the food in your kitchen so that you know that it will be there if you want it. Or if that seems too scary, go to a restaurant and order the particular food as often as you like.

oh, ok, I can do that

Once you've made peace with one food, continue on with your list until all the foods are tried, evaluated, and freed. If your list is quite large, which is possible, we have found that you don't have to experience each and every food listed. Rather, what is important is that you continue this process until you *truly know* you can eat what you want. You will get to a point where you don't have to experience the "proof" by eating.

If these steps seem like too much to handle right now, don't worry. Maybe you can call a cease-fire, that's okay—it's progress. The next chapter will give you some tools to help you loosen up with your food. Just as many peace treaties require a team of negotiators—and time—the next chapter will help you discover powerful allies to help keep the peace with food.

Beware of the I-Can-Eat-Whatever-I-Want, As-Much-As-I-Want, Whenever-I-Feel-Like-It Trap

This perception, or trap, actually distorts the premise of Intuitive Eating. Yes, make peace with food, and eat what pleases your palate. Yes, give yourself the freedom to eat unconditionally, and eat as much as you need to satisfy your body. But eating whenever you feel like it, without regard to hunger and fullness, might not be a very satisfying experience and might also cause physical discomfort. Attunement with your body's satiety cues is an important part of this process.

HABITUATION RESPONSE EXPLAINS WHY FOODS BECOME LESS ENTICING WITH EXPOSURE

One reason that having unconditional permission to eat is important is because of the habituation response. Habituation explains why we quickly adapt to a repeated experience—and subsequently experience less pleasure each time. It's a universal phenomenon that applies in many situations—such as when you buy a new car. At first, it's super exciting, but then the novelty wears off. Or when you hear a special person say, "I love you" for the first time. It's magical, but then it becomes routine, and even expected. Psychologist and author, Daniel Gilbert, aptly describes habituation as, "Wonderful things are especially wonderful the first time they happen, but their wonderfulness wanes with repetition" (Gilbert 2006).

Habituation is also one of the reasons why leftovers are less appealing, especially on days two and three. When you eat a food over and over, it simply loses its appeal. There is a good deal of research on food habituation, which shows that people habituate to a variety of foods, like pizza, chocolate, and potato chips (Ernst 2002). Scientists describe food habituation as a form of neurobiological learning, in which repeated eating of the same food causes a decrease in behavioral and physiologic responses (Epstein 2009).

Studies also show that the habituation response is delayed by eating novel foods and by stress and distraction. This works against chronic dieters, in particular. Dieting heightens the novelty and desirability for the forbidden foods. When they go off the diet, dieters often eat those forbidden foods in excess, in part because of the lack of habituation. When you combine low habituation with the fear of never being able to eat a particular food, it can become a powerful force in overeating, which we call Last Supper eating. It's difficult to tire of eating a food, which you think you may not ever eat again!

Part of the purpose behind having unconditional permission to eat, is not to "get sick" or burn out on a particular food—it's to experience habituation, in which the heightened novelty of eating a particular food wanes.

A recent study provided the first promising evidence of long-term food habituation (Epstein 2011). Two groups of women, non-obese and obese, were given the same food with their meals, daily, over a five-week period. This resulted in an increased rate of habituation and decreased energy intake in both groups of women.

CAN YOU REALLY BE ADDICTED TO FOOD?

There has been a lot of research speculation and media attention on food addiction. Scientists are curious, because the brain region (and neurochemicals) involved with substance abuse are also implicated in overeating. But there are many reasons, other than addiction, that can explain the reward aspect of eating.

Survival of the Species. This brain-reward system is believed to be necessary in order to ensure human survival. This involves the brain chemical dopamine, which triggers both a pleasurable feeling and motivation behavior. Engaging in activities necessary to survival (such as eating and procreating) triggers a rewarding feel-good experience.

Hunger Enhances Reward Value. Hunger by itself enhances the reward value of food, through triggering more dopamine-related activity. For example, if you discover you are hungry, you might find yourself suddenly interested and motivated to cook a meal. Dieting (which can be a form of chronic hunger) also has this effect.

Pavlovian Conditioning. The dopamine effect could be attributed to Pavlovian conditioning (recall the classic study, in which Pavlov's dogs salivated at the mere ringing of a bell. This anticipatory salivation occurred because the dogs were conditioned to receiving a treat each time, after a bell rang). This is not addiction.

Dopamine Deprivation. Many pleasurable activities trigger dopamine, including socializing, hiking, and playing games. The great majority of people we see in our practices, who binge-eat, are often leading very unbalanced lives. These unbalanced lives "deprive" them of the dopamine benefits. When needs are not being met, food becomes even more enticing, more rewarding.

Music Lights Up Dopamine Brain Centers. Recently, a new study showed that when people listen to music, it lights up the same region of the brain (nucleus accumbens), which has been implicated in the euphoric component of psychostimulants, such as cocaine (Salimpoor 2011). Just the anticipation of hearing the music lit up the dopamine brain centers. (Yet, we really don't think you can make the case for "music addiction"!)

cont.

Continued

Food Addiction Studies Are Limited and Flawed. The research on "food addiction" is too much in its infancy to be drawing any conclusions. In addition, the great majority of studies have been on animals. The limited research on humans has only been focused on brain-imaging studies with a very small amount of people and not much exclusion criteria (Benson 2010).

Yale Food Addiction Questionnaire. This has generated a lot of headline news. Yet, upon a closer look, the questionnaire seems to actually be measuring compulsive eating or rebound eating from chronic dieting (Gearhardt 2009). Here is a sampling of the questions:

- I find myself consuming certain foods even though I am no longer hungry. *(Classic compulsive eating or distracted eating can cause this.)*
- I worry about cutting down on certain foods. *(Chronic dieting and overeating can cause this.)*
- I have spent time dealing with negative feelings from overeating certain foods, instead of spending time in important activities such as time with family, friends, work, or recreation. *(Chronic dieting and compulsive eating can cause this.)*

(To read more questions and details on scoring the questionnaire see http://abcn.ws/dN8Fcl and Gearhardt 2009.)

Studies Show Eating "Forbidden Food" Decreases Binge Eating. Finally, there are three studies to date, in which binge eaters eat their "forbidden foods" as part of the treatment process (Kristeller 2011, Smitham 2008). Binge eating decreased significantly in all of these studies. If food addiction were an issue, you would not expect these types of results. Food addiction theory would predict increased binge eating, triggered by eating "addicting food." Yet, the opposite happened.

Chapter 8

PRINCIPLE 4:

Challenge the Food Police

Scream a loud "No" to thoughts in your head that declare you're "good" for eating minimal calories or "bad" because you ate a piece of chocolate cake. The Food Police monitor the unreasonable rules that dieting has created. The police station is housed deep in your psyche and its loudspeaker shouts negative barbs, hopeless phrases, and guilt-provoking indictments. Chasing the Food Police away is a critical step in returning to Intuitive Eating.

> *I felt so guilty eating an extra piece of birthday cake that when I felt nauseous for three days, I thought that I had earned and deserved this misery. To my surprise, I found out one week later that nausea was not my penance for my eating indulgence—I was pregnant!*
>
> —A chronic dieter

We have become a nation riddled with guilt based on how we eat. Even non-dieters experience eating angst. In a random survey of 2,075 adults, 45 percent said they feel guilty after eating foods they like! And nearly all of our clients also feel that way—guilty, guilty, guilty.

The thought of stealing or lying would instill a sense of guilt in most people. Yet, most dieters are able to create an equivalent level of guilt when they've eaten french fries or a hot fudge sundae. The quantity of any of these "bad" foods has almost nothing to do with the level of despair that is felt when they are eaten. The first bite often evokes a sense of having failed, or being bad. Eating a "bad" or "illegal" food then becomes a morality issue. The subsequent guilt that builds is enough to initiate a period of overeating that can destroy any previous moderate eating.

Foods are often described in moralistic terms, independent of dieting: decadent, sinful, tempting—all the words of food fundamentalism and

guilt in one of my primary drivers, for sure

eating morality. Historian Roberta Pollack Seid concluded in her book *Never Too Thin* that our beliefs about food resemble dietary laws of a false religion—we pay homage to dieting and its rules, but it doesn't work.

Since we are a nation that worships the lean body, it easily becomes virtuous to be eating foods associated with slimness and guiltlessness. It is no wonder that dieters have been found to think of food in terms of *absence* of guilt. A major finding in a 1987 study on chronic dieters at the University of Toronto found that the dieting experience appears to make the guilt-free aspect of foods a key attribute. One in four dieters categorized food using both "guilt" and "no guilt" labels, compared to one out of twenty-five non-dieters. Dieters primarily felt guilt for highly caloric, diet-breaking foods.

But dieters don't corner the market in the food guilt department. Nondieters, in the same study, associated guilt with poor nutritional quality of foods. And the media and food companies play a hand in this, tugging at our food consciences, whether or not we are dieting.

Food companies, magazines, and commercials are capitalizing on consumer eating morality with absolving themes:

- "Be bad. Snack well, they let you be bad, and still be good" (an ad for SnackWell's Fudge Drizzled Caramel Popcorn).
- Guiltless Gourmet (a food company that specializes in fat-free snacks)
- "It's like you dieted and went to heaven" (a magazine ad for Bailey's Light).
- "Butter Paroled, Margarine Charged" (an article in *Eating Well* magazine).

With these daily reminders it becomes difficult to view eating as simply a normal pleasurable activity; rather, it becomes good or bad, with the societal Food Police chastising each blasphemous bite of food. The Food Police are alive and well—both as a collective cultural voice and at the individual level, in the thoughts of our clients.

As you embark on your journey to Intuitive Eating you may encounter your fair share of societal Food Police—from the well-meaning friend, who comments, "How can you eat *that,* I thought you were trying to lose weight" to unsolicited commentary on your eating habits from a stranger. Just because someone makes an inappropriate comment does not make it true!

Yet, it can shed seeds of doubt as you begin to explore a new eating world that runs counter to the doctrine of fat-phobia orthodoxy in this nation.

Some years ago on a vacation, I (ET) experienced an unwelcome Food Police barb. I placed my order at the customized omelet bar, and requested an egg white omelet with mushrooms and *cheese*. The chef nearly gave me hell for my order; he reprimanded, "How can you order an egg white omelet with that fatty cheese, it's loaded with cholesterol." That unsolicited remark would have devastated most of our patients. I was on vacation, and did not feel like defending my consciously placed order. I knew full well what I was doing—I don't really like egg yolks, so why eat them? I'm not crazy about cheese, but since I was pregnant during this vacation, it was one way I was able to get my calcium in, since I'm not fond of drinking milk. It was our clients' worst fear personified.

We have found that regardless of the level of inappropriate comments from the collective Food Police—the inner Food Police that reside in the minds of our clients are even harsher. If our nation is being possessed by a food fundamentalism, then certainly no less than a Food Police exorcism will do.

FOOD TALK

In the world of dieting we develop a whole retinue of thoughts that can work against us. These thoughts can come from diet books, diet program commercials, and a generalized pervasive diet mentality in society. Self-awareness, or having the ability to think about our thoughts, distinguishes us from animals. It's also human, however, to let our busy lives lead us from one routine activity to the next without stopping to be aware of or examine our thoughts. Food thoughts and judgments run rampant through our minds, but how often do we take a moment to focus on them? We're not born with these thoughts. We hear the ideas behind them as we grow up, take them in, and sometimes then adopt them as "well-known" rules, which must not be defied.

Here is some of the "knowledge" and thoughts that prevail in the minds of our clients when they first come to see us:

- Sweets are bad for you.
- I shouldn't eat anything after 6 P.M.
- You should take in zero grams of fat.
- Walking three times a week won't do me any good.

- If I eat breakfast, it will just make me eat more throughout the day.
- Dairy products are bad for you.
- I shouldn't have any salt.
- Beans are fattening.
- Bread is fattening.
- Everything is fattening!

Even when these thoughts are evaluated, they stick like glue in the consciousness of the people who think them. Although there has been a great deal of evidence to refute these thoughts, they've become so well entrenched that it often takes years to loosen their hold and replace them with reality. The thoughts themselves can be very damaging and can affect subsequent behavior. These thoughts are called cognitive distortions, and we call the voices that speak these distortions the Food Police.

WHO'S TALKING

There are many psychological ways of looking at personality structure. Psychotherapist and M.D. Eric Berne tells us that the way we feel and the ways

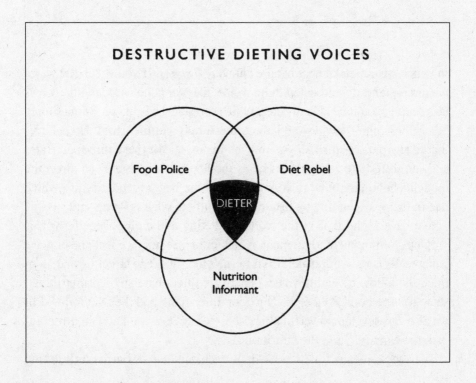

DESTRUCTIVE DIETING VOICES

Food Police

Diet Rebel

DIETER

Nutrition
Informant

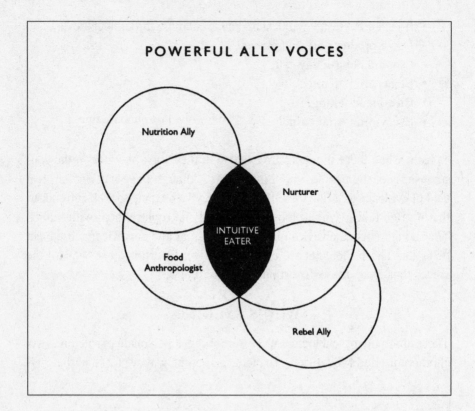

POWERFUL ALLY VOICES

Nutrition Ally

Nurturer

INTUITIVE
EATER

Food
Anthropologist

Rebel Ally

in which we act make up what are called *ego states*. If you watch the way a person is standing and listen to his voice, the words he uses, and the views he's stating, you'll be able to detect which ego state he is in. Dr. Berne simply labels these ego states as the Parent, the Adult, and the Child. He believes that at any particular time, you may be in any one of these three ego states and can shift quite easily from one to another. Each ego state can direct the thoughts floating around in your head. You can begin to identify just which one of them is speaking by listening carefully to what is being said.

We have found that in the world of dieting and eating, specific voices crop up from moment to moment, which influence how we feel and how we behave. We have extrapolated from Berne's theory of ego structure and identified the following eating voices. There are three that can be primarily destructive: the Food Police, the Nutrition Informant, and the Diet Rebel. But we also can develop powerful allies; these voices are: the Food Anthropologist, the Nurturer, and the Nutrition Ally.

Let's look at each food voice—how each can help or harm our thinking process in the world of eating. The diagrams on the previous pages give an overview of how they interrelate.

✦ The Food Police ✦

The Food Police is a strong voice that's developed through dieting. It's your inner judge and jury that determine if you are doing "good" or "bad." The Food Police is the sum of all your dieting and food rules, and gets stronger with each diet. It also gets strengthened through new food rules that you may read about in magazines or messages you hear from friends and family. The Food Police is alive and well even when you are not dieting (like a lobbyist positioning his issue during an election year).

Here are some common rules by which the Food Police may judge your eating actions:

- Don't eat at night (therefore if you eat at night, you are guilty of a violation).
- Better not eat that bagel—it's fattening, too many carbohydrates.
- You didn't exercise today, better not eat dinner.
- It's not time to eat yet—don't have that snack.
- You ate too much (even though it was based on being hungry).

It's important to remember that even when you reject dieting and begin to make peace with food, the Food Police will often surface. But it's not always obvious—just like a weed cut above the surface. A weed that is strongly rooted can easily flourish, even when there are no green tendrils peeking through the soil.

HOW IT HURTS: The Food Police scrutinizes every eating action. It keeps food and your body at war.

HOW IT HELPS: *It doesn't!* This is one voice that does not turn into an ally. By identifying its strong presence in your mind, however, you will learn how to challenge its power and loosen its hold on you.

Cyndi had a powerful Food Police voice that criticized every eating act. She woke up every morning praying for a "good" day, which meant eating only diet foods. But her Food Police voice set impossible standards. Her good day would begin with a light breakfast of grapefruit juice and a small bowl of cereal. On some days her growling stomach would beg for more food—just an extra piece of toast. Cyndi would "cave in" and have a piece of dry rye toast, and her Food Police would shout, "Now you have to skip lunch or dinner." When Cyndi was able to skip lunch, she'd get too hungry and find herself at the vending machine devouring whatever she could afford. Now, once she had officially broken her Food Police rule, she would overeat the rest of the day. In fact, Cyndi's vicious overeating cycle would begin anytime she disobeyed her Food Police. It wasn't until Cyndi began to challenge the Food Police voice that her overeating stopped.

The Nutrition Informant

The Nutrition Informant provides nutrition evidence to keep you in line with dieting. The Nutrition Informant voice may tell you to fastidiously count carbohydrate grams, or eat only fat-free foods, often in the name of health. While this may seem innocuous or even healthy, it's a facade.

The Nutrition Informant makes statements like:

- Check those fat grams, anything above one gram of fat is unacceptable.
- Don't eat foods with added sweeteners.

It's not unusual for someone to say, "I've rejected dieting, I truly believe I can eat what I want—I *want* to start eating healthfully." It's therefore possible to consciously reject dieting, but instead unknowingly continue to diet as a politically correct regimen for keeping your weight down.

HOW IT HURTS: This voice colludes with the Food Police. It operates under the guise of health, but it's promoting an unconscious diet. It can be a little difficult to identify, because its messages can mimic the sound advice of health authorities.

For example, Kelly declared, "I've made peace with food, I'm never going to diet again, but I'm ready to start eating healthfully." She was actually burned out on exploring "junk foods" which in and of itself was something she never thought she would accomplish!

Here's what happened. One afternoon at work, Kelly got hungry, so she honored her hunger and ate an apple, in the name of "healthy eating." But one hour later, she was hungry. Her Nutrition Informant voice chimed in with the Food Police telling her, "You shouldn't be hungry—you just had a healthy apple. Wait until you get home to eat." She waited until she arrived at home, and proceeded to devour her pantry out of ravenous hunger. Later, we talked about satisfying snacks including a bagel or bean soup. "But aren't those—fattening?" she asked. "The only snacks I thought I should eat were either fresh fruit or cut-up vegetables." Kelly's description sounded like the diet dogma of snacking, yet she did not see it as such, because she was focused on health and had sincerely rejected dieting. Yet, one of Kelly's Food Police rules had surfaced: "If you snack, you can't possibly be hungry later." This rule merged with the Nutrition Informant voice, which declared, "If you snack, it should only be raw veggies or fruit because they're good for you and healthy." While Kelly chose the apple in the name of health and nutrition, she had difficulty honoring her true hunger that surfaced only one hour later; because her Food Police and Nutrition Informant voices were overpowering (yet subtle, because she did not recognize them).

HOW IT CAN HELP: The Nutrition Informant becomes the Nutrition Ally when the Food Police are exiled. The newly emerged Nutrition Ally is interested in healthy eating with *no hidden agenda*. For example, if you were choosing between two brands of cheese that you like equally and you happen to have high cholesterol, the Nutrition Ally would advise choosing the brand with lower saturated fat. It's a choice based on health and satisfaction, *not* deprivation or dieting. We have found that the helpful version of this voice is one of the last to truly appear without being tied into the Food Police. (*Note:* We will address nutrition later in the book. Remember, however, that focusing initially on nutrition can undermine your attempts to be truly free from dieting. It's not that nutrition is not important, but rather that it can be self-defeating in the beginning stages of Intuitive Eating. Remember, we *are* nutritionists, and we honor health!)

One distinguishing factor between the Nutrition Ally and the Nutrition Informant is how you *feel* when you respond. If you make or reject a food choice in the name of health, but feel acquiescent or guilty, then you know the Food Police still have a strong hold on your Nutrition Informant who's guiding your decision.

The Diet Rebel

The voice of the Diet Rebel often bellows loudly in your head. It sounds angry and determined. Here are some typical statements of your internal Diet Rebel:

- You're not going to get me to eat that plain broiled chicken!
- I'll show you, you think I should lose five pounds, huh—I'll put on ten.
- Let's see how many cookies I can stuff in before Mom comes home.
- I can't wait until my husband goes out of town so I can eat whatever I want, without his chastising glares.

HOW IT HURTS: Unfortunately, these rebellious comments reside in your head, because you're usually too scared to confront your "space invaders" and tell them to bug off. Feeling powerless over their messages, you feel resigned to merely possessing the thoughts you wish you could say out loud, and then end up carrying out the "threats" just to spite them.

Janie had a strong Diet Rebel voice. Every time her mother put her on a diet as a child, Janie's sneak-eating would escalate. The Diet Rebel voice was Janie's primary guiding force as a child and as an adult. Janie would hang out at her friends' homes so she could eat as much of their treats as she could stuff in her mouth. Overweight as a child, Janie became morbidly obese as an adult. When her ex-husband carried on the parental diet messages, Janie's silent Diet Rebel became loud and angry. It was her "forget you" inner voice that directed her to go against any rules imposed upon her, which resulted in overeating. Janie's boundaries were being invaded everywhere she turned. In order to protect her autonomy, Janie's Diet Rebel was overpowering all other voices to help keep her independent. Yet it only ended up in private food riots of overeating.

Unfortunately, when the Diet Rebel rules the roost, self-destruction always ensues. Rebellious behavior often has no limits, and severe overeating is usually the result. How often does the diet rebel break forth in your thoughts? How often do you feel compelled to follow its directions, because you're so angry at the Food Police in your life imposing their dieting rules on you?

HOW IT CAN HELP: You can turn your Diet Rebel into the Rebel Ally. Use the Rebel Ally to help you protect your boundaries against anyone who invades your eating space. *Use your mouth for words instead of food* in a direct but polite way—it's surprising how powerful it can make you feel, while giving you a tremendous release.

- Ask your family members to stay out of your food choices or amounts. For example: "Aunt Carolyn, please don't push that second portion on me. I'm full, thank you." Or, "No thanks, Mom, I don't like macaroni and cheese. You know I've never liked macaroni and cheese."
- Tell your family and your friends and people on the street that they may not make comments about your body. For example: "Dad—my body is *my* business!" Or, "Joey, you have no right to comment about my weight."

luckily I don't struggle w/ this — supportive home & friend enu

The Food Anthropologist

The Food Anthropologist is simply the neutral observer. This is the voice that makes observations *without* making judgment. It's a neutral voice that takes note of your thoughts and actions with respect to your food world, without an indictment—just like an anthropologist would observe an individual or culture. It's the voice that will let you explore and discover. The Food Anthropologist will help pave the way to the world of Intuitive Eating. For example, noticing when you're hungry or full, what you ate, the time of day, and what you're thinking, are the actions of the Food Anthropologist. This voice simply observes and shows you how to interact with food both behaviorally and inwardly. The advantage to developing this voice is that only *you* know what you feel and think. No outside observer could possibly know this.

The statements of the Food Anthropologist are purely observational such as:

- I skipped breakfast and was ravenous at 2 P.M.
- I ate ten cookies. (No judgment here, just the facts.)
- I experienced guilt after eating dessert with dinner. (No condescending statements, just an observation of how you felt.)

One easy way to call your inner Food Anthropologist into action is to keep an Intuitive Eating journal. Sometimes simply noting the time of day and what you ate can give you some interesting clues about what drives your eating. Or note your thoughts before and after you eat. Do they affect how you *feel*? Does your feeling state affect how you behave or eat? If so, how? Consider this one big experiment, *not a tool for judgment.*

Many of our clients have had negative experiences with food journals because it was a requirement of past diets. But in those cases the food journal was used as evidence to convict bad eating! We use the Intuitive Eating journal only as a learning tool. Yet in spite of the fact that we stress this, our first-time clients still expect to get verbally beaten up upon their return visit for any "eating indiscretion" or violation. Remember this is not a tool of the Food Police, but a tool to help you access the Food Anthropologist.

HOW IT HELPS: The Food Anthropologist can help you sort through the facts rather than get caught up in the emotionally labile experience of eating. It keeps you in touch with your inner signals—biologically and psychologically. We often play the role of the Food Anthropologist with our clients until they can build their own voice. (It can be hard to be just neutral when you've had a critical voice harping on every food choice.) The Food Anthropologist can help find the loopholes in your thinking, similar to the way a sharp attorney can find the loopholes in a contract. But using this voice does take practice.

The Nurturer

cultivate this one! have definitely been hearing it more

The Nurturer's voice is soft and gentle and has the soothing quality that might be associated with the voice of a loving grandparent or best friend. It has the ability to reassure you that you're okay and that everything will turn out fine. It never scolds or pressures. It's not critical or judgmental. Instead it is (or can be) the vehicle for most of the positive self-talk in your head.

Here are some of the messages you might hear from the Nurturer in your head:

- It's okay to have a cookie. Eating a cookie is normal.
- I really overate today. I wonder what I was feeling that could have made me need more food to comfort myself?
- When I take care of myself, I feel great.
- I'm doing so well this week. There were only a few times that I didn't honor my hunger signals.
- I'm getting more in touch with myself every day.

Alice is a mother who usually knows just the right thing to say to her children to make them feel safe and secure. But for many years, Alice had not learned to speak to herself kindly about her weight problem. The voice of the Food Police punished her severely through all of her diets. On her journey to becoming an Intuitive Eater, Alice learned to counter the messages of the Food Police with the supportive messages of the Nurturer. She listened to herself speak to her family and realized that the voice she used when speaking to them was the same voice that she needed to comfort herself.

Alice learned to be understanding of the stumbling blocks in her path and to patiently reassure herself that she was in the midst of a process. When she would have difficulty honoring her hunger, she'd gently ask herself what was bothering her and what she really needed instead of food. When she found herself craving a food she had restricted on one of her many diets, the Nurturer gave her permission to eat that food.

HOW IT HELPS: When you get in touch with the Nurturer inside your head, you will experience one of the most significant tools to becoming an Intuitive Eater. The Nurturer will be there for you to help you to challenge the Food Police and support you through this process. The Nurturer provides coping statements for the harsh zingers that the Food Police and the Diet Rebel can throw.

The Intuitive Eater

The Intuitive Eater speaks from your gut reactions. You were born an Intuitive Eater, but this persona has probably been suppressed for most of your life by the voices of the Food Police (prevailing in your family and in society), the Diet Rebel, and the Nutrition Informant.

The Intuitive Eater is a compilation of the positive voices of the Food Anthropologist, who is able to observe your eating behavior neutrally, and the Nurturer, who holds you with supportive statements to get you through the tough times, as well as the Rebel Ally, and the Nutrition Ally. The Intuitive Eater knows how to argue the negative voices out of your head. For example, it knows how to challenge the distorted messages of the Food Police and how to get the Rebel Ally to speak out loud to fend off the boundary invaders.

The Intuitive Eater voice might say some of the following things:

- That little rumble in my stomach means I'm hungry and need to eat.

- What do I feel like eating for dinner tonight? What sounds good to me?
- It feels so good to be out of that dieting prison.

These statements all tell you about your gut reactions. They're instinctual and hit you out of nowhere, without your having to think about them. You'll find that you'll be in the midst of a meal and the Intuitive Eater voice knows that you're satisfied. Or you'll be doing some writing and a hunger pang will emerge. Or maybe your eyes lock onto the food on the menu that connects with your craving. When you have reached the last stages of your path to Intuitive Eating, the Intuitive Eater, rather than the dieter, will prevail most of the time. But there will be times when you find that you'll need to evoke one or all of the positive eating voices to help you get centered and in touch with your Intuitive Eater once again. There are no rigid rules in this process. Diets are rigid—Intuitive Eating is fluid and adapts to the many changes in your life. Go with the flow without trying to control it.

The integrated Intuitive Eater honors gut reactions, whether they are biological, satisfaction-based, or self-protective. *The Intuitive Eater is a team player* and can draw from the voices of the Nurturer, the Food Anthropologist, and the positive traits of both the Diet Rebel (the Rebel Ally) and the Nutrition Informant (the Nutrition Ally).

EATING VOICES:
HOW THEY EMERGE AND EVOLVE

Each of the voices may prevail at different times. Some of the voices were there at birth but may have become buried. Others were instilled by family and society. And some need to be learned and developed to become an Intuitive Eater.

You're born with the innate ability to sense when you're hungry and full. These are primitive signals and are the basis for the emerging voice of the Intuitive Eater, which is operating in the toddler as he or she starts eating solid food. The Intuitive Eater tells you what you like and what you don't like. If your parents are not sensitive to your signals, you may learn to mistrust them and ultimately lose touch with them.

If you happen to live in a family that has weight and eating issues, you may have your first experience with the voice of the Food Police when you are still very young. You may be told to stop eating so much or be re-

SUMMARY: HOW THE FOOD VOICES HELP OR HARM		
Voice	How It Harms	How It Helps
Food Police	Causes guilt and food worry. Full of judgment. Keeps you in the dieting world, and out of touch with inner cues of eating.	It doesn't.
Nutrition Informant	Uses nutrition as a vehicle to keep you dieting.	Once uncoupled from the Food Police, it becomes the *Nutrition Ally* and can help you make healthy food choices without guilt.
Diet Rebel	Usually results in overeating, self-sabotage.	When the Diet Rebel becomes the *Rebel Ally,* it can help you guard your food turf/boundaries.
Food Anthropologist	It doesn't.	A neutral observer that can give you a distant perspective into your eating world. Nonjudgmental. Keeps you in touch with your inner signals—biologically and psychologically.
Nurturer	It doesn't.	Helps to disarm the verbal assault from the Food Police. Gets you through the tough times.

stricted from eating certain foods. It doesn't take long before you internalize those negative messages, and create your own powerful Food Police. If on the other hand, you're lucky enough to have a family who is not invasive, making no food or body judgments, you may not encounter the Food Police until you start school, or until you become a teen reading magazines and listening to your friends talk. If the pressure to be thin is strong in your community, you are at risk of making the Food Police messages your own at any time in your life. And the Nutrition Informant constantly feeds nutrition information about food to the Food Police.

The voice of the Diet Rebel will crop up soon after you've encountered the Food Police. It usually goes hand in hand. The Food Police come in and invade your boundaries by interfering with your intuitive biological and food preference signals. In order to protect your private space, the Diet Rebel feeds you "forget you" messages that not only counter the Food Police but often send you off into a one-person food riot.

The Food Anthropologist will help give you a neutral perspective. For some individuals, interaction with this voice is often the first nonjudgmental, non-negative encounter with food.

The Nurturer can get you through outside abuse and your own self-defeating behavior if you have access to its positive voice. If your family has given you a sense that you are competent and adequate and has modeled positive ways of coping, you may easily find the voice of your Nurturer to combat the societal voices of the Food Police. If, however, your family has colluded with society and you have grown up with criticism and judgment, the Nurturer will have to be found elsewhere. Sometimes a grandparent, aunt or uncle, or dear friend may teach you how to speak kindly to yourself. For some, seeking help from a psychotherapist or dietitian may be the first experience with learning positive self-talk. However you learn to bring forth the voice of the Nurturer, this is a critical step in becoming an Intuitive Eater. You must make it available to yourself so you can buffer the negative voices which bombard you without notice and cause a barrier to your progress.

And finally, you find yourself back at that place where the Intuitive Eater is running the show. The Intuitive Eater integrates the voices of the Nurturer and the Food Anthropologist, the Nutrition Ally, and the Rebel Ally. The Intuitive Eater knows when your biological signals are calling; it tells you what you need and want, and with guidance from the other positive voices helps you make adult, neutral decisions about how you will take care of yourself.

Let's now take an eating situation and listen for the dialogue of voices that can affect its outcome.

You've been invited to dinner at the home of a gourmet cook. Many appetizers will be served during the cocktail hour, and later a spectacular dinner will be placed before you. Unfortunately, you arrive at the party in an overhungry state.

THE FOOD POLICE: You'd better be careful of what you eat. Everything is fattening. Don't touch the appetizers. If you even taste that little quiche you're a goner. And you can be sure you'll be tempted with lots of rich desserts. Watch out!

THE NUTRITION INFORMANT: You shouldn't have any cheese because there's too much fat in it, and the salt will make you feel bloated. You can only eat the raw veggies.

THE DIET REBEL: Nobody is going to tell me what I can eat at this party. I hate that stupid diet. I've had to succumb to cardboard crackers and diet cottage cheese. Well not tonight. I'm going to get my fill of these amazing foods. I don't care what happens to my diet. I don't care if I'm fat. I'll show my wife what she can do with comments about my weight.

THE FOOD ANTHROPOLOGIST: Look at the interesting array of appetizers. A lot of them look great. You're overly hungry—better eat something, or you'll probably overeat at dinner.

THE NUTRITION ALLY: I don't think I'll have any cheese or fried appetizers tonight. They're very rich and will make me feel too full for dinner. I'd rather have some crab and veggies now, so I can still have some hunger for dinner.

THE NURTURER: This food looks terrific. I want to taste *everything*. It's scary to feel such an overwhelming desire to devour these appetizers. That's okay, it's normal to feel this way when you're ravenous. This isn't the usual situation, and I'm human.

THE INTUITIVE EATER: I'm very hungry. But I think I'll pace myself, so I won't feel too full to enjoy the dinner later. Let's see, of all the appetizers, which look the best? Oh, I haven't had pizza in a long time—that looks good, and so does the baked brie. I think I'll try them both. The brie is great, but the pizza is kind of soggy—think I'll *throw it out* and taste the stuffed mushrooms.

(Halfway through dinner.) This is delicious, but I'm starting to feel full. One more bite, and I'll feel satisfied. I feel great getting to eat anything I like and leaving some of it (without feeling deprived).

THE REBEL ALLY (*TO THE HOSTESS WHO IS PUSHING SECONDS*): The dinner is delicious, but I'm quite full and couldn't eat another helping. Thanks, anyway.

SELF-TALK: SPECIAL ARSENAL FOR
CHALLENGING THE FOOD POLICE

Identifying the inner voices is useful for challenging the Food Police. But this powerfully negative voice requires more ammunition. The Food Police can throw many tricks that require special attention—especially in the thought process department.

When working with dieters in our offices, we have seen over and over that there is actually a middle step between the initial dieting thought and the subsequent eating behavior. We have found that the inner dieting myths (which are cognitive distortions), lead to feeling bad when the self-imposed dieting rules are broken. This concept is widely accepted and well explained by Dr. Albert Ellis and Dr. Robert A. Harper, highly respected pioneers in the field of rational-emotive psychotherapy, a system of psychotherapy which deals with the effect of our thoughts on our feelings and then our behaviors.

According to Ellis and Harper, we routinely flood our heads with crazy notions as well as sane and rational messages. These thought processes are called internalized sentences or *self-talk*. Negative self-talk often makes us feel despair. The feeling of despair can trigger sabotaging behaviors. Ellis and Harper believe that if we challenge the "nonsense" in our heads, we'll end up feeling better. When we feel better, we'll act better. In a review of hundreds of research studies of this type of therapy, it has been shown that if we can first change our *beliefs,* our feelings and behaviors will also change in a chainlike reaction. Therefore, it makes sense to examine our food or diet beliefs and the influence they can have.

Here's a favorite story that illustrates this principle. Let's say that you've been a dieter who has been carefully following your diet for several weeks. Your diet is low-fat and prohibits any kind of sugary, fatty desserts. You decide that you're going to visit your grandmother, whom you haven't seen for a while. You walk into Grandma's house and the first thing that strikes you is the enticing aroma of chocolate brownies hot out of the oven. Here are the *food beliefs* and *thoughts* that might fill your head:

- I've been so good on my diet the last few weeks.
- I haven't had any ice cream or candy or cookies.
- I'd sure love to have one of those brownies, but I can't—I shouldn't—I won't!

- If I have a brownie, I'll blow my diet.
- I won't be able to stop eating the brownies.
- Oh, maybe just one will be okay.

You eat the brownie.

- Oh, no—I shouldn't have done that.
- That was really stupid.
- I have no willpower.
- I'm going to be out of control.
- It's all my fault that I'm fat.
- Will I ever be able to lose weight?

Now, let's sense what you are *feeling*:

- Disappointment
- Fear of future deprivation
- Sadness
- Fear of being out of control   *my life at parties ...*
- Despair

Typical eating *behavior* that follows will be something like this:

- You slowly take a second brownie.
- . . . and a third brownie.
- Before you know it you've gobbled up the whole plateful.
- You collapse on the couch, stuffed and miserable, and fall right to sleep.

Now, let's see how challenging your basic food beliefs can change your feelings and your behavior. The *beliefs* and *thoughts*:

- I'm so glad I gave up dieting.
- I can eat anything I want, anytime I want.
- I'd sure love to have one of those brownies.

You eat the brownie.

- Boy, was that delicious.
- I'm satisfied with just this one.
- There's nothing like Grandma's home-baked chocolate brownies.

And now the *feelings*:

- Satisfaction
- Pleasure
- Contentment (no worry about future deprivation)

And the *behavior*:

- You leave the rest of the brownies on the plate.
- You put the plate of brownies on the kitchen counter.
- You're free to enjoy the afternoon with Grandma without another thought about the brownie.

Andrea is a college student who had been suffering from years of bouts of low self-esteem associated with her dieting failures. For a short time, she actually became bulimic when she saw no other way to control the bingeing that inevitably followed her dieting "falls from grace." Andrea was an expert at telling herself that carbohydrates were bad and that even a few grams of fat in a day would mar her "good" eating behavior (*belief*). As soon as these *thoughts* formed in her head, she *felt* bad the moment she would eat carbohydrates. The conflict between her restrictive thoughts and her craving for the forbidden food always created angry and hateful feelings. When she *felt* bad in her mode of shaky "willpower," she was off and running to her latest eating disaster (*behavior*).

As soon as Andrea succumbed to her natural desires to eat that food, the system of negative thinking led to negative feelings, which led to negative behavior.

Andrea has learned to check her food thoughts as soon as they arise. Old diet rules and thoughts get challenged immediately. Because she is free from distorted dieting thoughts, she feels better about herself and eating. Instead of feeling bad about wanting french fries or ice cream, she feels great about her new relationship with food. And you guessed it—her bingeing days are over.

NEGATIVE SELF-TALK (AND HOW TO CHANGE IT)

*... for there is nothing either good or bad but thinking makes it
so. To me it is a prison ...*

—Hamlet

When eating thoughts are irrational or distorted, negative feelings escalate exponentially. As a result, eating behavior can end up extreme and destructive. It's the classic case of perception becomes reality. Therefore to change our "food reality," we need to replace the irrational thinking with rational thoughts. This in turn helps to moderate our feelings and then behavior.

To get rid of distorted diet thoughts, you first need to identify irrational thinking. Ask yourself:

- Am I having *repetitive* and *intense* feelings? (This is a clue that you need to challenge your thoughts.)
- What am I *thinking* that's leading me to feel this way? (What are you saying to yourself?)
- What is true or correct about this belief? What is false? (Examine and confront the *distorted* beliefs that support this thinking. Your Food Anthropologist voice can be very helpful here.)

Once you have uncovered your distorted beliefs, you need to replace them with thoughts and beliefs that are more rational and reasonable. Here's one example, but the remainder of this chapter will show you how to do this in various ways:

Replace this distorted thought:

Every time I eat pizza—I'm much fatter the next day.

With a more rational thought:

I am salt sensitive. Since pizza is pretty salty, I'm most likely bloated. This isn't fat—it's just water retention. It's temporary.

Irrational beliefs often present themselves to us through negative self-talk. Let's examine the various types of negative thinking and how you can recognize their signs before they drag you into the ditches of overeating.

Dichotomous Thinking

When I furnished my first office (ER), I purposely chose gray fabric for the couches. I decided that it was a symbolic gesture to help my patients get away from the "black-and-white" thinking that usually coexists with the diet mentality. Here are some typical examples of dichotomous thinking: When you get on the scale in the morning and it drops a pound, you say that you've been "good." If it goes up a pound, you're "bad." When you're dieting, you think in terms of "all-or-none." You're not allowed to have any cookies, and if you eat one, you think and feel that you must finish them all. With dichotomous thinking comes black-and-white behaviors. Here are some typical eating examples:

- Eating none or eating all
- Never eating snacks or always eating snacks
- Always eating alone or partying all of the time

Dichotomous or black-and-white thinking can be dangerous and is often based on the premise of achieving perfection. It gives you only two alternatives, one of which is usually neither attainable or maintainable. The other then tends to be the black hole in which you inevitably fall after failing to get to the first. You set your sights so high, constantly chasing an ideal that you can grasp only moments at a time. When the standard for being okay is this lofty, you're destined to feel lousy most of the time. And we know that when you feel lousy, you're bound to end up going off the deep end in your eating behavior.

For example, Hillary is a client who set herself up for failure by thinking in a black-and-white manner. She would give herself permission to eat only when she felt ravenous. If she ate when just moderately hungry, she would consider it overeating. As a result of thinking that she had "blown it" when she didn't meet her "starving standard," she would feel awful and then go into a binge.

When you think in terms of how good or bad your eating is or how fat or thin your body is, you can end up judging your self-worth based on these thoughts. If you begin to feel that you're a bad person, you're likely to create self-punishing behaviors.

Rae is a young woman who set up perfectionist standards in her eating style throughout her high school days. She never allowed herself to eat anything with sugar, artificial sweeteners, salt, or fat in it. As a result, she consistently maintained a super thin, even unhealthy, weight. When Rae got to college and was away from the familiarity of home, she found that her standards were becoming impossible to keep up. As soon as she began to expand her food choices as a result of availability, temptation, and peer pressure, things began to fall apart for Rae. As a dichotomous thinker, her thoughts began to run like this:

- The only correct way to eat is the way I ate in high school.
- This new kind of eating is bad and will make me fat.
- I've lost my willpower to eat in the right way.
- The only way I can eat now is wrong.
- That's bad, I'm bad, and I deserve to feel bad.

agh this is totally my experience

Rae ultimately began to binge as a result of her dichotomous thinking and was willing to acknowledge that much of her bingeing behavior was done as a way to punish herself for her "bad" acts. The bingeing made her feel increasingly worse, but, ironically, this was okay with her as she felt that she deserved the punishment. Rae ended up gaining a significant amount of weight and is only now learning to change her thinking. She's stopped talking to herself negatively, is beginning to feel better, has stopped punishing herself with bingeing, and is slowly returning to a normal weight.

How do you get out of the dichotomous thinking trap?

Go for the Gray. Gray may seem to be a dull color, while black and white are dramatic extremes. In the world of eating, however, going for the gray can give you a rainbow of choices. Give up the notion that you must eat in an all-or-nothing fashion. Let go of your old black-and-white dieting rules. Allow yourself to eat the foods that were *always* restricted, while checking your thoughts to be sure that they support your choices.

You'll find that the thrill of being in the white area of diet restriction is gone, but so is the misery of being in the black area of out-of-control behavior. *go for sophomore summer*

Absolutist Thinking

When you think in this way, you believe that one behavior will absolutely, irrevocably result in a second behavior. This is considered magical thinking, because in reality, you can't and don't control life in this way. It leads you to believe that you "must" act in a certain way or else something "awful" will happen.

In the world of eating, absolutist thinking will lead you to statements like the following: "I *must* eat perfectly these next two months or else I won't lose enough weight for my daughter's wedding, and that would be *awful*." You don't really have any proof that eating "perfectly" will actually cause you to lose "enough" weight. You're not even sure what "enough" weight actually means. And you really can't define this "awful" state that you imagine. You end up feeling frantic trying to eat perfectly, and then, of course, eat imperfectly. Fearing that you won't lose enough weight makes you more anxious, and believing that will be awful turns you into a wreck. The result, of course, of all of these absolute thoughts and anxious feelings, is destructive, overeating behavior, which leads you to the opposite end of what you wished. You might even *gain* weight before the wedding and feel all the worse.

How do you get out of this kind of thinking?

Banish the Absolutes and Replace Them with Permissive Statements. Carefully listen for the "absolute" words that you use. Get rid of the *musts, oughts, shoulds, need to's, supposed to's*, and *have to's*. Every time you think that you *must* go on a diet, or you *need* to lose ten pounds before the reunion, or you *ought* to have a light lunch like a salad and tea, or you *shouldn't* eat before you go to bed, stop yourself and replace those thoughts. Those kinds of words and thoughts will only cause you anxiety about not being able to carry out the command. Thinking in this absolute way has no guarantee of resulting in the behavior you desire and is likely to create self-sabotaging behavior. In fact, it's fairly sure to make the result *awful,* which is just what you're trying to avoid.

Use words such as *can, is okay,* and *may.* Give yourself permissive statements such as:

- It's okay if I don't lose weight before the wedding.
- I can eat whenever I'm hungry.
- If I want, I can eat whatever foods I like.
- I may have anything that looks good to me.

Catastrophic Thinking

Each time that you think in exaggerated ways, you create miserable feelings for yourself, and, once again, compensate by extreme behaviors. The following are examples of catastrophic thoughts:

- I'll never be thin.
- It's hopeless.
- I'll never get a boyfriend or a job at this weight.
- My life is ruined, because I'm so fat.
- If I let myself eat candy bars and fries, I'll eat them forever.

This kind of thinking is a real setup. It makes a bad situation worse and ties all of your future successes in life to your ability to eat in a particular way or to losing weight. You tell yourself that all your happiness hinges on your eating and your body. If that is your premise, then you're bound to feel all the more unhappy than you are at the moment. You may be desperately unhappy about your weight right now, but you may become despairing by catastrophizing your bleak future.

Marion is a highly successful screenwriter who owns her own home, has many devoted friends, and two loving dogs. But Marion feeds herself a daily litany of catastrophic thoughts. Because she's overweight, she tells herself that she'll never get married, never have children, and never be happy. Looking forward to this negative self-created future only makes her feel miserable and causes her to overeat to comfort herself.

How do you get away from catastrophic thinking?

Climb Out of the Abyss. Replace your exaggerated thoughts with thinking, which is more positive and accurate. Treat yourself to hopeful coping statements. Marion is learning to nurture herself by telling herself that many overweight people find spouses who love them as they are. She's practicing positive self-talk that confirms her current as well as her future happiness. As a result, Marion is eating less and is accepting her weight. She knows that she'll never return to her episodes of negative self-talk.

Pessimistic Thinking or "The Cup Is Half Empty"

People who view the world in this way tend to see every situation in its worst-case scenario. They usually think that life is terrible, that they don't have enough of what they want, and that everything that they do is wrong. They're highly critical and blameful, not only of themselves but of others.

Bonnie walks into the office each week with a scowl. She complains about her husband and her job and says that her children are driving her crazy. She begins each session with accounts of how terrible her week has been and how badly she has "blown" her eating. Bonnie would evaluate the cup as half empty. This kind of negative thinking is insidious and often goes unnoticed by the participant. It needs to be pointed out on a regular basis, so the person can reevaluate her thought process and see that it only leads to a pervasive sense of unhappiness. It also perpetuates self-destructive behaviors. A person who thinks this way has great difficulty appreciating her small successes. She often even misses them and tends to condemn her progress.

How do you get out of this kind of thinking?

Half Empty	Half Full
1. I had a terrible week.	1. I had some success this week.
2. I overate so many times.	2. I had many times when I honored my hunger.
3. All I ate was sweets.	3. I had more sweets than I wished, but I had lots of other foods, too.
4. I feel so fat.	4. I'm feeling better about myself.
5. I'm such a failure.	5. I'm doing better little by little.

Make the Cup Half Full. The most obvious way to heal cup-is-half-empty thinking is to consciously catch each of your negative statements and re-place the words with more positive ones.

After you have done this consciously for a while, you'll find that you hear your own negative thoughts transform into more positive words. You will also become sensitive to how hard you've been on yourself. Once you begin to see the world in terms of the cup being half full, you'll find your daily dose of happy moments increases regularly. Soon you'll see much of your negative eating habits disappear along with the negative thoughts.

Linear Thinking

If you've been on even one diet, you'll know that diet thinking goes in one straight line. You begin at your initial weight, and all you can think about is getting to your goal weight. You follow a very specific plan that allows for no deviations. It's like trying to walk along the white line in the middle of the highway to get to your destination. If you put one foot in front of the other in perfect style, you'll successfully make it to the end. If you accidentally step off the line for even a moment, you're likely to be a highway disaster. We tend to be a society of linear thinkers. We want to get to the goal without appreciating the means. We're success-oriented and rarely stop long enough to just be and check out the scenery along the way.

Here are some examples of linear thinking that can set you up:

- All that is important is that I lose this weight.
- The faster I lose weight, the more successful I am.
- To be successful I must reach my goal weight by the specified target date.
- I will lose two pounds per week with no fluctuations.

How do you get out of this kind of thinking?

Switch to Process Thinking. The cure for linear thinking is *process thinking*, which focuses on continual change and learning, rather than just the end result. If you start thinking in terms of what you can learn along the way, and accept that there will be many ups and downs, you will go forward. By becoming a process thinker you will enjoy the opportunity to enrich many aspects of your life, while re-creating your relationship with food. Process thinking will help you become more sensitive to your Intuitive Eating signals, rather than endpoints such as how much you ate today.

Here are some examples of process thinking:

- This was a rough week. But I learned some new things about myself that will help me make changes in the future.

• What's most important is that I honor the positive changes I'm
making in my eating, not my weight loss!

• I ate more than I wanted to at the restaurant tonight, especially
the dessert. But I learned that by giving myself permission to eat
dessert, it took away the urgency to have sweets again later. Usually
I would have binged when I got home, alone.

SELF-AWARENESS: THE ULTIMATE WEAPON AGAINST THE FOOD POLICE

The next time that you see yourself eating in a way that feels uncomfortable, unsatisfying, or even out of control, give yourself the gift of remembering what you were thinking before you even took the first bite of
food. Examine that thought and challenge it. As you get more adept at
the Intuitive Eating process, you'll be able to catch these thoughts before
they make you feel bad or cause undesirable behavior.

Become self-aware. Pay attention to the food talk that inevitably arises
when you approach any eating situation. Listen for the different voices that
can either serve as your support or saboteur.

Banish the Food Police that keep you from making your peace with
food. Challenge the pseudo-nutrition thoughts that come from the Nutrition
Informant. Observe your eating through the eyes and voice of your Food
Anthropologist and allow it to guide you sensibly. Speak out loud the thoughts
of your Rebel Ally so you don't use food to take care of you. The real protection will come from your Nurturer who knows just how to soothe you and get
you through tough situations. And, finally, become acutely sensitive to the
positive voices that comprise your Intuitive Eater. It was there when you
were born. Discard the layers of negative voices that have buried it so deeply
that it seemed lost forever. By listening to its instinctual signals, you'll have
the opportunity to form a healthy relationship with food.

Chapter 9

PRINCIPLE 5:

Feel Your Fullness

Listen for the body signals that tell you that you are no longer hungry. Observe the signs that show that you're comfortably full. Pause in the middle of eating and ask yourself how the food tastes, and what your current hunger level is.

The vast majority of chronic dieters we have worked with belong to the clean-plate club. And most of them say that they've tried not to clean their plates. It may seem that an obvious step to normalizing your eating is to respect your fullness, rather than to habitually clean your plate. Yet, leaving food on the plate can be difficult to achieve, especially for the chronic dieter.

Dieting instills a license to eat at mealtime—when it is "legal." Ironically, this sense of entitlement reinforces a clean-your-plate mentality. This is particularly true for our clients who have sipped on over-the-counter liquid diets, such as Slim-Fast. (Liquid diet programs typically have you drink a "beverage-meal" for breakfast and lunch, and then "allow you to eat a sensible dinner" of "real" food.) Naturally, most of our patients practically licked their plates clean when given the opportunity to eat their one real meal. It's not that they overate; rather they ate *all* of their precise and "entitled" portions.

Other diet plans using regular food typically offer small portions at meals. This too, encourages you to eat while you can. Who would leave any morsel of food when quantities are meager? For example, even frozen diet meals hover at about three hundred calories (and often less), which usually leaves you less than satisfied. In fact, there is a trend of frozen diet entrees offering even fewer calories—closer to two hundred calories per package. This type of eating hardly fosters getting in touch with your inner eating signals, especially signals of satiety. Instead you eat it all.

Perhaps you've tossed your diet plans out years ago, but now carefully count fat grams. You may find however, that you clean your plate when it comes to eating fat-free foods. We've had several clients eat an entire package of *fat-free* chocolate cake (or other fat-free goodies) with carefree abandonment because of the entitlement factor. They would rationalize that "There's no fat so I can eat as much as I want." Unfortunately, fat-free is not necessarily calorie-free. But the calories wouldn't even be an issue if people were respecting their fullness level.

Of course, other factors can easily condition you to polish off every crumb on your plate, including:

- Having been taught to finish everything on your plate by well-meaning parents.
- Respecting economics and the value of food—thou shalt not waste. Remember, however, that either way the food can be wasted; in the case of chronically eating more than you need, it becomes an issue of w-a-i-s-t.
- Having an ingrained habit of eating to completion. Out of sheer habit you finish an entire plate of food, or a *whole* hamburger, or a *whole* bag of chips, regardless of how hungry or full you are. This is a reliance on external cues. You stop eating when the food is *gone,* regardless of the size of the initial portion.
- Beginning a meal (or snack) in an overly ravenous state. In this state, eating intensity is revved up and it's all too easy to bypass normal satiety cues.

Even if you don't clean your plate, it's still possible that you may be over-eating, or bypassing your comfortable satiety level. With our clients who don't clean their plates, we have often discovered that while there may still be food left on the plate, it took an *uncomfortable* level of fullness to get them to stop eating. The problem is the inability to recognize comfortable satiety or to respect fullness.

THE KEY TO RESPECTING FULLNESS

Respecting fullness, or the ability to stop eating because you have had enough to eat biologically, hinges critically on giving yourself unconditional permission to eat (Principle 3: Make Peace with Food). How can you or any dieter expect to leave food on your plate, if you believe that you won't be able to eat that particular food or meal again? Unless you truly give yourself permission to eat again when you are hungry, or have access to that particular food, respecting fullness simply becomes a dogmatic dieting exercise without roots. It won't take hold. The Intuitive Eater in training learns to stop eating when he or she has had just enough to fill the stomach comfortably without being overfull. It's easier to stop eating at this point and leave food behind, when you *know* you can eat it again, later.

RECOGNIZING COMFORTABLE SATIETY

We are surprised at how often our clients do not know what comfortable satiety feels like. Oh yes, they can usually describe with great detail how overeating or overstuffed feels. But knowledge of what comfortable satiety feels like is often illusive, especially to the chronic dieter. Yet, if you do not know what comfortable satiety feels like, how can you expect to achieve it? It's like trying to shoot at a target without ever seeing it, or to even know where it resides. When respecting fullness is the target—it could easily be missed if you are not looking for it, especially when you have been conditioned to clean your plate. Also, if you start eating when you are not hungry, it's hard to know when to stop out of fullness.

How do you *imagine* comfortable satiety feels? Here are some common descriptions offered by our clients:

- A subtle feeling of stomach fullness
- Feeling satisfied and content
- Nothingness—neither hungry nor full

The sensation is highly individual. And while we can describe it endlessly, it's akin to trying to tell someone what snow feels like. We can give you a good idea—but it's something that needs to be experienced at the personal level, so that *you* know what it feels like in *your* body.

HOW TO RESPECT YOUR FULLNESS

When you habitually clean your plate, your eating style easily evolves into autopilot—you eat until completion, until the food is gone. To break this pattern of eating, we have found it helpful to be keenly aware or hyperconscious of your eating. This means being conscious or mindful of your eating experience. While you may certainly be aware that you are engaged in the act of eating, we find that somewhere between bites one and one hundred, there is a significant level of unconsciousness. Quite often the food is not even being tasted! Likewise, it's all too easy to bypass comfortable satiety. Here are some examples:

- I wasn't aware of how much candy I would eat at the movies until suddenly, my hands were scratching at the bottom of an empty box.
- I wouldn't even consider splitting a meal when eating out until my boss asked if I would split an entree at her favorite restaurant. Begrudgingly I agreed. To my surprise I was thoroughly satisfied with half an entree, *knowing all too well that had I ordered the full portion I would have eaten it all, out of sheer habit.*
- Once I opened up a package of *any* food, I had to eat it all. God forbid I'd leave few tidbits. I know I'm not even tasting the food most of the time.

Conscious Eating

This initial step away from the blind autopilot eating mode is *conscious eating.* It's a phase where you neutrally observe your eating as if under a microscope. (Your Food Anthropologist voice will be very helpful here.) We have broken this stage into a series of steps, which begins with taking a mini time-out from eating. This will help you regroup and assess where you're at in your eating. It's like a time-out that athletes and coaches take during a game to help improve their play or strategy. Here's what to do.

Pause in the middle of a meal or snack for a time-out. Keep in mind that this time-out or pause is not a commitment to stop eating. Rather, it's a commitment to be in check with your body and taste buds. (If you thought that by pausing, you were obligated to leave food on your plate, you'd be reluctant to go though this step. In fact, many of our clients who initially appeared resistant to this step, later admitted that they were afraid that they would have to stop eating from that point on.) During this time-out, perform these checks:

TASTE CHECK: We find that this check is usually pleasurable, which is why we like to begin with it. Ask yourself how the food tastes. Is it worthy of your taste buds? Or are you continuing to eat just because it's there?

SATIETY CHECK: Ask yourself what your hunger or fullness level is. Are you still hungry, do you feel unsatisfied, or is your hunger going away and are you beginning to feel satisfied? In the beginning, this may seem like a hit-or-miss process. Be patient, and remember, you are getting to know yourself from the inside out. Just as you would not expect to get to know a person over one meal, how could you expect to understand your satiety levels in one meal or snack? It will take time. However, the more in tune you are with your hunger level, and the more you honor your hunger, the easier this step will be. Remember to be open to any answer. There can be considerable fluctuation in your fullness level depending upon the last time you ate and what you ate. If you find you're still hungry, then resume eating.

• *When you finish eating* (whatever the amount) *ask yourself where your fullness level is now.* Did you reach comfortable satiety? Did you surpass it? By how much? Use the Fullness Discovery scale to help you get in touch. Note: This is the same scale as the Hunger Discovery Scale on p. 126—only now we're focusing on fullness.

• *Discovering your fullness level will help you identify your last-bite threshold.* This is the endpoint. You know that the bite of food *in* your mouth is your last—finis! It may take you a long time to get to this point. The longer you have been disconnected from your body's sense of fullness, the longer it will take to identify this point. If you *honor your hunger* (Principle 2), it is much easier to know fullness. If, however, you do not eat from biological hunger, how could you expect to stop from biological fullness (or to even know what it feels like)? Please be patient with yourself.

• *Don't feel obligated to leave food on your plate.* If you find that you have a level of resistance for this activity, it may be from past dieting experience. You may be feeling obligated to leave food on your plate—which is a remnant of the diet mentality. Remember there is no commitment to leave food on your plate. The commitment, instead, is to getting to know your satiety level and your taste buds. It's perfectly normal, even when you discover your specific satiety level, to opt to overeat. That's okay. We have found that many clients continue to opt for more food—they are still testing the "unconditional permission" to eat. After awhile, when the newness

THE FULLNESS DISCOVERY SCALE

Time	Food	Fullness Rating										
		0	1	2	3	4	5	6	7	8	9	10

Empty   Set   **Neutral**   Full   Sick
Ravenous   Pangs   Satisfied   Stuffed

0   1   2   3   4   5   6   7   8   9   10

After you're finished eating, check out your fullness level. A level of 6 or 7 is just-satisfied to satisfied. At 8, you're full; at 9, you're stuffed; and at 10, you are beginning to feel sick from overfilling. Work toward ending your eating at a 6 or 7. Ultimately, you'll find that the last-bite threshold corrolates with this level of satisfaction.

Remember, the hungrier you are when you begin eating, the higher your fullness number is likely to be when you stop. But, if you start eating at a 3 or a 4, you'll be more apt to stop at a 6 or 7—satisfied but not overfull.

wears off and the deprivation feelings subside, you will find that it's quite easy to leave food on your plate. It does require, however, a degree of consciousness—checking in with yourself. But, if most of the time you can recognize your fullness, and respect it, it will make a considerable difference in your physical comfort level and peace of mind.

How to Increase Consciousness

It's very difficult to do two conscious things at once. While you certainly may juggle a zillion activities, your mind focuses primarily on one. That's why, for example, so many people lock their keys in their car. Their minds are focused somewhere else, such as getting into the office on time, or unloading the groceries. We find that to get the most out of eating, it needs to be a conscious activity, whenever possible.

• *Eat without distraction.* Value and enjoy the eating experience when possible. For example, Adelle, a fast-paced, hard-driven lawyer, always made the best use of her time, and would usually eat while doing something else. Adelle would read briefs while eating lunch at work and dine with a magazine at home. She took a step forward when she decided to try eating without distraction when at home (she was too busy at work to even consider "just" eating lunch). Adelle discovered that if she ate a meal or snack at home without engaging in reading, she would usually eat less. To her surprise she learned that she ate less, not because she was trying to eat smaller amounts, but because she would detect her fullness level much sooner. She was thrilled that "without trying" she was eating less food, feeling satisfied without deprivation, and not dieting. Adelle was willing to eat this way at home, but did not view it as realistic for work—and this was progress!

Many clients have taken the suggestion to eat without distraction as a hard and fast rule and feel guilty if they happen to read the newspaper with breakfast or have a snack watching TV. Remember, Intuitive Eating is not another diet with rules to be broken. As in every other aspect of Intuitive Eating, you are the one who has the internal wisdom about what works for you. You also know what doesn't work. Whatever the "other" activity may be, be honest with yourself about whether you are able to get the most satisfaction in your eating, while engaging in this activity or whether you're being distracted by it. *reading ↑ satisfaction, nothing else*

• *Reinforce your conscious decision to stop.* Many of our clients have *does that make me bad?* found that when *they* decide to stop eating, because they've reached the last bite threshold, it's helpful to *do* something to make it a conscious act, such as gently nudging the plate forward half an inch or putting their utensils or napkin on their plate. This simply reminds them of their decision. Otherwise it may be all too easy to innocently nibble on the remaining food, even though you had no intention of doing so. (If you have trouble with the idea of wasting food, try putting your leftovers away for tomorrow's lunch or dinner or giving them to a homeless person. If you're going to a restaurant, try bringing a small cooler to keep the food safe until you get home.)

• *Defend yourself from obligatory eating.* This usually means practicing saying, "No, thank you!" I never realized the significance of this act until I (ET) attended a very elegant cocktail party in which there seemed to be one waiter for each guest. The moment my hand was empty of food or drink, an all-too-eager waiter was there to offer more food or beverage. I found it was so much easier to say "yes," especially if I was in the middle of a conversation. It took much more energy, however, to say "no." The same is true if you attend any function in which there are well-meaning "food-pushers," from the gracious host to the obnoxious relative. A special caution to those of you who enjoy wine by the bottle at a good restaurant: A good server will often keep your glass full. Unless you are conscious of that, you may drink more than you intend. Remember, *you* are in charge of how much to eat and drink.

THE FULLNESS FACTORS

"I just ate two hours ago—I honored my hunger *and* respected my fullness, so how could I be hungry again so soon?" While the ebb and tide of satiety signals may seem puzzling, it's quite normal to have different degrees of hunger and fullness, especially when you begin listening to your body's eating cues. There are also several factors that affect fullness. These factors are both biological and learned. When you have a general understanding of some of these satiety factors, it makes it easier to trust your body and *feel your fullness.*

The ability to recognize comfortable satiety or fullness can ultimately determine how much food will be consumed in a meal. And the amount of food eaten in a meal is influenced by these fullness factors:

• *The amount of time* that has passed since the last time you ate. The more often you eat, the less hungry you will be. This has been found to be true in nibbling studies. These are studies in which people are given several snacks or mini-meals throughout the day. The nibblers are consistently *less* hungry than those fed identical calories divided into three meals. While the purpose of these studies was to examine the metabolic effects of snacking compared to traditional meals, the researchers have consistently noted that the nibblers were less hungry, even though calories and fat were identical in both groups.

• *The kind of food you eat.* The macronutrients, protein, carbohydrates, and fat influence subsequent food intake by their contribution to the total amount of food energy in the stomach. Other food factors such as fiber will also affect the fullness factor because of its bulk and water retention properties. Protein in particular seems to have a suppressive effect on intake beyond its contribution to total calories, according to several studies.

• *The amount of food still remaining in the stomach* at the time of eating. If your stomach is empty you will eat more than if some food is still present (from a prior snack or meal).

• *Initial hunger level.* If you begin a meal or snack in a famished state you are more likely to overeat and override satiety mechanisms.

• *Social influence.* Eating with other people can influence how much *you* eat. Studies have shown that:

—The more people gathered at a meal, the more people tend to eat.

—Eating with others increases the duration of the meal.

—Eating more on weekends is usually due to being around people.

—Dieters, however, have been shown to eat less when they know someone is "watching" them. The same can be true for non-dieters, when they dine with a "model" eater. In one study, when the model eater refrained from eating, so too did the non-dieter.

There is a tendency to ignore or be distracted from biological signals in social settings. We have found that the key to the social dilemma is to continue making eating a *conscious* activity with purposeful food choices.

Clearly, there are many factors that influence how full you feel from eating. With so many variables that exert influence on your eating, it should be no surprise then, that the amount of food that you desire to eat can and will fluctuate. A big key is to stay tuned in and remember conscious eating.

Beware of Air Food

Simply shoving some food in your mouth like a pacifier to ease hunger pangs may backfire, and the comforting effect will not be long-lasting. This is especially true for "air food"—food that fills up the stomach but offers little sustenance. Air food includes such low-calorie foods as air-popped popcorn, Pirate's Booty, rice cakes, puffed rice cereal, fat-free crackers, celery sticks, and calorie-free beverages. There's nothing inherently wrong with these foods. But if you eat them expecting to get full, it will often take massive quantities—and you might also find yourself on the prowl for something more substantial to "top off the meal." That's where having a balanced snack or meal, which includes a heavier carbohydrate, some protein, and/or some fat, is especially helpful, if you're looking for a little "staying power" or the stick-to-your ribs kind of feeling from eating.

If, on the other hand, you know you will be going out for a fabulous dinner or to a party, and want just a little something to take the edge off your hunger, lighter foods may serve your purpose just fine.

Foods with Staying Power

Snacks or meals with a little fiber, complex carbohydrates, some protein, and some fat will help increase satiety. Ironically, many of our chronic dieters shy away from the very foods that could help them feel more satisfied at meals—complex carbohydrates and fat. Here are some common unsatisfying food choices and suggestions for how you can round them out to be

Less Filling Foods:	Staying Power Boost: Add these types of foods to perk up your satiety:
Salad (no carbohydrates; little protein unless it's an entree)	Protein: tuna, chicken, garbanzo or kidney beans Carbs: crackers or whole grain roll Fat: salad dressing
Fresh fruit (no protein, can be low on carbs depending on quantity)	Protein/Carb/Fat: cheese and whole grain crackers; half sandwich; nonfat yogurt
Turkey breast (no fiber, no carbs, no fat)	Carb/Fat: whole grain pita; whole grain bagel; whole grain crackers; mayonnaise

more satisfying. (There's nothing inherently wrong with these light foods, they just may not provide staying power.)

WHAT IF YOU CAN'T STOP EATING?

If you discover after time that you are still eating even though you are not hungry, there's a good chance that you might be using food as a coping mechanism. This is not always as obvious and dramatic as some magazines and books suggest. Chapter 11 is devoted to this issue.

WHAT IF YOU FEEL
THERE'S SOMETHING MISSING?

If you've discovered what it feels like to feel comfortably full, and yet feel that something is missing, it could be the satisfaction factor. This is so important, we've devoted a whole principle to it—and discuss it in the next chapter.

Chapter 10

PRINCIPLE 6:

Discover the Satisfaction Factor

The Japanese have the wisdom to promote pleasure as one of their goals of healthy living. In our fury to be thin and healthy, we often overlook one of the most basic gifts of existence—the pleasure and satisfaction that can be found in the eating experience. When you eat what you really want, in an environment that is inviting, the pleasure you derive will be a powerful force in helping you feel satisfied and content. By providing this experience for yourself, you will find that it takes much less food to decide you've had "enough." *big challenge in college*

So, what is it about satisfaction that is so powerful? Abraham Maslow has taught us that we are driven by our unmet needs. We want what we can't have and will do whatever it takes to calm down the sense of deprivation that inevitably arises when our needs are not satisfied. Whether it is food or relationships or career—if we're not satisfied, we're not happy. In the seventeen years since *Intuitive Eating* was first published, it has become more evident that finding satisfaction in eating is the driving force of this process. We explain this to our clients by describing the following visual.

Imagine a wheel with many spokes. At the hub is satisfaction, surrounded by ten spokes. Each spoke represents an Intuitive Eating principle that influences satisfaction.

To be satisfying, a meal includes foods that you enjoy and that "hit the spot." Eating a salad, when you want a steak, will not lead to satisfaction. If you are served an appealing food or whole meal when you're not very hungry, your satisfaction will be diminished. You may eat anyway, but food tastes much better when you're moderately hungry. Conversely, if you eat when you're ravenous, your taste buds will barely have a chance to reg-

SATISFACTION: The Hub of Intuitive Eating

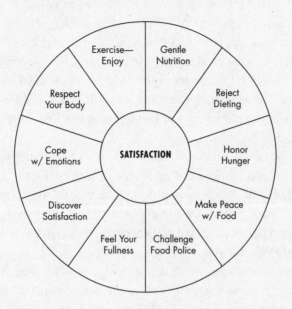

ister the exquisite tastes before you've bolted down the entire meal. Definitely not a satisfying experience! But when you begin to eat a delicious meal when you are moderately hungry, you are likely to find that you're comfortably full before the meal is finished. If you finish eating the whole meal, there will be diminished taste to the food, because the taste buds become desensitized to the nuances of the food, especially if you become overfull.

Now think about eating when you're in the middle of a fight with a family member. How delicious is the food you eat during that meal? You may not even notice that you've eaten! Or, think about an experience you've had when you've eaten to push down feelings. Again, not a very satisfying eating experience!

Honoring your hunger, making peace with food, feeling your fullness, and coping with your emotions without using food are four of the spokes on our imaginary wheel. Another spoke on the wheel involves *rejecting the diet mentality.* If you're still in diet mentality when you eat, it's likely that you're either not choosing the most satisfying food, or if you do choose it, you are judging yourself for eating it.

Respecting your body is yet another spoke on the wheel. Eating while you're wearing comfortable clothes, and eating without body bashing will free you to have more satisfaction in your meal. *Challenging the Food Police,* who chastise you for what you eat or for even eating at all, will also allow for optimal satisfaction. Later in this book, you will learn more about how exercise and nutrition fit into Intuitive Eating, but suffice it to say that a person who feels good moving or exercising, will also find that eating in a satisfying way will enhance this self-satisfaction. And when you're at a point in this process that you're craving all types of food—nutritious food along with the play food (see Principles 9 and 10)—your eating satisfaction level will be at its peak.

You may be taking a leap of faith when you give up diet mentality and jump headfirst into Intuitive Eating. If you're looking for the motivation to make this transition, think of finding satisfaction in your everyday eating experiences. After all, who wouldn't want to live a satisfying life that is built on a foundation of eating satisfaction? This chapter will crystallize finding satisfaction for you.

How many times have you eaten a rice cake when you really wanted potato chips? And how many rice cakes, carrots, and apples have you eaten attempting to get the same satisfaction you would have found with a handful of chips? If you feel truly satisfied with your eating experience, you will find that you eat far less food. Conversely, if you are unsatisfied, you will likely eat more and be on the prowl, regardless of your satiety level.

For example, one client, Fran, wanted a piece of corn bread with lunch, but she fastidiously refrained from eating it. Fran thought about having corn bread with dinner, but again stopped herself. That night, she ate six Weight Watchers desserts, and realized that what she was really seeking was corn bread—no amount of diet desserts would satisfy her corn bread craving. Ironically, the calories from the diet desserts far exceeded the calories from a single piece of corn bread. When Fran was eating the diet desserts she was chasing her *phantom food*—trying to fill the void created by denying the satisfaction factor from the food she originally wanted to eat.

THE WISDOM OF PLEASURE

Americans have gotten so focused on the alchemy of foods—whether as an adjunct to lose weight or seek health, that we have neglected a very important role that eating plays in our lives—provision of pleasure. The Japanese promote pleasure as one of their goals of healthy eating. "Make all activities pertaining to food and eating pleasurable ones," is one of their dietary guidelines for health promotion. How ironic this advice is for Americans, especially dieters, who have come to see food as the enemy and the eating experience as the battleground between "tempting" foods and the will-power to avoid them. Most dieters with whom we work have lost sight of how important it is to have a satisfying, let alone pleasurable, eating experience. For some, any experience that smacks of pleasure triggers feelings of guilt and wrongdoing. It's not too surprising, since we live in a society with strong puritanical roots and a tradition of self-denial. Dieting plays right into the puritanical ethic—make sacrifices, settle for less. Yet if you settle for food that is inferior, it will often leave you wanting . . . eating . . . overeating.

Jill is an example of a young woman who let the fear of eating pleasurable foods turn her into a restrictive eater. Her food choices were based primarily on their weight reducing powers. She was convinced that if she even tasted a pleasurable food, she would never again be able to control herself. Every time that Jill was in a dieting phase, she would find herself having strong cravings for forbidden foods. She chased her "phantom food," searching for a food that would quell her cravings. If she craved a chocolate cookie, she would spread sugar-free jam on fat-free saltines. When that didn't satisfy her, she'd go on to cinnamon-flavored rice cakes, then to fat-free "healthy" cookies (which she disliked since they "tasted like sweet-ened cardboard"), and lots of dried fruit. By the end of an evening, *Jill had eaten ten times more diet foods than she would have eaten had she just allowed herself to have the chocolate cookie.* And, not surprisingly, she would usually "succumb" to the chocolate cookie anyway at the end of her frustrating food chase.

After learning the Intuitive Eating process, Jill quit the phantom food searches and allowed herself to eat what she really wanted. She can now even order a hamburger *with fries* and finds that she ends up leaving half of her food because she's so *satisfied.* She's also found that she eats plenty of nutritious food along with enough play food to satisfy her whole spectrum of taste cravings!

DON'T BE AFRAID TO ENJOY YOUR FOOD

Like, Jill, our clients are initially afraid that if they let the pleasure of eat-ing into their lives, they might continue to seek food in an uncontrollable fashion. Yet letting yourself enjoy food will actually result in self-limiting, rather than out-of-control eating. Remember, as we explained in Chapter 7, deprivation is a key factor that leads to backlash eating.

Satisfied Now—Eat Less Later

For many of our clients, feeling a sense of satisfaction in a meal actually decreases their yearning for foods at a later time. We have had our clients compare having a full-course meal for dinner with just "picking" or scrounging. When they take the time to prepare a meal that attracts their sense of smell, taste, sight, and so forth, they invariably report a feeling of satisfaction and a decreased need for more food later in the evening. Those who come home and drop on the sofa with a box of crackers and a soda find themselves getting up at each commercial for yet another snack. They feel that they haven't really eaten and never seem to get satisfied. By the end of the evening, they feel overfull and frustrated.

Kelly is a busy person who often neglects her own needs. Sometimes, she'll be so busy with work and her child that she doesn't stop to prepare an entire meal for herself. On the days when she takes the time to figure out what she really wants to eat and ends up eating exactly what she wants for lunch or dinner, she finds that she has no desire for dessert. On the days when she diets all day and never feels satisfied, her dessert cravings at night are insatiable.

When you allow yourself pleasure and satisfaction from every possible eating experience, your total quantity of food will decrease.

HOW TO REGAIN YOUR PLEASURE IN EATING

As a result of dieting and the fear of giving it up, dieters have lost their pleasure in eating, and they don't know how to get it back. Here are the steps we use with our clients to help them achieve pleasure and satisfaction in their eating.

STEP 1:
ASK YOURSELF WHAT YOU *REALLY* WANT TO EAT

Satisfaction is derived when you take the time to figure out what you really want to eat, give yourself unconditional permission to eat, and then eat in a relaxing, enjoyable atmosphere.

[handwritten margin note: so it can be better to eat the cookie now rather than way too much later]

The problem for most dieters with whom we've worked is that they have figured out so many "tricks" to avoid eating that they no longer know what they like to eat! When you're about to begin a new diet, have you ever asked yourself what you *feel like* eating? That thought rarely enters a dieter's mind. After all, the basic premise of dieting is to be told what to eat— why would you begin to question your own needs!

Such was the case with a forty-year-old woman, Jennifer, who had been overweight and dieting all of her life. As a child she was put on diets by her mother and her doctors. When Jennifer first visited my (ER) office, she belligerently stated that she didn't want to hear another word about dieting. She had only come because her doctor had insisted, and she emphatically stated that she knew all there was to know about dieting. I told her that I didn't believe in dieting, but all I really wanted to know was what she liked to eat. Astonishment crossed her face. She could hardly respond, but when she did, she told me that no one in her entire life had ever asked her what *she* wanted to eat. She had been on diets since she was a child and had always been told what she *should* eat. She went deep into thought for a few moments and then said that she had no idea what she liked. In fact, this morbidly obese woman wasn't even sure if she liked food at all.

At the end of the session, I suggested that Jennifer spend the next week experimenting with food so that she could learn more about her taste preferences. During that week, Jennifer could only find ten foods that she actually liked and discovered that she could do without the rest! The following week, Jennifer's task was to eat only those ten foods and see how much she actually consumed. Again, she was surprised by the results. When she ate what she liked, she found that she was satisfied by much less and that her total food intake that week was lower than it had been in years. One night, all she had for dinner was a scoop of chocolate ice cream. In the past she would gulp down a huge dinner of foods she thought she *should* eat, even though she wasn't very hungry and would then finish the half gallon of ice cream, because she felt guilty about having any of it.

Jennifer was on her way to becoming an Intuitive Eater. In addition to appreciating that she could have exactly what she wanted anytime that she ate, she realized that eating when she was hungry would give her the most satisfaction. As a result of this revelation, she found herself eating only when she was hungry. She also found that eating past comfortable fullness was pointless, as the food no longer tasted good, her body felt miserable, and she could eat the same food again at her next meal if she liked. Soon it became automatic for her to eat smaller quantities than she ever had in her life. Since she felt good for the first time in her life, she was motivated to begin a program of regular swimming—not because she *had* to but because she *wanted* to feel even better physically! Her obesity had led to problems with her knees and virtual inactivity. As her weight began to normalize, Jennifer felt continually satisfied by her meals, without feeling deprived.

If you also have trouble figuring out what you truly like to eat, the next step will give you clarification.

STEP 2: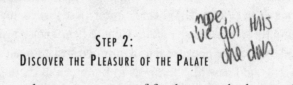
DISCOVER THE PLEASURE OF THE PALATE

Our clients are focused on every aspect of food except the here and now. They lament the past and worry about the future (what will I eat, how will I work off these calories), but very rarely do they focus on the actual experience of eating. Therefore they are not tasting—not experiencing or savoring food. It's almost as if the art of eating needs to be relearned without bias.

The Sensual Qualities of Food

To discover what foods you really like and how to increase satisfaction in your eating, explore the sensual qualities of foods. For most people, this means a conscious period of experimentation. Take your taste buds and palate for a sensory joy ride. Before you eat, consider:

• *Taste.* Put a particular food in your mouth to see which of your taste sensations gets stimulated. Roll the food on your tongue to see if it's predominantly sweet, salty, sour, or bitter. Is that taste pleasant, neutral, or maybe even offensive? Try this experiment at various times during the day to see if certain tastes are more pleasurable at different times. Some people are drawn to the sweet taste at breakfast and want waffles or pancakes. Something spicy, such as eggs with salsa, might be a turnoff early in the morning. Others can't think of something sweet until later in the afternoon.

• *Texture.* As you roll the food on your tongue and begin to chew it, experience the various types of textures that foods can provide. How does crunchy feel to you? Is it abrasive to have to break into a crunchy food, or is it a satisfying experience? What reaction do you have to a food that is smooth or creamy? Does it remind you of baby food, and is that appealing or annoying? Some foods are chewy and require a lot of work by your teeth and tongue. What is that like for you? Sometimes you might just want the flow of a liquid through your mouth and down your throat. Certain food textures might be appealing at different times of the day or even on different days.

• *Aroma.* Sometimes the aroma of a food will have more of an effect on your desire for it than does its taste or texture. Appreciate the various aromas that foods can emit. Walk by the bakery and smell the yeasty bread coming out of the oven, or inhale the coffee vapors as the coffee is dripping through the filter. If the aroma of a food is not appealing, you probably won't get your optimal satisfaction from it. If it smells great to you as it is cooking or served to you, however, it will probably increase your satisfaction.

• *Appearance.* Food artists who design commercial food sets or menus for restaurants know that foods that look appealing are alluring and make a person want to try them. Take a look at the food you're about to eat. Is it attractive to your eye? Is it fresh looking? Is its color interesting to you? Imagine a plate with a poached chicken breast, a boiled potato, and cauliflower—not too thrilling. You'll probably get less satisfaction from that meal than one that's more exciting to look at.

• *Temperature.* A steamy bowl of soup might just be the order of the day if it's cold and rainy outside. But chilly frozen yogurt is not usually desirable when you're shivering under an umbrella. Ask yourself what is the most appealing temperature of your foods. Do you like your hot foods boiling hot or temperate? Do you like your cold drinks with lots of ice or very little? Or is room temperature just fine for you for everything?

• *Volume or Filling-Capacity.* Some foods are light and airy, while others are heavy and filling. The filling capacity of your food choices can make a difference in how much food you need to satisfy you or how you feel after you're finished eating. Some days you might only be satisfied by a plate of pasta, which fills your stomach, while at other times, a lighter salad is more appealing. Even if something tastes and feels great on your tongue and in your mouth, if it makes your stomach feel queasy or too full, it will diminish the satisfying experience.

Respect Your Individual Taste Buds. Keep in mind that everyone has a different experience with taste and texture sensations. Not all foods will be desirable to you. People may rave about the best sushi in town, however, the thought of eating raw fish might be intolerable to you. If you have gotten sick on corn, regardless of the cause, corn might never seem appealing again. Your preferences may be lifelong or may change from time to time. Keep in touch with what is appetizing to you so that you can choose what is most satisfying.

Think About What You Really Feel Like Eating

Once you've gone through this hyperconscious experimentation with the sensory qualities of foods, the next time you feel like a meal or a snack, take a few moments to decide what you *really* want for a meal or snack. If you have trouble deciding what to eat, or need a little clarity, ask yourself:

- What do I feel like eating?
- What food aroma might appeal to me?
- How will the food look to my eye?
- How will the food taste and feel in my mouth?
- Do I want something sweet, salty, sour, or even slightly bitter?
- Do I want something crunchy, smooth, creamy, soft, lumpy, fluid, etc.?
- Do I want something hot, cold, or moderate?
- Do I want something light, airy, heavy, filling, or in-between?
- How will my stomach feel when I'm finished eating?

If you have a general knowledge of your taste preferences, it will lead you to the right place on the menu or in the supermarket. Checking in with yourself before a meal will give you the specifics of the moment.

A further critical key to finding satisfaction in your eating is to take a time-out *after* you've had a few bites of your food. Is the taste and texture consistent with your desire? Is the food satisfying enough to eat? If you continue to eat a food just because it's there, despite the fact that it's unappealing, you'll only end up feeling unsatisfied when you're finished and find yourself on the prowl for something else that will satisfy you.

STEP 3:
MAKE YOUR EATING EXPERIENCE MORE ENJOYABLE

Savor Your Food

Europeans seem to have a market on slow, sensual eating experiences. Businesses often shut down temporarily to allow for a long lingering lunch, so the meal can be savored and appreciated. Friends tend to gather together to enjoy the conversation and the food. Americans, on the other hand, often engage in desktop dining (fifteen minutes if you're lucky) while going over notes for a meeting, or zip through the fast-food drive-through while racing to pick up the kids from school. Who do you think has the most satisfying meal experience?

Alice is an executive in a company that stresses high productivity. Taking time to sit down for lunch is unheard of, and she's so anxious to get into the office in the morning to begin her calls to the East Coast, that she never allows herself to eat breakfast at home before she leaves. By the time Alice gets home in the evening, the frenetic pace of her day has become a part of her—she ends up gulping down her entire dinner before her husband and daughter get through their salads.

When you race through your meals as Alice does, you don't give yourself the opportunity to experience the sensual aspects of your food. You don't have time to appreciate the attractiveness of the different colors and shapes of the food. You can barely take in their aromas or feel their textures on your tongue and teeth—let alone taste.

To help you savor your food and get more satisfaction from your meals:

tips for college?

✓ Make time to appreciate your food. Give yourself a distinct time allowance for a meal. Even fifteen minutes is better than nothing.

✓ Sit down at the table or your desk. Standing at the refrigerator or walking around decreases attention and satisfaction.

• Take several deep breaths before you begin to eat. Deep breathing helps to calm and center you, so you can be focused on eating slowly.

• Pay attention to eating as slowly as you can. Remember that your taste buds are on your tongue, not in your stomach. Gobbling your food takes away your chance to really taste it.

- Taste each bite of food that you put in your mouth. Experience the different taste and texture sensations that the food can provide.
- Put your fork down, now and then, throughout the meal. This will help to slow you down.
- Remember Principle 5: *Feel Your Fullness.* Take a time-out in the midst of the meal to check your fullness level (see Chapter 9). Food won't taste as good or be as satisfying after you've reached the last-bite threshold.
- Finally, remember the three "S's" of **satisfying** eating:
  - eat **Slowly**
  - eat **Sensually**
  - and **Savor** every bite.

Eat When Gently Hungry Rather than When Overhungry

If you sit down for a meal when you're so hungry that you could eat a cow, you won't be able to sense the difference between a delicious steak and the cow itself! If you're overhungry, your biological need for energy supersedes your ability to eat slowly and taste what's before you. Likewise, if you begin to eat when you aren't really hungry, it can be difficult to decide whether what you're eating is really what you want and whether it's satisfying. When you're not very hungry, food is not as compelling. If you find this is true for you, this may be a sign that you're not ready to eat just yet. Wait a little while, until your hunger is somewhat more obvious, and you'll find that you'll have an easier time getting in touch with what you really want to eat.

Eat in a Pleasant Environment (When Possible)

Most people find that they get the greatest satisfaction from their meals by eating them in a pleasing setting. Restaurants spend a great deal of time and money creating environments that are appealing and will draw people back again and again. The aesthetics of a restaurant can be as important as the taste of the food. At home, the same thing goes. If you set your table in a pleasing manner (a placemat or table cloth, pretty china, and so forth), your food enjoyment will increase. But eating while standing or driving can diminish satisfaction. If you eat in the car, you are distracted by the traffic and by balancing food on your lap.

Avoid Tension ha ha ha

Keep heated fights off-limits at the table. One of the surest ways to decrease your satisfaction in eating is to try to eat when you're having an argument with a family member or friend. You'll probably end up eating faster and might even use your chewing as a way to show your anger. You definitely won't have your focus on the food and might eat everything before you without even noticing it—not a satisfying experience!

Provide Variety

Eating a variety of foods is not only nutritionally wise, but it will give you a much broader and more satisfying eating experience. Many clients take pride in keeping empty refrigerators and barren cupboards. They believe that if certain foods aren't around, they'll be less tempted to overeat. The reality is that a lack of appealing food choices creates a sense of deprivation and promotes a creative food foraging experience that never seems to produce a satisfying result. Give yourself the gift of keeping a variety of foods around, from soups to pastas to cookies or fruits and vegetables. You never know what you might feel like eating. Finding satisfaction in your eating will be a futile attempt if what you want isn't there.

Step 4:
Don't Settle

You are not obligated to finish eating a food just because you took a bite of it. Yet, how often have you tasted what appeared to be a mouthwatering dessert, only to discover it was mediocre—and yet you kept on eating? One of the biggest assets of being an Intuitive Eater is the ability to toss aside food that isn't to your liking. This can be easily done when you are truly tasting and experiencing food, combined with the knowledge that you can eat whatever you want again.

For the most part, adopt the motto: *"If you don't love it, don't eat it, and if you love it, savor it."* Order something else, find something different in the refrigerator, or eat the parts of the meal that you like, and leave the rest. For example, Barbara spoke of a meal served to her at a banquet that was comprised of salad, chicken, vegetables, and pasta. She took just one taste of the salad and left the rest when she found that the lettuce was soggy under a sea of dressing that she didn't like. The chicken and pasta were delicious, so she ate most of them. The vegetables were so buttery that they overwhelmed her taste buds, so she left them on the plate. In her old diet days, she would have eaten only the salad and vegetables, thinking that was the "diet" way to do it and would have left her meal unsatisfied, only to go home to search for something else to eat.

Melody is another client who is learning to discard what she doesn't find satisfying. One of Melody's favorite foods is a trademark muffin at a local restaurant. Every time she goes to the restaurant, she savors her muffin and feels satisfied. One day, Melody got the inspired notion to bake the trademark muffins from the restaurant's prepared mix. And bake she did. When she took a bite of the freshly baked muffin, she was sadly disappointed. It didn't taste anything like what she had eaten in the restaurant. Melody's connection with her Intuitive Eating allowed her to throw out the muffins, with the conviction that she would only eat them when she could get the "real thing."

STEP 5:
CHECK IN: DOES IT STILL TASTE GOOD?

Have you ever eaten a whole bag of cookies or a whole carton of Häagen-Dazs? If so, you can probably attest to the fact that the first couple of cookies or spoonfuls of ice cream tasted much better than those at the bottom of the barrel. Even the taste satisfaction of a large apple dwindles by the time you get down to the core. In studies of hedonics to food cues (hedonics is the branch of psychology dealing with pleasurable and unpleasurable feelings), researchers find that continued exposure to the same food results in a decrease of desire for that food. Researchers call this concept *sensory-specific satiety* (Epstein 2009). It does not take many bites of food to reach "taste satisfaction." Sensory-specific satiety is defined as a decrease in the subjective liking for a food that is eaten. This decline occurs within minutes of eating a particular food, which is highly influenced by the sensory aspects of food, such as flavor, texture, or aroma. We also see that in our clients.

Try your own hedonic experiment. Rate the taste pleasure you get from the first few bites of a food from one to ten—one being the least pleasurable and ten being the most. Then stop halfway through the food and check your taste buds. Finally, rate the food when you're down to the last bite. You're likely to find that the numbers diminish along with the food.

Routinely, check in with yourself to see if the food tastes as good as it did when you started. If it doesn't, consider stopping, as your satisfaction level is diminishing by the biteful. Wait until you're hungry again. Food will taste better and you'll be more satisfied. And, remember, no one is going to take that food away from your eating repertoire. You can have it for the rest of your life. So why waste your time and your food on a less-than-satisfying experience?

✴IT DOESN'T HAVE TO BE PERFECT✴

We've discussed how taking the time to figure out what you really want to eat, and eating in a favorable environment can lead you to more pleasurable, satisfying eating experiences. But what if this isn't always possible? There will be times when you don't have the option to get exactly what you want. You might be served a meal at a friend's or relative's house that offers little to say for it. Many a client has bemoaned meals made by a mother-in-law or an old friend who might boil the vegetables until unrecognizable or cook the chicken until it's the texture of an old shoe. At those times, remember the concept of *thinking in the gray* rather than in *black-and-white* (see Chapter 8). Intuitive Eating is not a process that seeks perfection, but one that offers guidelines to a comfortable relationship with food. Remember, most of your eating experiences will be more satisfying and pleasurable than you've experienced in years of diets. After all, it's only one meal— you will survive! It's how you jump back into taking care of yourself afterward that makes the difference.

Sometimes *honoring your hunger* is the best you can do. And for many of our patients, that alone is significant progress. But if survival eating occupies most of your experiences with food, your satisfaction factor will most likely be low.

RECLAIM YOUR RIGHT TO
PLEASURABLE, SATISFYING EATING

If dieting has been a significant part of your life for many years, you may need to make a serious commitment to reclaim your right to enjoy your food. You may have been so programmed to eat what you were told, especially foods that have little taste pleasure, that you hardly know where to begin to find satisfaction. *Knowing what you like to eat, and believing that you have the right to enjoy food, are key factors in a lifetime of maintaining normal weight without dieting.* If it takes you some time to accomplish all of this, be patient. After all, it's taken you many years to lose your ability to truly enjoy eating.

DISTRACTED VERSUS MINDLESS EATING

There seems to be a common perception that mindless eating is a condition in which you have no idea that you just ate, akin to "eating amnesia." Many of our clients eat while distracted—but don't consider themselves mindless eaters, because they are aware that they are eating while engaging in another activity, such as watching television.

Similarly, most car drivers would not readily identify themselves as *mindless drivers,* because they are aware that they are driving. However, if you describe someone as a *distracted driver,* it conjures up a clearer image—such as driving while talking on the cell phone or while applying makeup.

The problem, we believe, is a terminology issue. Unless you are trained in mindfulness, the description of "distracted" rather than "mindless" seems to resonate with more people. A recent study makes a good case about the effect of distraction on eating (Oldham-Cooper et al. 2011).

DISTRACTED EATING STUDY

Scientists divided people into two groups. The distracted group ate lunch while playing a computer game of solitaire. The non-distracted group ate the same type of lunch, but without the same distraction condition. The study's findings showed that distraction made a significant impact on the eating experience, both qualitatively and quantitatively. When compared to the non-distracted group, the distracted people:

- Ate faster
- Couldn't remember what they ate
- Ate more snacks
- Reported feeling significantly less full

The research also showed that distraction during a meal influenced meal size later in the day.

cont.

Continued

SATISFACTION AND SATIETY AFFECTED BY DISTRACTION

We are living in such a multitasking, high-urgency era, that even when not pressed for time, it seems that many people are in the routine of eating while distracted. The distracted conditions in the study are similar to how our clients eat, such as eating while checking e-mail, texting, surfing the Internet, tweeting—you get the idea.

The irony of eating while distracted is that you end up missing out on the eating experience, which often means that eating needs to be repeated. This is akin to having a phone conversation with a friend while you are checking e-mail. You might respond to the conversation at the right times, but something is missing, there is a disconnect—and usually the person on the other line can tell you are not 100 percent there. In the case of distracted eating—it is your body that knows.

ARTIFICIAL SWEETENERS

Artificial sweetener consumption has steadily risen since 1980. Currently, there are over four thousand foods which contain one or more artificial sweeteners, ranging from baby food to frozen foods and beverages.

People often assume that using artificially sweetened foods and drinks will help them lose weight. Yet, research suggests that the opposite may occur. A recent scientific review describes how consuming artificial sweeteners may lead to weight gain (Yang 2010):

- Artificial sweeteners may increase appetite, because they result in less satisfaction in eating.
- Calorie-free sweeteners offer only partial, but not complete, activation of the food reward pathways in the brain. This incomplete activation of the reward may contribute to increased food-seeking behavior.
- Artificially sweetened foods may encourage sugar cravings. The more often that someone is exposed to a flavor, the more this flavor becomes a preference. For example, people who are used to very salty foods often find unsalted foods to be bland and unfavorable.

cont.

Continued

Similarly, people who use artificial sweeteners become accustomed to the intensely sweet taste of artificially sweetened foods and beverages. This repeated exposure can lead to an increased preference for an unnaturally sweet taste.

- People tend to see artificially sweetened foods as lower in calories than foods that are naturally sweet or foods sweetened with sugar, leading them to overeat these foods.

Chapter 11

PRINCIPLE 7:

Cope with Your Emotions without Using Food

Find ways to comfort, nurture, distract, and resolve your issues without using food. Anxiety, loneliness, boredom, and anger are emotions we all experience throughout life. Each has its own trigger, and each has its own appeasement. Food won't fix any of these feelings. It may comfort for the short term, distract from the pain, or even numb you into a food hangover. But food won't solve the problem. If anything, eating for an emotional hunger will only make you feel worse in the long run. You'll ultimately have to deal with the source of the emotion, as well as the discomfort of overeating. *TRUTH*

Eating doesn't occur in a void. Regardless of your weight, food usually has emotional associations. If you have any doubt, catch a glimpse of food commercials. They push our eating buttons—not through our stomachs but through the emotional connection. They imply that in sixty seconds or less you can:

- Capture romance with an intimate cup of coffee.
- Bake someone happy.
- Reward yourself with a rich dessert.

Eating can be one of the most emotionally laden experiences that we have in our lives. The emotional rhythm to eating is set from the first day that the infant is offered the breast or the bottle to quell his crying. It's then reinforced each time a cookie is offered to soothe a scraped knee, or ice cream is eaten to celebrate a Little League victory. Nearly every culture and religion uses food as an important symbolic custom, from the American Thanksgiving feast to the Jewish Passover Seder. Each time a significant life experience is celebrated with food, the emotional connection deepens, from the I-got-the-promotion-dinner celebration to the annual birthday cake. Likewise, each time food is used for a little wound-licking or comfort, the emotional bond strengthens.

Food is love, food is comfort, food is reward, food is a reliable friend. And, sometimes, food becomes your *only* friend in moments of pain and loneliness.

Our patients are embarrassed that food can become so important—that food is their best friend. But if you consider how emotionally charged food is, it's no surprise that food can evolve into a special salve. When a dieter overeats during rough emotional times (whether periodically or chronically), it is usually obvious that food is used as a coping mechanism. For other dieters, it is not so clear.

Some of our clients are emotionally unaware—they have not yet learned to identify their feelings. It may not be obvious to them that they are using food to cope. Sometimes, these clients don't know why they are eating. Often the "why" is an uncomfortable feeling that has not been discovered. Or they may be engaged in a subtle form of emotional eating, such as boredom eating. Nibbling to kill time between classes or appointments is not emotionally charged, but the results can be the same as using food to numb strong feelings—*overeating*.

The eating experience itself, especially overeating, evokes feelings, and those feelings can affect your ability to eat normally. Some of the most detrimental feelings that overeating can stir up are guilt and shame. When our clients say, "I feel guilty because I ate _____" we ask these questions: Did you steal that food? Or did you steal money to get that food? They look aghast, and emphatically declare, "Of course not!" Feelings of guilt imply a crime or moral code was violated. Guilt may be an appropriate emotion when you have hurt another person or committed a crime, but guilt has no place in your eating world. Studies have shown that although you might have immediate emotional comfort from eating, the negative rush of guilt that bursts forth is powerful enough to completely wipe out the relief. If you replace the guilt with feelings of self-compassion, you'll be freed to concentrate on your underlying issues and find ways to understand them and deal with them.

Becoming an Intuitive Eater means learning to be gentle with yourself about how you use food to cope, and letting go of the guilt. As odd as this may sound, eating may have been the only coping mechanism you had to get through difficult times in your life. It may also have been an inevitable result of years of dieting and feelings of deprivation and despair that arose from dieting. *Dieting itself can trigger emotions, which ultimately lead to using food to cope with these feelings*—chalk up another vicious cycle due to dieting.

THE CONTINUUM OF EMOTIONAL EATING

Food can be used to cope with feelings in a myriad of ways. Using food in this way is not a component of biological hunger, but of emotional hunger. Emotional eating is triggered by feelings, such as boredom or anger, not by hunger. These feelings can trigger anything from a benign nibble to an out-of-control binge.

It's important to understand that this coping mechanism lies on a continuum of intensity that begins at one end with mild, almost universal sensory eating to the opposite end with numbing, often anesthetizing eating. The following diagram illustrates this spectrum:

sensory
gratification • comfort • distraction • sedation • punishment

Sensory Gratification

The mildest and most common feeling that food can call forth is pleasure. The significance of receiving pleasure from eating is emphasized in Principle 6: *Discover the Satisfaction Factor.* This concept is not only critical to Intuitive Eating, but is a normal, natural part of living. Don't underestimate the importance of pleasing your palate. As we explained in Chapter 10, by letting yourself enjoy and appreciate eating, you will actually reduce the amount of food you need to feel satisfied when biologically hungry. For example, allowing yourself to truly taste all of the special foods that appeal to you at Thanksgiving, without restriction, will usually offset overeating.

Comfort

Just the thought of certain foods has the ability to evoke feelings from a comfortable time or place. For example, do you ever crave chicken soup when you are sick, or macaroni and cheese on dreary days—because that's what your mom fixed on these occasions? Those are examples of comfort foods. It's normal to have a repertoire of comfort foods. If you want to curl up with a blanket in front of a fireplace and sip hot cocoa with your dinner that's fine. Occasionally eating comfort foods can be part of a healthy relationship with food, if you do it while staying in touch with your satiety levels and without guilt. If, however, food is the first and only thing that comes to mind to take care of you when you are feeling sad, lonely, or uncomfortable, it can become a destructive coping mechanism.

Distraction

If you go a little further on the continuum of emotional eating, food can be used to distract you from feelings you choose not to experience. Using food to cope in this way can become troublesome, as it can be a seductive behavior that blocks your ability to detect your intuitive signals. It also can inhibit you from discovering the source of the feelings and taking care of your true needs. Whether you're the teenager who sits in front of the TV with a bag of chips to distract you from the feelings of boredom in doing your homework, or you're the executive who goes through a whole bowl of peanuts on your desk to distract you from the anxiety of an arduous meeting, this kind of eating needs to be confronted. There is nothing wrong with occasionally wanting to distract yourself from feelings. Experiencing your feelings twenty-four hours a day can be tedious and overwhelming. *But food is not the appropriate distractor for temporary relief.*

Sedation

A more serious form of using food to cope is eating for the purpose of numbing or anesthetizing. One client calls this form of eating a "food coma." Another suggests that this kind of eating results in a "food hangover." In either case, eating to sedate yourself can be as emotionally dangerous as using drugs or alcohol for this purpose. It keeps you from experiencing any feeling for extended periods of time. It becomes impossible to sense your intuitive signals of hunger and satiety, and it deprives you of the satisfying experience that food can bring to your life. Most clients who use food in this way talk about feeling out of control, out of touch with life, and generally zoned-out. They also have trouble recognizing basic sensations of hunger and fullness.

Connie is a young woman who had an abusive childhood. She learned to use food at a very early age as a numbing agent. She continues to sedate herself through the anxiety, fear, and sadness of her present life. Connie's weight can escalate dramatically when she is regularly going into her "food comas." But even more frightening than her weight gain is the complete detachment from life that she experiences each time. She isolates from her friends, calls in sick to work, and feels completely hopeless about life itself. Connie is learning to utilize other coping tools so that she can improve the quality of her life.

When eating to numb and sedate is occasional and short run, it tends to have little detrimental effect. But this kind of eating can escalate into a habitual behavior before you hardly notice.

Punishment

Sometimes, eating for the purpose of sedation becomes so frequent and intense that self-blame ensues and ultimately triggers punishing behaviors. Clients find themselves eating large quantities of food in an angry, forceful manner that allows them to feel beaten up. This is the most severe form of emotional eating and can lead to loss of self-esteem and self-hatred. Clients who use food to punish themselves report no pleasure in their eating and actually begin to hate food. Fortunately, this type of eating behavior disappears when the Nurturer voice can be beckoned to give understanding and compassion. If there's no crime committed, no punishment need be tendered.

EMOTIONAL TRIGGERS

We've looked at general emotional reasons for eating; now, let's examine the specific feelings involved. A craving for certain foods, or simply a desire to eat can be triggered by a variety of feelings and situations.

Some people use food to cope when they have no idea that's what they're doing. They think that they're overeating "just because it tastes good" and deny or minimize that they're eating emotionally. If you find that you're doing quite a bit of eating when you're not biologically hungry, then there's a good chance that you are using food to cope. You may not have deep-seated emotional reasons to eat, but just getting through life's hassles with some of its irksome tasks and boredom might trigger you to seek food to make it all easier. The best way to gauge whether you're using food in this way is to ask yourself the following question: "If my body only needs a certain amount of food to feel satisfied, but I continue to eat after I'm full, then what other need am I trying to fill with food?" You may discover that the food is taking care of some of the feelings mentioned below.

Boredom and Procrastination

One of the most common reasons that our clients eat when they're not hungry is boredom. In fact, studies have shown that regardless of a person's weight, boredom is one of the most common triggers of emotional eating. One particular study divided college students into two groups. One group had the monotonous task of writing the same letters over and over again for nearly half an hour. The other group was engaged in a stimulating writing project. Students in each group were given a bowl of crackers to nibble on. Guess which group ate more? Regardless of weight, the "bored" group ate the most crackers.

In boredom eating, food is used as a way to fill time as well as a way to put off doing mundane work. For some people, the thought of the food and the actual experience of going for it and eating it, breaks the tedium. Here are some situations that produce boredom eating.

- Lying around the house on a Sunday afternoon when you've made no plans for the day.
- Having to get through an afternoon of studying, paperwork, or a writing project.
- Watching a boring night of television with nothing else to do but take food breaks.
- Killing time: waiting for a meeting to get started, waiting for a phone call, and so forth.

We also see this type of eating in our overworked clients—they feel they must always be *doing* something, being productive. The moment a tiny hole opens up in their schedule, they feel the need to fill it—often with food. (It's acceptable to eat, but not to rest!)

Bribery and Reward

Have you ever promised yourself that you could have a treat once you finished writing a term paper, or a contract, or cleaning the house? If so, you have experienced reward eating. It's not unusual to use food as a motivation to accomplish undesired tasks. For example:

- Children are bribed with treats such as candy or ice cream if they behave—at the mall, for a babysitter, and so on.
- People often reward themselves for working hard: at work, at home, or at school with an extra bagel or a muffin, for example.

Using food as a reward can be self-perpetuating, as there will always be ongoing tasks and challenges which can be made more tolerable if they're mitigated by food gifts.

Excitement

Food and the eating experience itself can serve as a way to add excitement when life begins to feel dull. At a subtle level, planning a special meal or making a reservation at a favorite restaurant can create a sense of excitement.

The notion of going on a diet can trigger excited feelings of hope. This is one of the reasons that dieting is so alluring. Our clients talk of how even contemplating a new diet gives them a rush of adrenaline—just imagining a new body and new life. When the diet fails, the excitement is replaced with despair. At this point, the experience of going to the store to buy large quantities of forbidden foods can be one way to re-create the excitement. And then the cycle continues—diet/overeating, diet/overeating. This is exciting, but at what cost?

Soothing

It's not hard to understand the soothing power that food can provide. It can be more appealing to go to the kitchen for cookies and milk than to sit on the couch and experience uncomfortable feelings. This is especially true if those cookies and milk remind you of a time that was pleasant and life felt less complicated. Habitually eating to soothe what ails you can evolve into a problem with food.

Food can have other symbolic meanings of comfort. Ellen is a sixteen-year-old who has battled with her father since she was a small child. She describes him as mean and nasty with a bitter personality. It was not surprising to hear Ellen talk about her obsession with eating large amounts of candy every day as a way to bring "sweetness" into her life. To her, the sweets countered the bitterness of her daily experiences with her father.

Love

Food can become connected to the feeling of being loved. There is certainly a romantic link with food—chocolate on Valentine's Day is a classic example. When dating, there's an unspoken ground rule that your relationship is elevated to a more intimate level when you have experienced a home-cooked meal for two.

Clients frequently tell of how their parents' only way to show love was through food. Their parents may not have been able to show physical attention or speak to them in loving ways, but food was always plentiful.

Frustration, Anger, and Rage

If you find yourself going through a bag of hard and crunchy pretzels when you're not hungry, it's a good bet that you may be feeling frustrated or angry. The physical act of biting and crunching can serve as a way to release these feelings for some people. One client, Nancy, a lawyer, discovered that she had a habit of subduing her anger at some of her clients by grabbing some hard food, whether it was carrots or crackers, and munching away.

Stress *not usually*

Many of our clients say they head for the nearest candy bar under stressful times. Yet, in most individuals, biological mechanisms associated with stress *turn off* the desire to eat.

The rush of adrenaline during stressful times sets in motion a cascade of biological events to provide immediate energy. As a result, blood sugar is elevated and digestion is slowed. These two elements alone tend to suppress hunger and heighten the sense of satiety when eating. The biological reactions are a form of self-preservation—to ready our bodies for "fight or flight." While this was quite useful for survival in an acute situation—*fighting off* a man-eating tiger or *fleeing* from danger required immediate energy—a growing body of research suggests that in our modern day, this mechanism may actually contribute to obesity when it becomes chronic. It may be stressful to *fight off* rush-hour traffic or to *flee* from a deadline, but you don't need the extra blood sugar that the stress reaction provides. Chronic stress also raises cortisol, which is a steroid hormone produced by the adrenal gland and secreted into the bloodstream. Prolonged higher levels of cortisol can increase abdominal fat, which is associated with a greater amount of health problems. These biological problems are only compounded if you cope with stress by eating. Studies have also shown that people who have been dieting are especially vulnerable to overeating during stressful times. Stress becomes one more reason to "blow" the diet. Dieting itself can also be a source of stress.

Anxiety   maybe

Worries, of any magnitude, from an upcoming final to waiting to hear if you got the job, can trigger an urgent need to eat to relieve anxiety. Sometimes generalized anxiety can be described as that uncomfortable feeling that you are unable to put a finger on; our clients say it feels like butterflies in your stomach. With the focus on the stomach, so goes the food.

Mild Depression   maybe

It's not uncommon for many people to turn to food when they are mildly depressed. In mild depression, weight gain is often seen, especially in dieters. In one particular study, 62 percent of the dieters and 52 percent of non-dieters stated they ate more when feeling depressed.

Being Connected   a lot in college (aka the dining hall)

The need to feel part of a group or to feel a connection to others can be very powerful for some people, and can even affect how and what they eat.

This experience was poignantly described by Mathew, when he was talking about the dinner he had eaten one night with some friends. Although he didn't like the food served, he ate it anyway. He made the choice to feel connected but dissatisfied with the food rather than feeling different. How many times have you eaten to be part of the crowd—from running out to get ice cream to sharing a pizza?

* * *

| *Loosening the Reins* | *oh dear yes that's it*

Frequently, clients who are highly successful in every aspect of their lives, except in their eating, discount their accomplishments. They feel as if their food problems indicate they are truly failures in life. We have found that in most cases, overeating is the only mechanism that such a person has for letting go and letting loose of the tight reins of control in his or her life. A good example is Larry, a wealthy businessman who is the chief executive officer of a large business. He dresses impeccably, keeps his car perfectly washed and waxed, and lives in a beautifully decorated house in an affluent neighborhood. He maintains rigid discipline with his children and has high expectations for his wife as well. He never drinks or uses drugs, he keeps perfect records of his household finances, and he has an immaculate appointment book that maintains his punctuality. Larry's only outlet from his self-imposed militaristic control is overeating—it is his way of letting out some steam.

COPING WITH EMOTIONAL EATING

Whether your response to emotional hunger is mild emotional eating or out-of-control bingeing, there are four key steps to making food less important in your life. Ask yourself:

1. *Am I biologically hungry?* If the answer is yes, your next step is to honor your hunger and eat! If you are not hungry answer the following questions.
2. *What am I feeling?* When you find yourself reaching for food when there is no biological hunger, take a time-out to find out what you are feeling. This is not such an easy question to answer, especially if you are not in touch with your feelings. Try the following:

- Write out your feelings.
- Call a friend and talk about the feelings.
- Talk about the feelings into a tape recorder.
- Just sit with the feelings and experience them if you can.
- Talk to a counselor or a psychotherapist.

3.) *What do I need?* Many people eat to fulfill some unmet need, which is related to the emotional or physical feeling being experienced. If you are a chronic dieter you can be particularly vulnerable. Eating to assuage an unmet need can be used as an excuse to eat. Here is a simple example:

Molly is a freelance writer who was working into the wee hours to meet her deadline. Around three o'clock in the morning she found herself walking downstairs into the kitchen. She realized that she was not hungry, yet she was about to devour a bowl of ice cream. When Molly asked herself what she was feeling, she discovered frustration, exhaustion, and a sense of being brain-dead. She realized that she was trying to feed both her fatigue and her frustration. But what she really *needed* was rest—no amount of food would replace sleep. She decided to call it a night and go to bed. But before Molly made that decision, she told herself she could have the ice cream tomorrow if she still wanted it. She also realized the ice cream would taste better if she experienced it fully awake rather than half asleep. The next day Molly finished her story and had no desire for the ice cream— she removed the need.

4. *Would you please . . . ?* It's not unusual to find that when you ask the question, "What do I need?" the answer can be found simply by speaking up and asking for help. Laurel Mellin, innovator of the successful Shapedown weight management program for families, has found that overweight kids often have trouble speaking up for their needs. We also find this to be true for many of our clients. The "Would you please" step originated from Laurel Mellin's work, and we find it extremely helpful for our clients.

Danielle, a full-time stay-at-home mom, learned that she was using food as a momentary time-out. Eating was her only retreat between baby cries. Danielle discovered that what she needed was not food, but time just for herself. To obtain this she used the "Would you please" step. She asked her husband to give her thirty minutes of uninterrupted quiet time after he came home from work. Having gained this, food was no longer important.

MEETING YOUR NEEDS WITHOUT FOOD

There are various ways in which we learn to handle the unending emotions that life can trigger. Some people learn from early on that it's okay to express their feelings or to ask for a hug. Others aren't lucky enough to be taught how to take care of themselves in productive, nurturing ways. The first task in learning how to cope without using food is to acknowledge that you are entitled to having your needs met. But basic needs are often discounted, including:

- Getting rest.
- Getting sensual pleasure.
- Expressing feelings.
- Being heard, understood, and accepted.
- Being intellectually and creatively stimulated.
- Receiving comfort and warmth.

Seek Nurturance

Feeling nurtured can allow you to feel comfort and warmth so that food loses its number-one position in this role. There are many routes and avenues available for nurturing yourself and receiving nurturing from others.

- Rest and relax.
- Take a sauna or a Jacuzzi.
- Listen to soothing music.
- Take time to breathe deeply.
- Learn to meditate.
- Play cards with friends.
- Take a bubble bath in candlelight.
- Take a yoga class.
- Get a massage.
- Play with your dog or cat.
- Develop a network of friends.
- Ask friends for hugs.
- Buy yourself little presents.
- Put fresh flowers in your house.
- Spend time gardening.

- Get a manicure, pedicure, facial, haircut, etc.
- Buy a teddy bear and hug it!

Deal with Your Feelings

If you receive a steady flow of comfort and nurturing you'll be better pre-pared to face the feelings that have been so frightening. Acknowledge what is troubling you—allow your feelings to come up. This will reduce your need to push them down with food. Here are some suggestions of how to deal with your feelings.

- Write your feelings in a journal.
- Call a friend (or several).
- Talk about your feelings into a tape recorder.
- Release anger through pounding a pillow or a punching bag.
- Confront the person who is triggering your feelings.
- Let yourself cry.
- Breathe deeply.
- Sit with your feelings and discover how the intensity will dimin-ish with time.
- If you have trouble identifying your feelings or coping with them, it may be helpful to talk with a therapist, especially if it is a persistent issue.

Find a Different Distraction

Many people use food as their primary distraction from their feelings. It's okay to get away from the feelings from time to time, *but you don't have to use food as an excuse.* Many teenagers tell us that they come home from school every afternoon and plop in front of the TV with a bag of chips and a soda. When asked why they do this, they say that they're avoiding the boring feelings of having to do their homework. When it's suggested that they first have a snack to take care of their biological hunger and *then* watch some TV to distract themselves for a while before settling down to homework—they exclaim that their parents would never let them. *As long as they're eating, they can legitimately procrastinate from homework, but having other distractions is not allowed!* This is also true for many worka-holic clients. It's socially acceptable to take a time-out to eat (coffee break), but to just sit at the desk, even while entitled to a break, is not allowed. They fear that it will appear as if they are doing nothing. Others use food to distract themselves from loneliness, fear, and anxiety. Since it would be overwhelming to try to feel your feelings twenty-four hours a day, give yourself permission to take a break from them for a while. Take the assertive stance of distracting yourself in an emotionally healthy way. Try the following:

- Read an absorbing book.
- Rent a movie.
- Talk on the telephone.
- Go to the movies.
- Take a drive.
- Clean out your closet.
- Put on some music and dance.
- Peruse a magazine.
- Take a stroll around the block.
- Work in the garden.
- Listen to an audio novel.
- Do a Sudoku or a crossword puzzle.
- Work on a jigsaw puzzle.
- Play with the computer.
- Take a nap.

HOW EMOTIONAL OVEREATING
HAS HURT *AND* HELPED

As you begin to examine your use of food as a coping mechanism, it's helpful to take a look at how food has actually helped you. The notion that overeating can have benefits may sound crazy to you, especially if you're feeling distressed by this behavior and your weight. *But if there were no upside to overeating, you probably wouldn't continue it.* Take a piece of paper and divide it in half. On one half, make a list of "How Using Food Serves Me" and cite all the benefits you receive from overeating. Title the other side, "How Using Food Disserves Me" and examine the ways in which food has become harmful or destructive to you. A list might look like the following:

How Using Food Serves Me	How Using Food Disserves Me
• It tastes good.	• My cholesterol is high.
• It's reliable—it's always there.	• My clothes don't fit.
• It keeps me from feeling bored.	• I'm uncomfortable walking and exercising.
• It soothes me.	• I feel overfull and uncomfortable.
• It numbs my bad feelings.	• I'm numbed to the joys of life.

As you look over your list, you might be surprised to learn that the use of food is not just a negative experience for you. In fact, it may give you some valuable perks. But if you're feeling bad and guilty about using food to cope, it will be hard for you to recognize that its benefits may equalize its burdens. By recognizing that there are indeed some benefits to using food, you'll begin to own your eating experience, rather than feeling out of control.

WHEN FOOD IS NO LONGER IMPORTANT

Many clients have talked about having strange, uncomfortable feelings when they're no longer using food to cope with their emotions. At the same time, they're feeling happy and secure in their new Intuitive Eating style and have stopped struggling with food and their bodies. There are a couple of reasons for the conflicting feelings.

• You no longer have the "benefits" of using food. While coping with food can be destructive, one client noted that on tough days she knew she could always go home to her chocolate. Now, instead, she's "stuck" with experiencing her feelings. You might even need to go through a grieving period for the loss of food as comforter and companion.

• You may also notice that you're experiencing your feelings in a deeper, stronger way. Since you're no longer covering them up with food, they may have a profound effect on you. This is a point at which some people decide that it would be helpful to get counseling as a way to process these long-buried feelings.

Sandy is a client who experienced the loss of using food as a coping mechanism. By acknowledging what food used to do *for* her as well as *against* her, Sandy was able to understand that her uncomfortable feelings were normal and appropriate. Sandy had either dieted or used food to cope all of her life. She talked about feeling very frustrated when she would stop eating after finding the threshold bite and truly not wanting any more food. She knew that she'd had enough, didn't want to feel uncomfortable by eating more, yet felt unhappy that she wouldn't be able to continue to have the taste sensations that the food provided. She also talked about feeling angry that she no longer had food to turn to when she was feeling bad. Eating isn't as exciting as it used to be when Sandy would restrict and then overeat. Soon, however, after mourning the loss of being able to *use* food, she was able to leave these feelings behind and feel mainly the exhilaration of being an Intuitive Eater who copes without using food.

A STRANGE GIFT

You may go for a long time without using food to cope, when all of a sudden emotional eating catches you by surprise. If this occurs, it's not a sign of failure or that you've lost ground; instead, it's a strange gift. Overeating is simply a sign that stressors in your life at that moment surpass the coping mechanisms that you have developed. Some of these stressors are divorce, a job change, a move to a new city, the death of someone close, marriage, or the birth of a child. These may be new or unexpected experiences for you. As a result, you haven't had the opportunity to develop coping skills to deal with them. So, you revert back to eating as the familiar way to take care of yourself.

Overeating can also occur when your lifestyle becomes unbalanced with too many responsibilities and obligations, with too little time for pleasure and relaxation. Consequently food is used to indulge, escape, and relax (albeit so briefly). When you find this happening, it may be a signal for you to reevaluate your life and find ways to put more balance into it. If you don't make these necessary changes, food remains important by filling an unmet need.

In both of these situations, overeating becomes a red flag to let you know that something isn't right in your life. Once you truly appreciate this, eating will not feel out of control—rather it's an early warning system. Recognize how lucky you are to have this mechanism to alert you that something is out of kilter in your life! (At first, our clients think this notion is a bit absurd, until they realize the truth behind it in their own lives.) Those people who have never had an emotional eating problem often have no ostensible warning of excess stress in their lives. If you can see that your eating problem can have benefits as well as negative effects, you won't get into a pattern of self-defeating behaviors that become destructive and difficult to reverse.

USING FOOD CONSTRUCTIVELY

Once you learn new ways of coping, think about how food can continue to nurture you in a constructive way. You have a right to feel good—and that means not just not feeling stuffed, but also feeling satisfied with your food choices, being healthy now, and reducing future health risks. Your relationship with food will become more positive as you begin to let go of food as a coping mechanism and bring it into your life as a nonthreatening, pleasurable experience. In Chapter 14 we discuss how you can eat healthfully without falling back into the diet mentality. But first you need to learn how to respect your body and appreciate how it feels when you include movement in your life.

Chapter 12

PRINCIPLE 8:

Respect Your Body

Accept your genetic blueprint. Just as a person with a shoe size of eight would not expect to realistically squeeze into a size six, it is equally futile (and uncomfortable) to have the same expectation about body size. But mostly, respect your body, so you can feel better about who you are. It's hard to reject the diet mentality if you are unrealistic and overly critical about your body shape.

Body vigilance begets body worry, which begets food worry, which fuels the cycle of dieting. So what do you do, just forget it? Crawl into a dark cave, hide from the world, and eat everything in sight? No. But as long as you are at war with your body it will be difficult to be at peace with yourself and food. For every disparaging glimpse in the mirror, the Food Police gain power, and with that comes vows of just one more diet.

Has all the self-loathing because of your body helped? Has dwelling on your imperfect body parts helped you to become leaner, or merely make you feel worse? Does chewing yourself out every time you step on the scale make your weight any less? We have yet to find one client who says that focusing on his or her body in such negative ways is helpful. Studies have shown that the more you focus on your body, the worse you feel about yourself. Yet the body torture game goes on—Mirror, Mirror, on the wall, who's the slimmest of them all?

It's hard to escape the body torture game when the whole country is playing it. In the name of fitness, a lean and hard shape has become the body icon for modern times. Self-proclaimed fitness gurus insist that you can "sculpt" your body as if it were a lump of clay, that you can change your genetic shape with an aerobic huff and puff. We are ardent advocates of being fit and recognize the health benefits of exercise, but we feel we must point out where unrealistic expectations are being painted. It is widely accepted in the research community that you cannot spot-reduce (lose fat in just one specified place). So how could it be that you can simply sculpt your body by working on certain body parts? Yes, you can build specific muscles through strength and resistance training. Yes, you can lose overall body fat through aerobic exercise. But you cannot personally select where that fat will be lost. It's possible therefore to build muscle underneath fat layers—but this is not the concept of body sculpting that most have in mind. Most clients we speak with take body-sculpting classes in hopes of chiseling off the fat.

The fashion world has also shaped the ideal look for women into various versions of thin—from the sixties Twiggy figure to the waif look first embodied by supermodel Kate Moss. Even the full-bodied fashion look turns out to be too thin by medical standards. When clothing giant, Guess, hired model Anna Nicole Smith, she made headlines in the fashion and news media because she was "big." Her weight was actually in the lower range of ideal according to 1990 U.S. height and weight charts! If a normal weight is considered "big," what does that say to the average woman? This hardly fosters realistic body-shape expectations.

If the ideal body type for women is sandwiched between the spandex-fitness look and fashionable waifness, most bodies don't stand a chance. No wonder body dissatisfaction has become the norm in this country. Repeatedly we seem to be sold the message: If they could do it, you can do it; just try harder (after all, even if you are lean, you could still be leaner). With such standards, it's no wonder that women and increasingly men, too, are at war with their bodies. Whether you are male or female, fat is considered the enemy.

There is no doubt that there are unrealistic pressures to be thin with contributions from the media, advertisers, fashion industry, beauty industry, and on and on. We could groan and point fingers at the causes leading to increasing body dissatisfaction. Yes, there is a myriad of cultural factors that lead to unrealistic body expectations. But we want to get past the cause-and-effect analysis, and instead focus our energy on how you can get past body vigilance. Besides, plenty of good books have been written on this topic (see the reference list at the back of this book).

BODY IMAGE:
A WAIST IS A TERRIBLE THING TO MIND

Most of our clients are adept at being overly critical or hating their bodies. And putting an end to body worry and self-loathing is no easy task. Most of us have trouble accepting a compliment, let alone the idea of accepting our bodies. We have found that the notion of accepting your body was too far of a stretch to our clients as a beginning point. They feared that if they accepted their current body size, it would mean complacency, giving up, and getting even bigger. It's one thing to lose the battle of the bulge, they'd say, but to totally give up would mean ultimate failure. At least there's honor and dignity in continuing the fight. Our clients also argued that embracing the notion of body acceptance felt hypocritical. After all, the reason they sought our help is because they did *not* accept their current body—they wanted a change.

What a paradox. Our experience has shown us that if you're meant to get to your *natural* ideal weight, you need to loosen up on yourself, put weight loss on the back burner, and treat your body with respect.

Remember, repeated diets and a disparaging attitude toward your body have not helped—it's part of what got you to where you are right now. When you are caught in the I-hate-my-body mind-set, it's all too easy to keep delaying good things for yourself, waiting until you have a body that you think is more deserving. But that day never comes (especially when your standards are unreachable). So, you put off treating yourself better. Many aspects of your life literally get weighted down. "I'll join the health club after I lose ten pounds," "I'll go on a special vacation after I reach my goal weight," "I'll start going out with my friends when I just get some of this weight off"—and so the empty promises go. And life gets a little emptier during these times.

Body image expert and psychologist Judith Rodin notes in her book *Body Traps*, "You don't need to lose weight first in order to take care of yourself. In fact, the process actually happens quite in the reverse!" We also have found that if you are willing to make weight loss a secondary goal, and respecting your body a primary goal, it will help move you forward.

We are not saying disregard your body—we are urging you instead to respect and appreciate it. This does not mean that you throw in the towel. This does not mean that you should disregard your health. In fact, respecting your body *means* taking care of your health. There is a growing movement that shifts the focus to health, rather than to weight—it's called Health at Every Size (HAES). Instead of focusing on numbers (weight), the emphasis is on healthy living and behaviors. For example, physical activity is vital for health, for everyone. Yet, lean people may conclude that they have no reason to be physically active since their body weight is considered to be normal. To learn more see "Health at Every Size" on page 181.

Respecting and appreciating your body is the beginning of making peace with your body and your genetics. It is probably the most difficult thing that you will do. If you could place your priorities on making peace with your food and body (becoming an Intuitive Eater), it will allow you to loosen up. Otherwise, it will be a constant tug-of-war.

It's normal to feel panicky when thinking about respecting your body. But by doing so it will allow you to go through the Intuitive Eating steps much more easily. Ironically, we observe a marked difference in our clients who are able to respect their bodies versus those who are not. Those who are able to get to a place of respect for their bodies have more patience for the Intuitive Eating process. This patience allows them to explore further, and move forward quicker.

Those who have trouble respecting their bodies often find themselves in conflict. When they feel loathsome toward their bodies they struggle with an intense desire to diet and "just get the weight off." Then they vacillate with intermittent feelings of peace when working through the Intuitive Eating process. It is those moments of peace that give them hope, however, to continue Intuitive Eating.

WHY "RESPECT"

We chose the word *respect* as a launching point for working through your body issues. It's a tough place to begin for most of our clients. Just keep in mind these points, which will ease you into the idea of body-respect: You don't have to like every part of your body to respect it. In fact, you don't have to immediately accept where your body is now to respect it. *Respecting your body means treating it with dignity and meeting its basic needs*. Many of our clients treat their pets with more respect than their own bodies—they feed them, take them out for walks, and are kind to them. Finally, if you are someone who has used food as a way to cope with your emotions over a lifetime, your present body shape may be representative of the way you took care of yourself when you knew no other way. Rather than demeaning the results of this coping mechanism, respect yourself for surviving.

Respecting your body is a critical turning point in becoming an Intuitive Eater. It's not easy. Our culture has a built-in bias against large body sizes while placing a premium on appearance. It's important to recognize that these biases exist, because it may seem like you are a salmon swimming up against the cultural norm. After all, it's all around us in both subtle and blatant forms, from the thin actresses in diet soft drink ads to glaring magazine covers such as a cover from an issue of *People* magazine's "Diet Winners and Sinners of the Year: Here's the Skinny on Who Got Fat, Who Got Fit and How They Did It." It takes a conscious effort to move away from this societal norm. Just because seeking a slender body is the societal norm does not make it right!

How to Respect Your Body

Think of respecting your body in two ways: first, by making it comfortable, and second, by meeting its basic needs. You deserve to be comfortable. You deserve to get your basic needs met. Or the more miserable you feel, the more miserable you'll be.

Consider these basic premises of body respect:

- My body deserves to be fed.
- My body deserves to be treated with dignity.
- My body deserves to be dressed comfortably and in the manner to which I am accustomed.
- My body deserves to be touched affectionately and with respect.
- My body deserves to move comfortably.

Let's explore how you can offer more respect to your body (and to yourself). It's an easy concept to understand, but far more difficult to implement. The following ideas and tools have helped our clients begin a new relationship with their bodies.

Getting Comfortable. Let's get personal here. When is the last time you bought new underwear? Don't laugh. All too often we have clients who feel that they don't deserve new underwear (let alone, new clothes) until they reach a certain weight or clothing size. Think about what that means at a basic level. Wearing panties, a bra, or briefs that are constantly pinching or riding up is highly uncomfortable. How can you be comfortable in your body when you have an unpleasant reminder constantly binding your body? How can you be at ease, when your body is constantly pinched and squeezed by poorly fitting garments? Even an old car still needs a new set of tires. While initially you may snicker at the simplicity of changing your underwear, its had a significant impact on many of our clients. "I just had a baby a few months ago. My maternity underwear was laughably big, but my regular panties fit too snugly. They were a constant reminder that I was too big. I felt miserable, until I invested in underwear that fit. The funny thing is that I didn't want to spend the money—even though I had shelled out plenty on a weight loss program that did not work. I was amazed at how a simple act made such a difference in feeling better about myself."

Cassandra was in her fifties and hadn't bought new bras in years. (The ones she had were of very high quality and quite expensive, so they lasted.) Sadly, the underwires in her bras were jabbing and scarring her, but she didn't feel she deserved to buy new bras until she lost weight. Yet every day she was miserable. Her first step toward respecting her body was buying new bras and tights. She learned that wearing a tortuously tight undergarment would not make the process happen any quicker. When she was more relaxed in her underwear, she was able to be more relaxed about her eating.

The comfort principle goes beyond undergarments. How you dress can be a step toward a newfound respect for your body. We are not saying to be a slave to the fashion industry, however. Rather, dress in the manner in which you are accustomed. If you are used to dressing in a tailored suit ensemble, why should you stop just because you body is not where you currently want it to be? You should not have to settle for leftovers or dowdy clothes. There's nothing wrong with dressing in worn-out jeans and an oversized shirt, *if that is what you are used to and are comfortable in*. If however you prefer wearing dress pants and a casual blazer and settle for worn-out jeans, it may affect how you feel about yourself and your body. It's an issue of being consistent. All too often weight loss programs have urged you to "get rid of your fat clothes," otherwise, they warn, you are issuing an invitation for failure. By following this dictum, however, you are setting yourself up to feel uncomfortable and more body-phobic. Instead, dress for your here-and-now body; be comfortable.

so I should go shopping? ☺

Change Your Body-Assessment Tools. We have found that most of our clients who weigh themselves frequently have difficulty living in their present body—they get too worried about the numbers. Our advice: Stop weighing yourself. Remember, the scale is the tool of a chronic dieter.

Also, beware of substituting a tight pair of jeans as a pseudo-scale or body-assessment tool. Hanging on to a small piece of clothing, and trying it on daily or weekly can equally undermine how you feel about yourself and your body. Jamie, a young account executive for a public relations firm was doing quite well with Intuitive Eating. She quit dieting, honored her hunger, respected her fullness, and so forth. Jamie had also gotten rid of the scale. But she began to assess her progress by trying on a tight miniskirt. Every time she tried the skirt on she felt bad about herself. It conveyed the message, "You haven't made enough progress. You need to lose weight." Jamie eventually got rid of the skirt and her bad feelings about her body. *Even a slender person will feel uncomfortable in a pair of pants that feel too tight.*

Quit the Body-Check Game. Most of our clients are embarrassed to admit this, but when they enter a room with other people, they play the silent game of body-checking. The game of body-checking revolves around the theme: How does my body compare to the rest of the crowd? Perhaps you've played this game (and maybe are not even quite aware of it):

Am I the biggest one here? Who's got the best body? How does my body rate compared to the others? This can be a dangerous game, especially when played with people you don't know.

We've had clients admire and envy a stranger's body shape. "Oh, if I only had *her* body. She must work out daily. Look at her eat—only low-fat food. I should be able to do that. Something is wrong with me. I need to try harder." These are big assumptions. You do not know how someone acquired her current body shape. You may not be on a level playing field. You don't know if the person is truly eating! The person may have had surgery (such as liposuction), many suffer from an eating disorder, may have just finished a quickie diet with fast results, and so on. You can't judge the shape of someone's body and assume he or she "earned" it. The person may put on a "false food face" socially. The individual you are admiring may also be miserable in her body! Or this person could just be naturally lean— with no effort at all.

In one session, Kate described a party that she had attended and how good a particular woman's body looked. Kate thought that she should be able to get those kind of results, too, if she just tried harder. Little did Kate know, however, that the acquaintance at the party was a client of mine (ET), who happened to be bulimic! (Of course Kate would never know this from me because of strict patient confidentiality.) Kate had been admiring a woman with an eating disorder who was fighting for recovery. The bottom line is, you never know. Even if it was a friend or relative, you still don't know. We have worked with clients whose own spouses and roommates did not know that they had an eating disorder.

Playing the body-check game may lead to more dieting and more body dissatisfaction, illustrated in the Case of the Dueling Dieters:

Both Sheila and Cassie had been on their share of diets, and they silently competed in the body-check game. This began to change when Sheila became an Intuitive Eater. Sheila had made substantial progress over six months, even though it was slow. Fortunately, Sheila accepted this process and was feeling good. Meanwhile, her neighbor, Cassie, had just finished another crash diet. Cassie was proud of her weight loss and paraded her body around. Sheila was beginning to wish her body had changed also.

That night, Sheila and Cassie went out together for dinner with their husbands. Sheila ate want she wanted, had a good meal, left some food on her plate and overall, felt satisfied. Meanwhile, Cassie proudly nibbled like a bird, while she preened her body and boasted how easy her current diet was. Next to Cassie, Sheila felt as if she were overeating. But she kept listening to her Intuitive Eater voice that told her to respect her body, that her body deserved to be fed, that she should be patient. Her voice gently reminded her that Cassie was on a path to diet destruction—the weight loss euphoria wouldn't last long. Sheila knew this all too well from her old dieting days.

Sheila's private body competition with Cassie made her feel inferior about her own body and progress. Nonetheless, she continued the journey of Intuitive Eating. One month later, Cassie had gained back all her weight and was binge eating in spurts. One year later, Sheila was at her natural weight and Cassie was on another diet. But Sheila had come very close to going back on a diet because of playing the body-check game.

Don't Compromise for the "Big Event." Whether it's a class reunion or wedding, it's natural to want to look your best at important occasions. It's a subtle form of body-checking. But if you succumb to the pressure by "dieting down" to squeeze into that special outfit, it will only backfire. You'll only add another notch on the belt of yo-yo dieting; this time however, it's yo-yo dieting with a cause.

Remember, there will always be important occasions in your life. One particular client was attending the Grammy Awards because her husband was up for an award. Of course she wanted to look not just good, but great. It became clear, however, that she would not be at her ideal body weight for this prestigious event. She was feeling desperate and considered a quick fast to get her weight down. She was asked, "When will the dieting stop?" There will always be an important award or event, always a "legitimate" reason to diet. At that moment she saw the future futility of crash diets triggered by competitive body-checking. She decided to respect her current body. She kept her usual standards of dress and wore a custom-made outfit. This time, however, the outfit was designed for her here-and-now body. She did not have to squeeze into a gown and worry about every move she made. She still maintained her other routine standards—stylish hairdo, glittery accessories, and so forth. The only thing different was that this time she felt comfortable rather than self-conscious.

It's all too easy to cross over into the dieting mentality if you rationalize that the specialness of an event makes it okay to diet. The more you exert pressure on yourself to be a certain body size, the more you are bound to create problems. Jesse would always panic when a special occasion arose, whether it was a wedding or her company's annual awards banquet when she had to give a keynote speech. First, she would worry about what to wear, which would lead her on an intense shopping foray. Eventually, she would buy a stunning dress that was just a little too small. Jesse always shopped for her "future body," rather than her here-and-now body. But she knew she could "make weight" for the big day, just like a boxer weighing in for the big fight. As the big day drew near, Jesse would feel more pressure. She'd try her dress on daily and chastise herself for not fitting into it. Then the meal skipping would begin. On the big day itself, Jesse would allow herself a light breakfast. She would forgo eating the rest of the day to make sure she looked good and fit into her dress. Yes, the dress would fit. But by the time Jesse reached her destination she would invariably overeat (discreetly, of course) at the special function. Her body was famished, and she'd rationalize that she earned it. But by the end of the night, her overfull stomach would "remind" her she was too big. She'd spend the event worrying about her body rather than having a good time.

How much time and energy have you spent getting your body ready for the big event? What if the energy was directed on recognizing your inner qualities, such as wit, intelligence, or listening ability? What if you came prepared for a function by spending your time thinking of ways to engage in meaningful conversation, or getting to know someone new? You'd probably have a better time! Gladys almost skipped her twenty-year class reunion because she was too big and had nothing to wear. She could not bear the thought of shopping for a larger dress size. Eventually, Gladys decided to put her body worries aside and attend her reunion. Instead of worrying about her body, Gladys focused on finding out what her chums had been doing over the years. She even danced the night away with old friends. (She had not danced in years!) Gladys's reunion experience had far exceeded her expectations. She found her "old self"—the witty and charming person that loved to have fun and dance. Over the years, Gladys's private body war had only served to isolate her, and keep her from doing the activities she enjoyed. The sad irony is that Gladys came so close to avoiding her reunion because her body was not ready for the big event.

It might have taken Gladys a lot longer to rediscover her wonderful self.

Stop Body-Bashing. Every time you focus on your imperfect body parts it creates more self-consciousness and body worry. It's difficult to respect your body when you are constantly chastising yourself for looking the wrong way. How often do you have these kinds of thoughts?

- I hate my thighs.
- My arms are too fat and wobbly.
- My butt is disgusting.
- I hate my double chin.
- My stomach is gross.

Many of our clients are surprised at how often they degrade their bodies in one day. How many times a day do you chide yourself about your body? Try keeping count for a day or a few hours. It is surprising how often you can be triggered to worry about your body, whether it's a quick glimpse in a store window reflection or passing a mirror. Each disparaging thought lands another nail in the coffin of body dissatisfaction. Surrounding yourself with these body thoughts will only make you more unhappy and frustrated. It can also bleed over into how you feel about yourself in general.

Instead of focusing on what you don't like about your body, find parts of your body that you like or at least tolerate. Start simply. Perhaps you like your eyes or smile. We've had clients who could find only one body part that they did not dislike, such as their wrist or ankle. That's okay; it's a beginning. Every time you catch a maligning body thought, disarm it. Replace it with a kind body statement that you believe, such as, "I like my smile."

Instead of:	Replace with This Positive Statement:
My puffy jowls are disgusting.	I like my hair.
My thighs are too big.	I like my muscular calves.

If you find saying that you "like" some part of your body is too difficult, try respectful statements.

Instead of:	Replace with This Respectful Statement:
I can't stand my cellulite-dimpled legs.	I'm lucky I have legs that can move my body.
My body is so out of shape, it's horrible.	My body got me to school. I've been supporting my family while finishing my degree, so it was hard to work out optimally.

Don't Engage in "Fat-Talk." Fat-talk is a public form of body-bashing, in which you participate in conversations disparaging your own body, or the bodies of others. Studies show that refraining from this type of discussion is helpful in reducing body dissatisfaction, dieting, and eating disorder symptoms. See "Friends Don't Let Friends Fat-Talk" on page 180.

Respect Body Diversity, Especially Yours. It's ironic that we are celebrating cultural diversity, but as a culture we still have trouble with the idea of body diversity. We come in all shapes and sizes, yet we somehow expect that we should all be one-size-fits-all, as long as it's thin. As long as we feed into this cultural stigma, it will be a long time before societal norms will change into a healthy acceptance of body diversity.

There are many factors that contribute to obesity, including genetics, activity level, and nutrition. You cannot assume, for example, that just because someone is overweight he or she earned every ounce with a spoon in one hand and a fork in the other. Several studies have documented that obese people do not necessarily eat more than their lean counterparts. Yes, there are compulsive eaters. Yes, there are those who are not active. But we cannot assume that someone with a large body overeats and does not move. Many classic studies on twins have shown that genetics plays a powerful role in determining body build.

Obesity is still the last bastion where overt prejudice exists. Some call it weightism, others call it fattism—but by any name there is the prejudice against people with bigger body sizes. Today it would be unconscionable to make a racial slur, yet body-size slurs abound. When you see a big person on the street do you cast judgment and disdain? If you are that harsh on a stranger, how can you create a kinder environment for yourself? If you have trouble being kind and respectful to your body, perhaps you can begin with others.

A scientific review by Yale's Rudd Center for Food Policy and Obesity shows that weight stigma has serious medical and psychological consequences (Puhl 2009, Rudd Report 2009). Weight bias creates shame, the impact of which creates an environment in which an overweight person is more likely to delay medical care and to seek preventive health care services.

Beware of stereotyping overweight people. Remember that fat people are not any less intelligent, capable, well-adjusted, or more gluttonous than thin people. Try beginning with a place of neutrality and compassion. Check your body bias at the door.

While we have spent a great deal of time (and many words) on respecting bigger body sizes, it's important to recognize that some people are naturally born with a leaner body type, although they are in the minority. Similarly, we cannot assume that because someone is slender they have an eating disorder or are obsessed with dieting.

Be Realistic. If maintaining or obtaining your weight requires living on rice cakes and water while exercising for hours, that's a glaring clue that your goal is not realistic or that you have an eating disorder. If your parents are extremely heavy, chances are you will never be model-thin. Remember, genetics are a strong determinant of body size.

Do Nice Things for Your Body. Your body deserves to be pampered and touched. Schedule massages as often as you can, even if it's just a fifteen-minute neck rub. Try a sauna or a whirlpool. Buy luxurious smelling lotions and creams to rub on your body. Take bubble baths with bath oils and salts. (Try this in candlelight with classical music!) Doing these things for your body shows that your respect it and want to make yourself feel good.

YOUR NATURAL BODY WEIGHT

One of the first questions that we are invariably asked is, can you help me lose weight? Or, how much should I weigh? That answer varies from individual to individual, and no one can really say what a specific ideal weight is. In fact, the 1990 edition of U.S. Dietary Goals threw out the recommendation that Americans reach or maintain an *ideal weight,* because no one knows exactly what that number is!

The 2010 *Dietary Guidelines for Americans* used body mass index (BMI), which is a ratio of weight to height, to determine overweight categories. Initially, scientists created the BMI as a screening tool for large populations. But BMI has been criticized because it does not take into account muscle composition. Notably, muscle weighs more than fat. That's why many professional athletes have high BMI values that would classify them as overweight, when, in fact, they are actually lean. Yale scientist and obesity expert, Kelly Brownell, says that the BMI is not particularly relevant—whatever the cutoff (Brownell 2006). Much more important than a number is how to improve the health of the nation. If the factors necessary to improve health can be changed, everyone benefits, no matter his or her BMI.

We agree. That's why, in part, we use the concept of *natural healthy weight.* This is the weight your body will maintain with *normal/intuitive* eating and *normal* movement.

The problem with most of the people we see is that their eating relationship is *not normal,* due to years of dieting. If you fluctuate between periods of dieting and overeating, it is likely that you are not at your natural healthy weight. If you've been coping with life's ups and downs with food, it's also likely that you're not at your natural healthy weight.

But your healthy natural weight may not match what you have in mind. The weight that many people wish to achieve or maintain often has more to do with aesthetics than health. According to the National Institutes of Health, many people in this country who do not need to lose weight are trying to—and it may be in part from chasing an unrealistic body size.

A recent study demonstrated that a woman's ideal body image is 13–19 percent *below* expected weight. Examining the weights of Miss America contestants and *Playboy* centerfolds drew this conclusion. Over the years from 1959 to 1988, their weights and body sizes got *thinner.* That level of thinness overlaps with one of the criteria for anorexia nervosa—body weight below 15 percent of expected. If the cultural ideal for women overlaps with eating disorder criteria, American women are not only chasing an unrealistic body goal, but are engaged in a potentially dangerous pursuit.

If you have a weight number in mind that comes from a time when you were dieting, this sheds information on how low your body weight was able to go under duress—which is *not* realistic. The more extreme the method used to lose weight, such as fasting, the less likely that you were at a healthy weight as a result of that diet. Remember that research shows that the actual process of dieting, losing or recycling the same fifteen pounds, is probably more harmful than the actual body weight itself. And studies show that dieting predicts that you will gain even more weight than when you started, regardless of age.

SAYING GOOD-BYE TO THE FANTASY

One of the hardest facts many of our clients face is that their weight expectations are not realistic for their bodies. Our clients do not like to hear this. For some, it shatters a lifelong dream. But we refuse to perpetuate an unobtainable goal. We will not be partners in helping someone destroy his or her metabolism or health. It would be like giving a match to a smoker.

For example, Kathy is a thirty-year-old actress who has been told to lose weight by her agent. She reported healthy eating habits, with no use of food emotionally, and she said she worked out daily for one hour. After a soul-searching session, it was concluded that Kathy not only did not need to lose weight, but doing so would be detrimental to her metabolism and psyche.

Her weight for her height was appropriate, although higher than society's expectations. She was actually relieved to hear this; she decided she would change agents, and keep looking for jobs until someone would cast her as she was—a healthy person.

Many of our clients discover in hindsight that had they *accepted* the initial body weight that was the cause of their first diet, they would be happy with that very same weight today! Instead, they've dieted their bodies to a bigger size. So often we hear: "If only I knew then what I know now. I thought I was heavy in high school, now I'd kill for *that* body weight."

You may need to mourn for the lost body you never had or will have, and evaluate what this means to you. What price have you paid (energy, time, emotional investment) chasing one diet after another to seek your fantasy body shape? By saying farewell to the fantasy, you open the door to being at peace not only with your body, but with other facets of your life.

FRIENDS DON'T LET FRIENDS FAT-TALK

"Friends don't let friends fat-talk" is the motto of Fat Talk Free Week, which is a national campaign to eliminate negative body talk and ultimately to prevent eating disorders. Examples of fat-talk include: "I'm too fat to go out," "I can't eat that cookie—it will make me fat," or "You look so good, did you lose weight?"

Fat Talk Free Week challenges the unrealistic thin ideal for women, and is based on the work by Eric Stice's research team at the Oregon Research Institute (2009). Fat-talk is insidious in everyday conversations and perpetuates body dissatisfaction. Stice's team created an effective method which demonstrated impressive results from adolescents to college-aged women, with significant reductions in:

- Body dissatisfaction
- Dieting attempts
- Eating disorder symptoms

Notably, there was a 60 percent reduction in the risk of developing an eating disorder. Remarkably, the effects were achieved with a relatively short intervention, consisting of just three to four hours! What is particularly encouraging is that these effects appear to be long lasting (three years at follow-up).

cont.

Continued

Why is this method so effective? Chalk it up to *cognitive dissonance*. Cognitive dissonance is the feeling of discomfort that results from holding two conflicting beliefs, or when a belief is incongruent with a person's actions. When there is a discrepancy between beliefs and behaviors, something must change in order to eliminate or reduce the dissonance. Stice's team created several types of activities to create cognitive dissonance related to body dissatisfaction and body image acceptance. The activities consisted of written, verbal, and behavioral exercises, conducted in four weekly group sessions, called the "Body Project."

HEALTH AT EVERY SIZE

Health at Every Size (HAES) is a concept embraced by many different disciplines. It focuses on health, rather than on how much a person weighs. HAES promotes improved health behaviors for everyone, regardless of size (Bacon and Aphramor 2011).

Unfortunately, the weight-focused war on obesity has contributed further to food and body preoccupation, yo-yo weight loss and regain, distraction from other personal health goals, reduced self-esteem, eating disorders, and weight stigmatization and discrimination. In 2011 the Succeed Foundation commissioned a Body Image Survey, the findings of which prompted a scientifically supported campaign in the United Kingdom, aiming to improve body image and prevent the onset of eating disorders. Their survey revealed the following:

- 30 percent of women say they would trade at least one year of their life to achieve their ideal weight and shape.
- 46 percent of the women have been ridiculed or bullied because of their appearance.

HAES encourages the following (which are compatible with Intuitive Eating):

- Accepting and respecting the natural diversity of body sizes and shapes.
- Eating in a flexible manner that values pleasure and honors internal cues of hunger and satiety.
- Finding the joy in moving one's body and becoming more physically vital.

cont.

Continued

Research to date indicates that using a HAES approach is associated with statistically and clinically relevant improvements in health, including improvement in blood pressure, blood lipids, physical activity, and body image. There were also reductions in metabolic risk factors and eating disorder behaviors. Notably, not a single study found adverse changes. This latter finding is important, because some people have expressed a concern that *not* focusing on weight would result in worse health outcomes. Not so.

Chapter 13

PRINCIPLE 9:
Exercise—Feel the Difference

Forget militant exercise. Just get active and feel the difference. Shift your focus to how it feels to move your body, rather than the calorie-burning effect of exercise. If you focus on how you feel from working out, such as energized, it can make the difference between rolling out of bed for a brisk morning walk or hitting the snooze alarm. If when you wake up, your only goal is to lose weight, it's usually not a motivating factor in that moment of time.

If you were to classify your attitude toward exercise, would it be "just do it" or "just forget it"? Many of our clients fall into the latter category. They are burned out. Working out often went hand in hand with the negative experiences of ineffective dieting. Our clients were *not* enjoying exercise for two key reasons. Either they had started exercising when they initiated a diet, or they abused their bodies with unrealistic amounts of exercise, which led to injuries. Regardless, both felt guilty for not doing enough.

If you began an exercise program while simultaneously starting a diet, it's likely that your energy (calories) intake was too low. When you don't have enough energy, exercise is not invigorating, let alone fun. It becomes a chore, pure drudgery. When you are underfed from dieting, it's increasingly difficult to exercise, especially if carbohydrates are inadequate (which is often the case with our chronic dieters).

Carbohydrates are the preferred fuel of exercise. As you can see in the table, *Carbohydrate Power Chart,* running two miles uses the amount of carbohydrates found in three slices of bread. If you regularly limit carbohydrate foods (such as potatoes, bread, and pasta) and then add exercise, you are burdening the body with a carbohydrate deficit. Remember, for normal

hmm, am I getting enough carbs?

biological functions, the body *must* have carbohydrates. If you do not feed your body enough carbohydrates, it will dismantle its muscle protein to create vital energy. This has been demonstrated even in studies on endurance athletes. Endurance athletes who did not get enough carbohydrates for their exercise activity burned branched-chain amino acids (a component of protein) to help create vital energy to fuel their bodies.

Keep in mind that even very fit and motivated athletes have difficulty working out if they are low on carbohydrates! This effect was illustrated in a study of elite college swimmers by exercise physiologist, David Costill of Ball State University in Indiana. He found that swimmers who did not eat enough carbohydrates were *not* able to complete their workouts. If elite athletes had trouble working out because they didn't eat enough, why would you expect to be any different?

If you have never enjoyed exercise, let alone experienced the "runner's high" euphoria from working out, there's a good chance it was because of dieting, or the diet mentality of limiting foods. When a diet fails, exercise often stops because it was only done as an adjunct to dieting. You're left with memories of feeling bad, which makes you less likely to want to exercise in the future.

CARBOHYDRATE POWER CHART	
Activity	Equivalent (slices of bread)
Running	
2 miles	3
6 miles	10–11
26 miles	33–37
Swimming	
200 meters	1
1500 meters	6
Cycling—1 hour	15–17

Adapted from: Costill, D.L. "Carbohydrates for Exercise: Dietary Demands for Optimal Performance." *International Journal of Sports Medicine* 9:5 (1988).

No wonder the chronic dieter has difficulty with consistent exercise. Who wants to continually subject his body to something that does *not* feel good? Yet clients often blame themselves for not having enough willpower, or not possessing the admirable "just do it" mantra of exercise. This is like feeling guilty for not having enough willpower to "will" a car to operate on an empty tank of gas. Yet to reap the many positive results from exercise there needs to be a consistent effort.

Many of our clients have been burned out both mentally and physically from "crash exercising." Like crash diets, crash exercising doesn't last long. This typically occurs when someone is determined to get in shape and lose weight quickly. They start with too much activity in a short time period and end up either very sore, or not enjoying exercise, or both.

Others feel intimidated for not having a lean enough body to go to the gym or work out. It's a one-two intimidation punch. First, because they don't feel thin enough next to all the other hard bodies. Second, they get a glaring self-conscious reminder from floor-length mirrors plastered on every empty wall.

There are other reasons that chronic dieters don't feel like starting or continuing to exercise:

- Bad experiences growing up including: being forced to run laps or do calisthenics as a punishment, being teased for being uncoordinated, not getting picked for teams.
- Rebelling against parents, spouses, and others who pushed exercise, like a "good" diet: "You should go run, you should go to the gym," and so forth.

BREAKING THROUGH EXERCISE BARRIERS

Rather than insisting that our clients immediately embark on an exercise regime, we wait until *they* are ready. Postponing activity a few weeks, even a few months will not make a big difference in a lifelong commitment. So, don't worry if you don't feel like strapping on your shoes and running a few laps, especially if you have leaned toward being an exercise abuser. There are several keys to breaking through the barriers that prevent you from exercising.

Focus on How It Feels

We have found that one key to consistent exercise is to focus on how it *feels*, rather than playing the numbers game of counting calories burned. Instead of just biding your time or gritting your teeth when working out, explore how you feel throughout the day (including during exercise and immediately after). How do you feel regarding:

- Stress level—Are you able to handle stress better? Are you less edgy? Is it easier to take situations in stride, roll with the punches?
- Energy level—Do you feel more alert? Is there a little more spunk in your attitude? If you exercise in the morning, does it wake you up instead of feeling groggy?
- General sense of well-being—Do you have an improved outlook?
- Sense of empowerment—Do you feel more determined? Do you say "I can do it" and seize the day?
- Sleep—Do you sleep more soundly and wake up more refreshed?

If you are in a period of inactivity, it's especially important to note these feelings. They will serve as your baseline. Compare the difference between when you did and did not exercise. Note how you felt. When you can really feel the difference between exercising consistently and being inactive, the positive feelings can be a motivating factor for continuing. Why would you stop doing something that feels good? Instead, if you exercise with the dieting mind-set, you get used to stopping and starting, just like each new dieting attempt. In fact, it has been shown that 70 percent of those who begin an exercise program quit during the first year (Miller 1994). Remember, *exercise is much more than a calorie-eating machine.*

Decouple Exercise from Weight Loss

It's well accepted that physical activity is the one consistent element associated with long-term health. Exercise does play a significant role in metabolism and preserving lean muscle mass. Yet exercise alone accounts for only a minimal amount of weight loss. If your prime focus is on weight loss, it won't motivate you to exercise for long. It will only serve as a time card to be punched by a bored assembly-line employee. And when the payoff isn't quick enough, it becomes discouraging. Researchers also say that it's about time we decouple exercise from weight loss, because it minimizes its myriad of significant health benefits (Chaput et al. 2011). Movement is important for its own sake and should be considered as a way to promote health, increase quality of life, and fight off diseases.

Using weight loss as the ultimate reason for physical activity could also drive you to exercise abuse. Even then you still may not be happy with your body.

PHYSICAL ACTIVITY IS THE ULTIMATE STRESS BUFFER

Exercise helps to protect the body from the health-damaging effects of chronic stress. Chronic stress can create a hormonal imbalance, which increases fat deposition and appetite. This hormonal imbalance results in increased production of cortisol in the body, while also rendering insulin as less effective (which is known as insulin resistance). Increases in cortisol are also associated with elevated neuropeptide Y release (which, you may recall, increases appetite).

But regular physical activity can counteract this effect by improving the effectiveness of insulin and mood. Additionally, regular movement improves sleep patterns, which is often disrupted during stressful times. Notably, sleep deprivation is associated with weight gain, insulin resistance, and disturbed appetite regulation.

Focus on Exercise as a Way of Taking Care of Yourself

Whether young or old, regardless of weight, everyone benefits from being active. It makes you feel good and helps prevent health problems later in life. Specific benefits include:

- Increased bone strength.
- Increased stress tolerance.
- Decreased blood pressure.
- Reduced risk for chronic diseases, including heart disease, diabetes, osteoporosis, hypertension, and some types of cancers.
- Increased level of good cholesterol (HDL); decreased total cholesterol.
- Increased heart and lung strength.

- Increased metabolism—helps maintain lean body mass, and revs up energy production in the cells.
- Reduced risk for "silent" stroke (Gandey 2011).
- Improved satiety cues and appetite regulation (Chaput et al. 2011).
- Improved mood (Chaput et al. 2011).
- Improved learning and memory (Chaput et al. 2011).
- Prevents or delays cognitive decline associated with ageing (Chaput et al. 2011).

Don't Get Caught in Exercise Mind Traps

If you've had a diet mentality for a number of years, there's a good chance that versions of it have permeated into do-not-exercise traps. Let's identify and refute them:

can walk on days I can't swim!

The It's-Not-Worth-It Trap. We know many people who wouldn't walk unless they could get in one hour—anything under that "doesn't count." Therefore, a fifteen-minute walk break during lunch doesn't count. Instead, they do nothing. We commonly see clients discount their workout because they didn't reach their prescribed quota. It "didn't count" because they only exercised three times in a week, rather than five. All the more reason to be focused on how exercise feels, rather than doing it by the numbers.

Besides, over the long term, it all counts. We like to take the power out of numbers, whether those numbers refer to pounds, calories, or even minutes exercising. In this case, however, we use numbers to show how even the smallest amount of exercise does matter.

Activity	Time Spent in 1 Year
5 minutes of taking the stairs at work twice daily/five times a week	43 hours
10 minutes of walking your child to school three times a week	26 hours
15 minutes of mowing the lawn one time a week	13 hours

Couch-Potato Denial. The classic image of a couch potato is a person lei-
surely reclined on the couch with the remote control in one hand and a
snack or two in the other. However, it's all too easy to lead a "hectic couch-
potato lifestyle" without ever laying your body on a sofa. Your life may be
very hectic, but *being busy is not the same as physical activity*. Most of us
spend time "running around" in our car! Unless you are Fred Flintstone,
there is no fitness element to driving. Any of the following could be a component of couch-potato existence:

- Spending hours *sitting* in transit to work (either car, train, bus,
  or taxi).
- Sitting behind a desk all day (pushing papers and fax and telephone buttons is no different than fiddling with the remote control).
- Working at a computer all day.
- Arriving home exhausted; sitting and reading the mail or paying
  bills, eating, then going to bed.

The key is to find ways to incorporate physical activity into your everyday life. Remember, hectic schedules and mental exertion may keep your
mind active, but that is not the same.

The No-Time-to-Spare Trap. Ask most people if exercise is important,
and you'll hear an overwhelming yes. Yet, it often gets shoved aside as
other details in life vie for your time and attention. This is especially evident when you consider that less than 10 percent of adults in this country
regularly engage in physical activity (Miller 1994).

The question we often ask our patients who are in this time-crunch dilemma is, "How can you make movement a nonnegotiable priority?" This
is not intended as a rigid guideline, rather a new way of thinking of exercise so that it won't slip through the cracks. In fact, we often substitute the
word "movement" for "exercise," as a way to help people see that one of
the most important aspects of maintaining good health is to move your
body! It's not about going to the gym to exercise, it's about finding a realistic way to provide regular, joyful movement in your life.

If this seems like an impossible task, you may need to evaluate your
standards and priorities. Your life may be chronically overscheduled. Can
you continue living this way? If so, what price are you paying? Are you
taking care of yourself? Are you happy? Do you feel good? Ironically,

many of our overscheduled clients attribute the fact that they don't work out to laziness, when in reality, they are truly too busy! If time is rare and precious, then you certainly cannot afford to be sick. All the more reason to invest in making time to take care of yourself.

An option you may want to explore is hiring a personal trainer, if you can afford it. "When I make an appointment with somebody, including my trainer, it automatically becomes a priority on my schedule," said one client. Be sure however, to check out the credentials. Minimally, a personal trainer should be certified through either the American College of Sports Medicine (ACSM) or the American Council on Exercise (ACE).

★*The If-I-Don't-Sweat-It-Doesn't-Count Trap.* It's easy to believe that the only way to be fit is to engage in activities that make you sweat profusely. But you don't have to invest in sweat equity to reap fitness dividends. It is well accepted that you don't have to perform rigorous workouts to obtain health benefits. You can reap benefits from simple activities such as gardening, raking the leaves, or walking. These no-sweat activities make a physical difference. In a landmark scientific paper, which reviewed over forty-three studies, the CDC and ACSM concluded in 1990 that *simply moving* thirty minutes over the course of most days of the week could reduce the risk of heart disease by half!

All you need to do is accumulate thirty minutes of activity a day, most of the week. The thirty minutes of activity do *not* need to be all at once. (This particular conclusion surprises many people.) For example, the activity could be divided into three ten-minute sessions, or two fifteen-minute sessions and so forth. In fact, a recent study demonstrated that as little as two minutes of exercise each day significantly alleviated shoulder and neck pain (ACSM 2011). And another encouraging study found that short sporadic activity (defined as incidental, nonpurposeful physical activity that is accumulated through activities of daily living) was significantly beneficial (McGuire et al. 2011). Every little bit counts!

GETTING STARTED ON A LIFELONG COMMITMENT

Get Active in Daily Living

Kids are naturally active—squirming, running, and jumping. But as we get older our physical activity declines in spite of fast-paced living.

Unlike children, we need to consciously look for ways to increase our routine activity. Begin by asking how you can become more active in your daily living. For example, consider parking your car down the block from where you work to build in a ten-minute walk. When you factor in the return walk, you've just built twenty minutes of walking into your day. Add a ten-minute walk break during lunch and you've met the minimum level for physical fitness and its health benefits. Do this five times a week and you've walked 130 hours or about 400 to 500 miles in one year! Remember, ordinary activities do make a difference. (Of course conventional exercise can also be included, such as running or aerobics.)

Get rid of energy-saving devices and invest in human energy that will help you increase your daily activities.

- Use a hand-push lawn mower, rather than a power-operated one.
- Take the stairs rather than the elevator or escalator.
- Walk your dog (or even consider getting one)!
- Ride your bike to work if you live close enough.

Make Exercise Fun

For some people this means exercising with a friend, family member, or trainer. It might be the one time of the day you can talk freely with a friend, uninterrupted. Or perhaps your days are so crazed with demands from other people that a little solitude would add to your exercise enjoyment.

One sure way to take the fun out of exercise is to get injured. Do be sure to start slowly in whatever activity you choose. Some further suggestions:

- Be sure to choose activities that you enjoy. Consider playing a team sport such as volleyball, basketball, or tennis.
- Do engage in a variety of activities—you need not dedicate your life to just one sport. By diversifying, you'll also decrease your chance of injuries and increase your enjoyment factor.
- If you exercise at home on stationary fitness equipment, add fun by getting a DVR and recording your favorite television show or movie or reading a fun book or magazine (rather than work-related papers).
- Make your walk more enjoyable with an iPod or portable CD player. Listen to recorded books or your favorite music.

Make Movement a Nonnegotiable Priority

Ask yourself, "When can I consistently make the time to work out?" Make an appointment with yourself to work out, and honor it as you would any other meeting or appointment.

If you travel a lot:

- Pack your walking shoes. (It's an interesting way to get to know a new city.)
- Pack a jump rope. (It's a lightweight piece of equipment that delivers a cardio-wallop in a short amount of time.)
- Choose hotels that have workout facilities. (They are increasing in number.)
- Take advantage of airport layovers, and walk around the airport. (It usually feels good after hours of sitting.)

Be Comfortable

Workout attire need not be fashion-show material, but it is important to wear clothes that breathe and allow you to move. This also means dressing for weather. Heavy sweats can make you uncomfortably hot when you wear them to disguise your body. An oversize lightweight T-shirt and leggings will usually do for women. Or bike shorts with an oversize shirt works well for both men and women.

Don't forget about comfortable shoes as well. Not only will they feel good, they are an investment in injury prevention.

Include Strength Training and Stretching

Strength training helps rebuild muscle wear and tear from dieting. This is also important because our lean muscle mass declines as we get older. Americans lose an average of about 6.6 pounds of lean muscle mass for each decade of life. Therefore, someone who has been dieting for years is losing her muscle tissue from both the process of ageing *and* dieting. Remember, muscle is metabolically active tissue that helps keep your metabolism revved up. In fact, Bill Evans and Irwin Rosenberg, Tufts University researchers and authors of *Biomarkers,* estimate that our metabolic rate decreases 2 percent each year from the age of twenty, and they attribute this downward shift of metabolism to decreasing muscle mass.

Ordinary activity, and even vigorous activity such as running, does not leave you immune to muscle-wasting due to age. A ten-year study following master runners (minimum age of forty) showed that while they maintained their fitness from running, they lost an average 4.4 pounds of muscle from their untrained areas. Their muscles stayed the same size in their legs but decreased in their arms. There was an exception, however, for three runners who did upper body weights. They were able to *maintain* their lean body weight in their upper body. Therefore you don't have to lose your muscle mass.

Stretching helps prevent injuries, improve muscle performance, and keeps the tendons flexible, the latter of which is important as you age. Aging often results in substantial loss of tendon flexibility, which limits motion and increases risk for injury.

The American College of Sports Medicine (ACSM) recommends that strength training and flexibility become an integral part of a fitness program for *all* healthy adults (Pollock et al. 1998). Specifically, they recommend:

- Strength training at least twice a week.
- One set of eight to twelve repetitions of eight to ten exercises for conditioning of each major muscle group.
- Stretch at least two to three days per week.

BEYOND PHYSICAL FITNESS

Is there anything wrong with wanting to work out more, to feel good? No. Just be careful that you do not fall into the dieting–weight loss trap, where you become a slave to working out and counting calories burned. We have found that increasing exercise can be a way to channel anxiety while becoming an Intuitive Eater. Intuitive Eating can feel foreign, and progress may feel slow in the beginning, especially when the world around you is dieting. Exercise allows you to feel that you are actively *doing* something to improve your health. You *feel* benefits.

It's one thing to invest several hours in exercise if you are training for a marathon or because you are an athlete. It's a problem, however, when exercise consumes you, and begins to interfere with your everyday living.

Exercising more isn't necessarily better. How do you know if you are reaching the outer limits of exercise? Signs of *exercise abuse* include:

- Inability to stop, even when you are sick or injured.
- Feeling guilty if you miss a single day.
- Inability to sleep at night—a sign of overtraining.
- Paying exercise penance for eating too much, such as running an extra three miles because you ate a piece of pie.
- Being afraid that you will suddenly get fat if you stop for a single day

RR—REMEMBER REST

The hardest lesson that I (ET) learned as a competitive marathoner was that rest was equally important as training. It's also hard for our clients to recognize this tenet of training. Similarly, if for some reason you are unable to work out on a particular day, it does not mean that you will be suddenly out of shape or gain weight.

Some clients fear that once they stop exercising they will not continue. That's the all-or-none thinking commonly seen in dieters. There's an easy way to prove to yourself that no exercise today does not mean no exercise forever. Simply resume exercise when you are able. The more you reinitiate an exercise program after a break from it, the more confidence you will have in your ability to continue exercising, even if it's been a few days. After a while it stops being a big issue or worry. Besides, this time it's different. You are not dieting, therefore it will be much easier to resume training.

Remember, a few days or weeks of no exercise will not make or break your health or weight. After the big 1994 Los Angeles earthquake, Diane, a client, had to stop exercising. But for the first time, Diane knew that although three weeks had passed, it wasn't a big deal. She knew she'd be lacing up her walking shoes again in the near future. Diane missed the stress relief; she missed the freedom from the kids. But she also knew that she had a house to rebuild. After the earth settled, she got back to her routine walking. Her missed exercise did not become a crisis, and neither did her health.

Sometimes taking care of yourself means choosing *not* to exercise. For example, if you only got four hours of sleep and exercising meant rising at five in the morning, it's probably best to take that day off. Remember, rest is important. Likewise, if you feel a cold coming on, or you're feeling worn-out, take a day off. Listen to your body. Rest will also help keep exercise feeling fresh and fun.

MINDFUL EXERCISE

You can integrate exercise recommendations for health while being attuned to the experience of your body. This type of physical activity is called "mindful exercise," a concept championed by psychologist and researcher, Rachel Calogero and Kelly Pedrotty (2007). Mindful exercise is processed-based and has four components:

- Enhances the mind-body connection and coordination, and does not confuse or deregulate it.
- Alleviates mental and physical stress, and does not contribute to and amplify stress.
- Provides genuine enjoyment and pleasure, and is not used for punitive reasons.
- Is used to rejuvenate the body, not to exhaust or deplete it.

Approaching physical activity with mindfulness helps you to experience your body. When you pay attention to how your body feels, before, during, and after exercise, it helps with attunement. The primary focus is to connect with how your body feels during exercise and to listen to your body's signals indicating fatigue, pain, and when to stop.

When the pursuit of exercise is about feeling good, not about calories burned, or used as a penance for eating—it becomes enjoyable and sustainable.

Chapter 14

PRINCIPLE 10:
Honor Your Health with Gentle Nutrition

Make food choices that honor your health and taste buds while making you feel well. Remember that you don't have to eat perfectly to be healthy. You will not suddenly get a nutrient deficiency or gain weight from one snack, one meal, or one day of eating. It's what you eat consistently over time that matters—progress not perfection is what counts.

the idea of perfection is what trips me up

> *We will not be healthier, both psychologically and physically, about our food until we learn to love it more, not less . . . with a relaxed, generous, unashamed emotion. In the process, it may be that we will have to redefine fundamentally the concept of "eating well."*
> —Michelle Stacey, author of *Consumed: Why Americans Love, Hate, and Fear Food*

I keep thinking that someday I'm going to walk in here and you're going to tell me the food party is over." We hear this fear a lot. It's one of the reasons that nutrition is discussed with our clients much later in the Intuitive Eating process, rather than sooner. It's also the reason that *honor your health* is the last principle of Intuitive Eating. You can hardly talk about health and taking care of yourself without discussing nutrition. But our experience has shown us that if a healthy relationship with food is not in place, it's difficult to truly pursue healthy eating. If you've been a chronic dieter, the best nutrition guidelines can still be embraced like a diet.

We don't want to give the impression that just because nutrition is reserved for the last principle of Intuitive Eating, that it's not important. We certainly value health. Don't worry though; we are not going to pull the food carpet from under you.

The role of nutrition in preventing chronic disease has been clearly established by the scientific community. But the emerging importance of nutrition has served to breed a nation of "guilty" eaters—feeling the need to apologize for eating a traditional Thanksgiving meal or a fatty dessert.

FOOD WORRY

Our whole country needs a food attitude adjustment. You don't have to be a chronic dieter to be worried about food. Almost daily there is a new headline or cover story on a nutrition related topic, from killer biotech foods to research proclaiming that margarine is no better than butter (and may be even worse). At best, the dueling headlines get you confused, and at worst, they contribute to a growing food phobia. With special-interest groups massaging the media, the fear is magnified. (The recent food-poisoning scare related to spinach, lettuce, and cucumbers—foods not ordinarily associated with food-borne illness—is probably the best example of this.) Add the food companies that climb onto any nutritional bandwagon that furthers their economic cause, and you get one nation of confused and worried consumers.

The medical nutrition research, as it's reported in the media, easily creates the impression that food will either kill or heal you, or make you fat. This fuels the fire of magical thinking with food. No wonder some people erroneously believe that drinking a mixture of apple cider vinegar, honey, and cayenne pepper will burn off fat or that special food combining will raise metabolism. Sadly, this isn't so.

Ironically, nutrition stories that blow the whistle on misleading food-product ads unintentionally create more fear in food. The message to the consumer is that you can't trust the food companies, or the food label—you've been duped. If you are worried about what's in your food, how can you begin to enjoy it? If you believe that a magical food or pill is around the corner to solve your weight issues, why would you even look inward for the answers? If you don't trust what's in your food, and have trouble trusting your body's inner signals for eating, how can you begin to eat healthfully without guilt or trepidation?

In tandem with the growing anxiety over food selection, there is a new type of eating disorder emerging called orthorexia, which is characterized by an unhealthy and rigid obsession to eat healthfully. While not officially recognized as a medical diagnosis, physician and author, Steven Bratman, M.D., called attention to this problem in his book, *Health Food Junkies—Orthorexia Nervosa: Overcoming the Obsession with Healthful Eating.*

A Young Case of Orthorexia. A few years ago, a ten-year-old who was terrified of eating trans fats came in for nutrition counseling. Part of her treatment
was to sit down and eat a Ding Dong during one of her sessions in the office.
Can you imagine a dietitian eating a Ding Dong with her client? But this girl
needed the opportunity to create a healthier relationship with food by observ-
ing a health professional she respected eating a Ding Dong. She began to realize that she wouldn't end up with a clogged artery from eating one Ding Dong!

Contrary to popular belief, nutrition science is not set in stone. Research
is a slow, evolutionary process of gathering and validating data, the process
of which often overturns widely held theories. Here are a couple of landmark examples:

- The cause of 80 to 90 percent of ulcers is a bacterium, called H.
  pylori. But up until that discovery in 1982, food was thought to be a
  contributing cause, resulting in a diet prescription of bland eating.
- For decades, polyunsaturated fats (PUFA) have been heralded as
  "heart healthy," but a critical analysis of the data showed that a particular type of PUFA may actually increase heart disease risk
  (Ramsden et al. 2010).

Similarly, you might believe that eating rich, fatty foods would automatically lead to heart disease or obesity. Or perhaps you believe that to be fit,
you need to eat a "perfect" diet of spartan cuisine. Not so. If you keep in
mind that the science of nutrition is regularly evolving, you won't get stuck
in the belief that you have to choose a perfect array of foods. After all, if
information is regularly changing, there can be no "perfect way to eat"!

Before getting into specific nutrition information that may be of interest
to some and may be a section to postpone for others, let's take a look at
what we can learn from other cultures.

Americans Are Number One in Worrying about Food

"Food worry" has not served the health status of Americans. In fact, it may
have an opposite effect. Food psychologist Paul Rozin and his research
team from the University of Pennsylvania, conducted a study of four countries and found that the French are the most food-pleasure oriented and the
least health oriented (1999). In contrast, Americans had the worst of both
worlds: They had the greatest worry over their health and eating, and greater

dissatisfaction with what they ate. Americans scored the highest on worrying about the fattening effects of food.

Rozin concluded that the negative impact of *worry and stress* over healthy eating may have a more profound effect on health than the actual food consumed. Indeed, it is widely accepted that stress triggers a biological chemical assault in our bodies, which is harmful to our health (McEwen 2008).

France and the Pleasure Principle of Health

More information about the French reveals that the U.S. currently has twice the incidence of overweight people compared to France, for both adults and children. The French have a longer life expectancy, take less medication, and have a markedly lower rate of heart disease (see table: Health Indicators in France Versus the United States). Yet the French eat a diet that appears to be less than healthy. This is popularly known as the French paradox. Notably, France has the highest per-capita dairy fat consumption (think cream, butter, and cheese) of any industrial nation (Guyenet 2008).

Less publicized, but just as important, the French have fewer eating disorders and don't engage in dieting as much as Americans. Despite this fact, in 2010, the *New York Times* reported that Jenny Craig plans to open diet centers in France. Unbelievably, the CEO of Jenny Craig, France, believes that Americans have credibility for weight loss! We hope that France's strong aversion to Americanized foods will protect the French people from going down that dieting path.

While it has been speculated that wine consumption and eating smaller portions of food may explain the French paradox, we believe it could be the relationship that the French have with food. The French have a more positive attitude toward eating—it is viewed as one of life's pleasures, not as poison. Food is not revolting; instead it's something to be revered. Perhaps this is why our clients who have traveled to France, *even before working with the Intuitive Eating process,* describe that they had discovered how much they enjoyed their eating experience and their celebration of food without the worry.

The French pay more attention to the sensory qualities of food, eat for a significantly longer period of time, while eating less—thus creating a more satisfying food experience. Even when the French eat fast food, they take more time to eat, compared to the eating pace of Americans (Rozin et al. 2003). They also cultivate the pleasures of the palate at a very early age. For example, public child-care centers in Paris provide three-course meals for their tots. Can you imagine an American toddler sitting down to braised lamb served with cauliflower au gratin, and enjoying every bite? That's a typical entrée for the French toddlers, who joyfully ate that meal on the day that National Public Radio interviewed the dietitian responsible for the 270 public day-care centers in Paris (Beardsley 2009).

Interestingly, research has shown that the medical practices of French versus American physicians reflect their culture. Consequently, American physicians prescribe more medication, while the French physicians are inclined to suggest rest, vacations, or a stay at a spa (Rozin 1999).

HEALTH INDICATORS IN FRANCE VERSUS THE UNITED STATES

These statistics are rounded to the nearest whole number.

	United States	France
[a]Incidence of obesity and overweight people ages ≥15 years	62%	32%
[a]Life expectancy (rounded to the nearest year)	78 years	81 years
[a]Dollars (U.S. equivalent) spent on medication per capita	$897	$607
[b]Heart disease death rates (per 100,000 people): Women	79	21
[b]Heart disease death rates: Men	145	54
[c]Incidence of dieting (percent of total population)	26%	16%
[d]Use of light foods and beverages (percent of total population)	76%	48%
[d]Consumption of low-fat products (percent of total population)	68%	39%
[e]Duration of minutes eating at McDonald's	14 minutes	22 minutes

[a]OECD Factbook 2010. [b]OECD Health Data 2009. [c]Calorie Control Commentary, 14(1):1–2, 1992. [d]Adapted from Calorie Control Council National Surveys. [e]Rozin 2003.

What We Can Learn from Nutritional Outliers

Despite all that we currently know about nutrition, there are instances in which even the most "unhealthy" food intake does not have a negative effect on people's health.

The Roseto Effect. A remarkable discovery by physician Stewart Wolf found a strikingly low incidence of heart disease and deaths from heart attacks, spanning three generations, in a small Italian immigrant community, located in Roseto, Pennsylvania (Stout et al. 1964, Wolf et al. 1994, Egolf et al. 1992). Even more astonishing was the discovery that it wasn't diet that was protecting their heart health. To the contrary, Rosetons embraced westernized foods and cooking, at the expense of their Italian-Mediterranean culinary roots. For example, Rosetons:

- Shunned olive oil, and used lard instead, as the main fat for cooking.
- Dipped their bread in a lard-based gravy, rather than olive oil.
- Ate an Italian ham, including its one-inch rim of fat.
- The average Roseton diet was high in fat, containing 41 percent of calories from fat.

The distinguishing protector of their heart health and longevity was found to be social cohesion and social support. This paradoxical discovery became known as the Roseto Effect, and it inspired author Malcolm Gladwell to write his best-selling book, *Outliers.* Once again, as with the French, the effect of positive emotional experiences can have a greater impact on health than which foods people actually eat.

Olympic Swimmer—Poster Boy for Junk Food Diet

Champion swimmer Michael Phelps made global headlines—not just for his record-shattering, perfect eight-for-eight gold-medal performances in the 2008 Olympics. The quality of his food choices also captured the rapt attention of the media. For example, Phelps's typical meals included the following foods:

- Breakfast: Fried egg sandwiches, loaded with cheese, fried onions, and mayonnaise.
- Lunch: One pound of enriched pasta. Large ham and cheese sandwiches, with mayonnaise on white bread.
- Dinner: An entire pizza and one pound of pasta.

And while his large caloric intake (around twelve thousand calories) was no surprise to sports nutritionists—the quality of Phelps's diet was criticized.

A full two-page photo spread in *People* magazine, with Phelps in his Olympic Speedo, surrounded by the foods he typically eats, is quite an image. Phelps appears as if he is a poster boy for eating a diet of nutritionally inferior foods. This visual aid has helped many of our patients. When patients see this photo spread and examine it carefully, they are asked, "If foods that some people call junk food could automatically make someone unhealthy—why can Phelps perform so well and look so healthy, eating foods like these?"

The point in this example is to remove the power of the widely perceived belief that eating a particular food will automatically make you unhealthy and unfit—that food is either good or bad. There seems to be a prevalent fear that "I'm one bite away from_____" (fill in the blank: a heart attack, getting cancer, or gaining weight). Unless you have a lethal food allergy or a medical condition, such as celiac disease—one bite of food, one meal, or one day of eating will not make or break your health or waistline. Phelps is a good example of the latter.

Paul Rozin, the food psychologist, believes that a key contributing factor to the good-food/bad-food belief, is the increased availability of studies reported by the media. These studies have not been accompanied by education of the basic concepts of probability, risks and benefits, and the difference between cause and association. The average consumer takes these findings as facts, especially when deleterious effects of eating a certain food are reported. In order to take the uncertainty out of every bite, people tend to develop a reductionist belief—that food is either good or bad. Rozin says this type of belief establishes a goal, which is both extremely unhealthy and unattainable.

WHAT ABOUT NUTRITION BY THE NUMBERS?

New York Times columnist Michael Pollan profoundly struck a chord with the simplicity of his advice in his best-selling book, *In Defense of Food:*

An Eater's Manifesto, published in 2008. He explored a very complex topic of nutrition science, politics, and the industrialization of food, yet managed to describe how to eat healthfully in just seven words: "Eat food. Not too much. Mostly plants." There are no numbers to strive for—no grams, calories, or any nutrient quotas.

Consider that for nearly two decades, there has been nutrition information on just about every food label, thanks to the 1990 Nutrition Labeling and Education Act. Yet, the incidence of obesity and eating disorders in the United States has steadily risen ever since. There's even more nutrition information available today, thanks to the Internet.

Pollan popularized the term "nutritionism," a paradigm created by Dr. Gyorgy Scrinis, which describes how the overly reductive focus on nutrients in food undermines how we think about food, *how we view the experiences of our own bodies, and how we understand the relationship between food and our bodies* (2008). Ultimately, the nutritionism ideology has only served to add a lot of anxiety to grocery shopping and food selection.

We agree—our experience has shown that the more a person focuses on a number, the more it interferes with the process of listening to the body.

Eating healthfully should feel good, both physically and psychologically, ultimately resulting in a satisfying experience. But we've lost sight of that feeling, due to the food and fat phobia that's sweeping the country. Michelle Stacey, author of *Consumed: Why Americans Love, Hate, and Fear Food,* concludes that Americans need to change their eating attitude to enlightened hedonism: a balance between information and pleasure, an educated hedging of bets. That's how we approach nutrition and food.

We amend Pollen's recommendation to do the following: *Enjoy* eating food. Not too much—*not too little.* Mostly *what satisfies you.*

MAKING PEACE WITH NUTRITION: ACHIEVING AUTHENTIC HEALTH

Critics express concern that encouraging people to eat what they want will lead them to eat with abandon, resulting in poor nutrition and weight gain. The underlying belief is that self-monitoring is essential for keeping appetite under control. It is thought that without this vigilance, people would make nutritionally poor choices, including eating to excess. Yet, several studies show that eating restraint is associated with weight gain. Instead, Intuitive Eating is associated with improved nutrient intake, eating a wider variety of food, reduced eating disorder symptomatology, and lower body mass. (For more details see The Science Behind Intuitive Eating, Chapter 17.)

Eating Healthfully Feels Good. When you remove the clutter of guilt and morality from eating, it allows you to really feel the physical sensations that you derive from eating. Many of our clients unknowingly create a somatization of guilt from their eating experience. This occurs when the *feelings* of guilt arise, in tandem, with the unpleasant *physical sensations* of eating without attunement. It becomes an intertwined union of uncomfortable feelings from guilt *and* the discomfort from eating, joined into one physical experience. When you know you can truly eat whatever food or meals you want— without guilt, why would you choose to feel physically uncomfortable?

Here is one of my (ET) favorite stories that illustrates how eating healthfully simply feels good. My son was in his rebellious teenage phase and had spent an entire day at an amusement park. When he came home, he rushed into the kitchen and said, "Mom, I ate junky today, will you make me something extra healthy for dinner?" This was not a boy trying to please his mom (or score points). Nor was he uber health conscious—he just knew how it *feels* to eat healthy and was seeking that experience for his next meal.

What Is Healthy Eating? We define healthy eating as having a healthy balance of foods *and* having a healthy relationship with food. Of course there is a nutritional difference between eating an apple versus a piece of apple pie. Having a healthy relationship with food means you are not morally superior or inferior based on your eating choices. Eating selection is not a reflection of your character. Throughout this book, we've focused on the healthy relationship part, because there's been a big whopping gap in American eating that leaves out this important concern.

Intuitive Eating is a dynamic attunement process of your mind, body, and food. The majority of Intuitive Eating principles (1–8), deal with attunement to your inner world, which is informed by the inner workings of your mind and body. The inner world includes your thoughts, feelings, beliefs, and physical sensations arising from within your body (such as hunger and satiety cues).

Achieving "authentic health" is a process of dynamic integration of your inner world and the external world of health guidelines, which include exercise and nutrition. You decide, if and what, of the external world you'd like to integrate, ultimately, to achieve "authentic health." The external world includes health policy (usually a consensus from experts, based on a body of research).

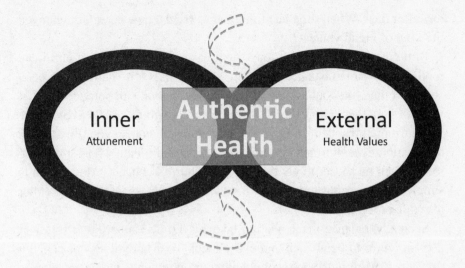

Intuitive Eating: The Dynamic Integration Between Inner Attunement and External Health Values to Achieve Authentic Health

Adapted with permission from Catherine Cooke-Cottone, SUNY Buffalo

The external world can also include philosophical preferences, such as a desire to eat locally grown foods with a low carbon footprint. If you are truly inner-attuned, you can integrate this value, while paying attention to hunger, fullness, satisfaction, and so forth. If, however, you enter this realm too soon, there is a risk for the new mind-set to be embraced as another rigid set of rules.

Food Wisdom Tenets

No doubt you've heard for years of the nutritional merits of variety, moderation, and balance. There's a reason these nutrition mantras have been chanted for decades: They work! It's one of the best ways to hedge your bets for healthy eating. But "eat a variety of foods" sounds like "wear a sensible pair of shoes"—practical but easily ignored advice. A study looking at diet diversity has gotten those sensible shoes tap dancing in the spotlight of health. According to this study reported in the *American Journal of Clinical Nutrition,* people who omitted several food groups had a higher chance of dying! Adults who ate foods from two or fewer food groups were associated with an excess mortality risk of 50 percent in men and 40 percent in women. But how often do you eat the same meal day after day? When's the last time you've tried a new cereal, or changed the kind of bread you eat?

In the world of dieting, it may seem easier and safer just to eliminate foods rather than to balance them into your meals. Or perhaps you've been so afraid that you couldn't eat just moderate amounts of some foods that you just shun them altogether. But where has that gotten you? Here's where the nutritional tenets of moderation and balance can help you. First of all, moderation does not mean elimination. If you eliminate whole groups of foods it can be harder to get the nutrients your body needs. Moderation is simply eating various amounts of food without going to extremes of either too little or too much.

Secondly, balance is intended to be achieved over a period of time—it does not have to be at each and every meal. Your body does not punch a time clock. Most nutrition recommendations are intended to be an *average* over time, not for a single meal or a single day, and with good reason. You will not suddenly get a nutrient deficiency if you did not eat enough in one day. Similarly, you will not make or break your health from one meal or even one day of eating. It is consistency over time that matters. Our bodies are remarkably adaptable. Here are a few examples:

- If you eat too little iron, the body starts to absorb *more* of it.
- If you take in too much vitamin C, the body begins to excrete more of it.
- If you eat too little, the body slows its need for calories.

We'd like to suggest another tenet, progress not perfection. You don't have to eat perfectly to be healthy. Much of what you eat is primarily for your nutritional health, and a smaller amount is simply for pleasure. Regardless of your food choice, however, all foods can offer satisfaction.

In Matters of Nutrition, Consider: Taste, Quantity, and Quality

Taste. Eating nutritiously does not have to be about deprivation, although that's what many Americans fear. The problem is that healthy eating for many people has been clouded with regrettable food experiences. How often have you heard, for example, "You'll get used to it," which really means that the food tastes so bad you have to condition yourself to like it! Or, how many times were you told as a child, "Eat your vegetables, then you can have dessert"—which really means that vegetables are so difficult to eat that you deserve a reward for choking them down. Or maybe you've experienced:

- Inferior "new healthy foods"—from food companies scrambling to capitalize on the latest nutrition trend—from fat-free to gluten-free. The introduction of rubbery fat-free mozzarella to cream cheese that resembles a caulking agent, hardly fosters enthusiasm for healthy eating.
- Pretending—this is where you close your eyes (and taste buds), and pretend that what you are eating is a terrific substitute for what you'd *really* like to be eating. For example, whipping a few ice cubes in a blender with a diet hot chocolate mix and calling it a milk shake—hardly! Or adorning applesauce with graham cracker crumbs and pretending it's apple pie—James Beard is probably rolling in his grave!

The combination of taste atrocities in the name of healthy eating, with the emerging fear of food in the U.S., prompted Julia Child to take action in the late 1980s. She spearheaded a revolutionary project through the American Institute of Wine & Food (AIWF) called Resetting the American Table: Creating a New Alliance of Taste and Health. This venture joined together opinion leaders from both the culinary (taste) world and the health community, with the mission to move Americans toward healthier eating, without having to give up the pleasures of the table. (ET: Early in my career, I was fortunate to be included on this task force, which had a big influence on how I work.)

Julia's task force had two key conclusions:

- Negative, restrictive approaches to eating do not work.
- People need to be steered toward a healthy diet they can live with, *without guilt* (the italics are our emphasis).

Ultimately, the key message from the task force was, "In matters of taste, consider nutrition and in matters of nutrition, consider taste." If a food aficionado can consider nutrition without compromising his or her gastronomic palate, so can you! We call this approach *gentle nutrition.* Taste is important, but health is still honored, without guilt.

Quantity Issues—Not Too Much—Not Too Little

Portion Control Is Not an Issue for Intuitive Eaters. Many public health policy makers attribute the inflated size of food portions to be a key contributor to obesity. But if people were truly attuned to hunger, fullness, and satisfaction, it wouldn't matter if they were served a twenty-pound steak or a gallon of ice cream. That's because Intuitive Eaters would stop eating when comfortably satisfied—there would just be a lot more leftovers.

Researcher Brian Wansink makes a strong case, with cleverly designed studies, that eating while you are distracted (also known as mindless eating) increases the quantity of food eaten. So, if you are inclined to eat with distraction, such as watching television, reading, texting, or surfing the net, you will be more likely to overeat (see "Distracted versus Mindless Eating" on page 146 for more details). Eating without distraction is especially important for emerging Intuitive Eaters. But, of course, it doesn't need to be done perfectly. Only you can determine where you are in this process.

Eat Enough-Not Too Little. Clearly you need to eat. Remember that to stoke your metabolic fire, you need wood, not just kindling. For many of our clients, this means eating more of some foods than they are used to, especially carbohydrates. You may be thinking, "Forget eating more, I'll just exercise." But, as we explained in Chapter 13, exercise will not prevent metabolic damage from under eating, even for athletes. Scientists at the University of British Columbia in Canada studied fourteen competitive female rowers. Half of them were weight-cyclers. During the study, the weight-cyclers lost about ten to eleven pounds during the four weeks leading up to their national championships. Consequently, their metabolic rates plummeted by about 7 percent. They also lost over six pounds of fat-free body mass (primarily muscle). In this particular study, the rowers were fortunate and were able to get back their previous metabolic rate, *when they began eating more.* If athletes can lose precious muscle from under eating, why would you be any different? Remember, the more muscle you have, the higher your metabolic rate. It is one reason that men need more calories than women—they naturally have more muscle.

How do you make peace with feeding your body? This is a scary prospect for most of our clients. To help you overcome this fear, keep reminding yourself that by feeding your body you are feeding your metabolism.

Quality Issues

Some people are eager to hear what the nutrition community is recommending in the realm of food to promote optimal health. Take out of the following sections what suits you, and be sure to let go of any guilt feelings that might emerge if you find that this information triggers any discomfort. Remember, we are not pulling the rug out from under you and suddenly telling you what we think you *should* eat. We are simply providing information for those who would like to learn more about nutrition.

Eat Enough Fruits and Vegetables. Three years after Michael Pollan's book was published, the USDA revamped the iconic food pyramid and replaced it with a new concept, called *My Plate*. One of its six key messages seems to reflect Pollan's plant-based advice: Make half of your plate *fruits and vegetables*.

People who eat higher amounts of fruits and vegetables have lower risks of many chronic diseases, especially cancer. In almost every study looking at plant food and people (over two hundred studies to date), plant food is associated with lowering the risk of cancer. These foods are loaded with antioxidants and fiber, which offer many other health benefits. There is a growing body of research that shows fruits and vegetables have special

Phytochemical	Plant Food	Potential Benefit
Limonene	Citrus fruits	Helps increase enzymes that get rid of cancer-causing agents
Sulforaphanea	Cruciferous vegetables: broccoli, cauliflower, brussels sprouts, and cabbage	Helps amplify the body's own defense against chemicals that can lead to cancer
Allyl sulfides	Leeks, garlic, onion, chives	Increases the production of enzymes that make it easier for the body to excrete cancer-causing compounds
Ellagic acid	Grapes	Scavenges carcinogens and may prevent them from altering the body's DNA

food factors, called phytochemicals that have added health benefits. See the chart on the previous page.

There are hundreds and maybe even thousands of phytochemicals. Research is just scratching the surface on their health benefits. This is one reason why we can't rely on getting all of our nutrition in a bottle. You can't manufacturer compounds that have yet to be identified and put them into a supplement!

One problem we've seen with our chronic dieters is that they've been "veggied out." For example, nearly every diet regimen prescribes celery and carrot sticks as the safe and approved snack of choice. If that's your case, ask yourself how you can incorporate vegetables (and fruit) in a manner that's *pleasing* and does not smack of a weight loss diet, such as adding grated carrots to a favorite pasta sauce. Think of possible ways in which you can eat fruits and vegetables as a built-in component to a meal, such as:

- Vegetable lasagna
- Ratatouille
- Potato cakes spiced with various chopped vegetables
- Stir-fried vegetables on rice
- Stuffed baked squash
- Stuffed peppers
- Stuffed baked potatoes
- Fajitas (they're usually loaded with vitamin-rich peppers)
- Pancakes topped with a fresh fruit medley
- Fruit compote
- Fruit smoothie

One client, Sally, was averse to fruit, though she didn't know why; she just had trouble eating it. But one day she found she was having no difficulties whatsoever. What had changed? Two things. First, she was rid of her diet mentality and second, she began eating fruit in a "non-diet" manner. All of her past diets had prescribed eating a spartan single fruit for a snack or with a meal, such as a plum, an apple, and so forth. When she tried fruit salads of all sorts, her interest in fruit was renewed.

Frankly, we've never seen anyone get into trouble eating fresh fruits and vegetables (unless that's all they eat). In fact, emerging research results also show this to be true. John Potter, a physician and researcher out of the University of Minnesota, has been studying a group of people who were told to eat up to eight servings a day of fruits and vegetables. His preliminary data suggests that people eating more fruits and vegetables actually like it and *feel better on it.*

Eat Enough Fish. There is a bounty of research that shows a multitude of benefits from eating seafood—from improved mood to lower risk of chronic diseases. This health benefit prompted the 2010 U.S. Dietary Guidelines to include a recommendation for eating fish.

Drink Enough Fluids—Primarily Water, Rather than Sugary Beverages. Water actually doubles as both a beverage and a nutrient. Water is essential for living—we can only survive a few days without it. We included it, because it often gets overlooked. The need for getting plenty of fluids is no secret, but many of our clients wind up short in this department. The traditional eight 8-ounce cups of fluid a day is the same as drinking a half gallon (that's the size of your typical milk carton). Other fluids, such as milk and tea, can help meet your water quotient. Even solid foods, like fruit, provide water.

The Issue of Processed Foods. Generally, the less a food is processed, the more nutrients are retained, and less sodium and sugar are added. If possible, choose the following types of foods to eat more often:

- Nutrient dense foods—these foods naturally provide more nutrients per bite. These include: whole grains, beans, fish, avocado, nuts, and calcium-rich foods such as milk, cheese, yogurt, and calcium-fortified soymilk.
- Protein-rich foods—eat a variety of these foods. They include beans, seafood, chicken, turkey, nuts, and lean meats, eggs, and dairy. In addition to its role in building and maintaining muscles and hormones, protein helps provide a feeling of fullness.
- Quality fats—fat is also a nutrient, required by the body. Notably, when the essentiality of fats was first discovered, they were called "vitamin F" (Evans et al. 1928). Too bad this nomenclature didn't stick—if it had, it would help remind people that we do need some fat in our diet. We need fat in our diet to help absorb fat-soluble nutrients, such as vitamin A and vitamin E. The brain is made up of mostly fat and functions best with omega-3 fats, which are found in seafood, fish oil, algae, and seaweed. Other quality fats include: olive oil, avocado, nuts, seeds, flaxseed oil, and canola

oil. And for satisfaction purposes, fat is the molecule that gives flavor to foods and promotes satiety.

• Whole foods—these are the unprocessed foods, which are high in fiber and include, for example: brown rice, oatmeal, millet, beans, quinoa, fresh fruits, and vegetables.

The Fat-Free Trap

The low-fat message has gone to extreme levels for many chronic dieters, and has created the fat-free trap. Because fat has become the national enemy, it has spawned a profitable cottage industry of fat-free foods—from fat-free cheese to fat-free potato chips and ice cream. While this may seem advantageous to the American diet, we've seen problems, especially for chronic dieters.

One of the most common problems we see is the idea that "it doesn't count, I can eat as much as I want." The problem with this thinking is that it can actually lead to overeating. Instead of responding to satiety levels, it often becomes an eating affair of "I'm going to eat it all." When inner satiety cues are bypassed, it perpetuates further dissonance from your body. In addition, *fat-free does not mean calorie-free.* Ironically, many of our clients discover that if they were to have the real version of a food, they'd end up eating much less, because it's more satisfying, and they would remain in touch with satiety cues.

Eating fat-free foods is *not* the epitome of healthy eating. Sugar is naturally fat-free, yet one would hardly want to base a diet on sugar for health. Yet that's what many people are doing when they are building diets based primarily on processed fat-free foods. Many of the fat-free products are high in sugar (especially the desserts), and low in whole grains. For example, Rice Krispies cereal proclaims on its label that it's always been fat-free. But it's also always been low in fiber. If your prime mission in eating is selecting processed fat-free foods, you could easily end up with a nutritionally weak diet. There's nothing wrong with eating fat-free foods as an adjunct to a healthy diet. But you cannot assume that just because you've been eating 100 percent fat-free foods, your diet is healthy.

What's on Your Plate? We've talked about how important it is to make peace with food. There's a useful tool that extends this principle to nutrition for meals. Visualize your plate as a lopsided peace sign (see figure below). As you can see, the plate is mainly filled with carbohydrate-rich foods (grains, fruits, and vegetables). This tool serves two purposes. First it gives you an easy-to-remember guide for healthy eating, and helps to serve as a reminder to keep the peace with food. Remember, this is just a guide, not a rigid edict. There are days when your intuitive signals send you to a different balance of foods than is on this diagram. It's important to look at the big picture, rather than judging your overall nutrition by one particular day.

PLATE METHOD

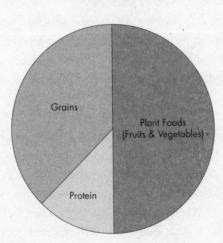

Grains

Plant Foods
(Fruits & Vegetables)

Protein

So Where's the Chocolate Group? As we have said, we're not going to pull a fast one. There are no forbidden foods, because deprivation doesn't work. All of the above guidelines are intended as a balance over time—which means even if you eat a candy bar, it will eventually average out. When you have let go of the diet mentality and have made peace with food, you will discover that you sometimes have a desire for food that has no nutritionally redemptive powers. We call this food *play food*. We prefer this term to one of the most commonly used terms to describe what's considered unhealthy foods—junk food. The term *junk food* implies that there is no intrinsic value in this food—in fact, that it probably should be thrown in the garbage can. But we feel that this thinking is unwarranted. There are times when a piece of red velvet cake or a stick of licorice is just the food that will satisfy your taste buds. And eating these types of foods doesn't mean you are an unhealthy eater. Here's a favorite story I (ER) like to tell that illustrates this point:

One day, when my son was a teenager, he asked me, "Mom, what happens to people who don't eat as healthfully as you do?" His question sparked a sense of pride in me that, as a nutritionist, I had taught him the virtues of healthy eating. My response to him included some lofty comments about how people who didn't pay much attention to nutrition probably had a higher incidence of heart disease, diabetes, cancer, and so forth. But before I could get the words fully out of my mouth, he pointed to me with his best adolescent "got you" finger and said, "but sometimes I see *you* eating french fries and other junk foods!" I had to stop and laugh for a moment and then said, "You're right, honey. Much of what I eat considers my health, and sometimes I eat things just for pleasure." I explained that for true satisfaction in my eating, those foods that he called junk can be part of a balanced diet. From that point on, the term *junk food* has been replaced with *play food* for its role in the world of eating satisfaction.

But how can eating play foods be healthy? This is where you pull together all the Intuitive Eating skills, which means, in a nutshell, listening to your body. This is key. For example, if you were to eat chocolate all day long, there's a very good chance that by the end of the day, you would experience the following physical feelings: nauseous, heaviness, dullness, and so forth. The question to you is, do you want to continue feeling this way? The truth is, if you listen to your body, you will not feel good eating this way. Even kids exposed to gobs of Halloween candy do not want to indulge for long. And when you know that you can truly have the food again (chocolate, or whatever else), it doesn't not take too much to satisfy you.

One client, Joe, was extremely fond of chocolate. He had truly made peace with food and was also at the stage of honoring his health. He was grocery shopping and discovered a new *triple* chocolate ice cream dessert, which was very rich. He chose not to buy it, not because it was loaded with fat, but because he did not want to experience what he calls headache food. He did not feel deprived; he knew he could have chocolate whenever he wished, and instead bought a small bag of M&Ms, and was satisfied.

Making Informed Food Choices

Clients often ask us if there is any value in knowing the nutrient content of food. The answer to this question can be tricky. If you have any remnant of diet mentality lingering in your mind, looking at a food label might trigger some of your old diet thoughts. If, on the other hand, your food choices are based on hunger and deriving satisfaction from your meal, then having a general sense of the nutrient content of foods—such as fiber, fat, and sodium can help guide your eating decisions.

For example, if you know that including high fiber foods in your meals will be beneficial to the functioning of your gastrointestinal tract, and you notice that one type of whole wheat bread is higher in fiber than another, then by all means choose the higher fiber product. Using nutrition information in this manner helps to honor both your palate and your health.

Or suppose you discover for the first time that a particular canned soup is very high in sodium, and you're concerned that it might have an adverse effect on your blood pressure. You may feel that you could take or leave the soup, because you don't enjoy it that much and wouldn't feel deprived by choosing a lower sodium soup. You might also decide that, if you were going to eat something high in sodium, you'd rather have pizza! Or perhaps you discover that a beverage you drink contains a high amount of sugar, and you would equally enjoy mineral water—then, by all means, opt for the mineral water.

There may come a time in your journey back to your Intuitive Eater, when eating with regard to nutritional quality becomes a priority for you. The key to knowing if you're ready for that decision is based on the following;

- In making your food choices, are you considering the sensual qualities of the food, while, at the same time honoring how you will physically feel when you eat this food?
- Do you have a medical condition that will be helped by paying attention to nutrition?
- Does thinking about nutrition feel neutral to you, rather than stirring up any old diet thoughts?
- Are you able to choose a food that may not have a high nutritional value, but will simply give you pleasure, without any old guilt feelings?

If you can answer "yes" to these questions, then making choices based on health and nutrition will not betray your ability to be an Intuitive Eater.

How to Keep the Pleasure in Healthy Eating

If we are to change our eating attitudes to enlightened hedonism, we need to balance information with the pleasure of eating. The information part comes from two sources, listening to your body and the nutrition guidelines we shared in this chapter. Listening to your body means not only staying in touch with satiety levels, but also assessing the following questions:

- Do I really like the taste of these foods, or am I being a diet/ health martyr?
- How does eating this food or type of meal make my body feel? Do I like this feeling?
- How do I feel when eating consistently in this manner? Do I like this feeling—would I choose to feel this way again?
- Am I experiencing differences in my energy level?

If eating healthfully is a pleasurable experience, *and* it makes you feel better, you are more likely to continue honoring your health with your food choices. The key, however is *not* to turn the idea of healthy eating into an all-or-none prospect based on deprivation. Deprivation does not work in the long run.

It's hard to enjoy eating a meal when the people around you are engaged in dieting talk, "fat talk," or body bashing. To keep the pleasure in eating, consider your Intuitive Eating Bill of Rights:

1. You have the right to savor your meal, without cajoling or judgment, and without discussion of calories eaten or the amount of exercise needed to burn off said calories.
2. You have the right to enjoy second servings without apology.
3. You have the right to honor your fullness, even if that means saying "no thank you," without explanation, to dessert or a second helping of food.
4. You have the right to stick to your original answer of "no," even if you are asked multiple times. Just calmly and politely repeat "No, thank you, really."
5. It is not your responsibility to make someone happy by overeating, even if it took hours to prepare a specialty dish.
6. You have the right to eat pumpkin pie for breakfast (or cereal for dinner!), regardless of judgmental comments or rolled eyes.

Remember, no one, except for you, knows how you feel, both emotionally and physically. Only you can be the expert of your body. This requires inner attunement, rather than the external, well-meaning suggestions from family.

Don't Let Yourself Be Put on a Food Pedestal

At first our clients think we must be perfect in our eating habits, after all, we are dietitians. We are not food and nutrition goddesses and do not want to be placed on a pedestal. Some of the best information we've passed onto our patients is not about how nutritiously we eat, but rather that we ate a whole piece of tiramisu and enjoyed each bite. Or how we got stuck with our food down, so to speak, and gobbled the nearest candy bar. And in spite of these times, we balance out our nutrition. We still honor our health, and our taste buds, and our humanness.

Many of our clients have been elevated to a place of specialness among their friends, colleagues, and family members, because they *appear* to eat so well. "She is the health-conscious one." In the beginning, it's fun to garner the extra attention, because they have attached a value to this identity. After a while, however, most of our clients no longer want this notoriety. It adds more pressure. When you are on this food pedestal it can intensify feelings of deprivation. It often means sneaking around to eat, which doesn't feel good or creates fears of "getting caught." My goodness, to get caught "cheating" on your diet! Horrors!

I'll (ET) never forget attending a dinner, hosted by a professional group at an incredible French restaurant. I was a stranger, seated among twenty people at the same table (I was a guest of one of the members). As the meal was winding down, the server presented us with a bounty of beautiful desserts. When the last dessert was described, someone asked, "Let's see what the nutritionist thinks—which one of these desserts is the *healthiest* to choose?" This was a food pedestal moment. As I opened my mouth to speak, all heads turned toward me, and I replied, "What's more important is whatever dessert is the most *satisfying*!" There was a very loud and collective sigh of relief!

Our clients usually feel relieved when they voluntarily dethrone themselves as the food-fitness czars. What this means is they are no longer closet eaters—they no longer put on a false food face. If they feel like ordering dessert with a meal, they will. It's their opportunity to show how appearing to be a perfect eater does not equate to the value of optimal health and fitness. Remember, balance is the key!

Chapter 15

Raising an Intuitive Eater: What Works with Kids and Teens

We are often asked if it is possible to teach children Intuitive Eating. The answer is not only is it possible to help children return to the Intuitive Eaters they were at birth, but it is often easier than with adults. Children are less dubious than adults and far more open and eager.

Let's begin with prevention. When an infant is born, this child is equipped with the innate ability needed to know how to eat.

I (ER) was fortunate enough recently to visit a friend's daughter, who had just given birth two weeks before to her beautiful baby girl. Alexis was just getting comfortable with the overwhelming task of figuring out how to take care of her newborn. Which cry meant that she was sleepy, which one said that there was a diaper that needed changing, and which one let her know that the baby needed to eat? Now, if you have ever observed a hungry baby, you know that her most recognizable cry is the one of hunger. If the child is ignored when she's hungry, she'll scream and scream until offered the breast or bottle. The hunger signal is acutely available for the majority of babies, and there is a natural instinct to make the need for nourishment known. I was sitting and talking with Alexis, when little Lily made the noises that let her mother know that she was hungry. To sit and watch this beautiful connection between mother and child was a true gift. Lily nursed on one breast and then the other, and when she was full, she turned her precious head away and fell asleep. Alexis was in awe of how intuitive her infant's feeding experience was.

If there is attunement to the wide array of obvious and nuanced messages that the child offers, the child will grow up with a sense of self-confidence that his needs are appropriate and will be consistently met. When the child is hungry and is quickly fed, many important messages will be conveyed. The first message is that hunger is a natural, normal, and "correct" sensation. As time goes on, the feeling of hunger will be coupled with the drive to find food. An attuned response to the child's hunger will elicit a sense of safety, eliminating any fear of deprivation. If, instead, this primary need of the child is not met at the appropriate times, the child will begin to fear that there won't be enough food. In response, this child is in danger of muting hunger signals, rather than trusting that the hunger signal is a reliable message throughout life.

Imagine an infant who is put on a feeding schedule, something that was a common recommendation from generations past. The parent was advised to place the baby on a schedule of eating, ranging from every two to three hours to every three to four hours. Many parents responded positively to this recommendation, as regulating the feeding schedule would allow them to plan the whole day in advance. Of course, most parents did not adopt this method out of selfish needs. They were counseled that a regular feeding schedule would be best for the child. Unfortunately, this is not usually the case, as this method has the potential to create a number of problems. If the child got hungry and cried half an hour before the scheduled time, the parent was prompted to wait to feed her. If, on the other hand, the child wasn't yet hungry at this time, she might be coaxed to eat anyway. Since hunger and fullness signals were not consistently being reinforced, the hungry, screaming baby or the not yet hungry baby was on his way to mistrusting these powerful messages. For the hungry infant, the potential fear of future deprivation can take root. For the infant who was encouraged to eat before hunger had sufficiently arrived, confusion and resistance to eating can emerge. For a child who was fed on schedule, rather than on demand, moving on to the toddler years can initiate a disordered relationship with food. If an abundance of food becomes available to a child who had experienced a feeling of deprivation in infancy, the child might be prone to develop a natural tendency to overeat. When the next meal is offered, one of two possibilities might occur. The child is likely to be too full and refuse to eat or might go beyond this fullness signal and take in even more food, storing up for the next potential famine. For the child who had been cajoled to eat as an infant, the freedom to eat more independently as a toddler can also present two possibilities. He might continue to eat when he's not yet hungry, or he might exert his independence by refusing to eat.

Fortunately, feeding schedules are rarely recommended today, and conscientious caregivers tend to respond regularly to the child's hunger signals.

But, what about fullness signals? Have you ever tried to continue to feed an infant after she turns her head away from the breast or bottle, because you're afraid that she hasn't had enough nutrition or that she's not growing quickly enough? When that child's tummy is full, she will naturally balk at being force-fed. We have seen, with horror, toddlers who were regularly persuaded to eat more than they needed, throughout their first couple of years. Eventually they either gained far more weight than was healthy or ended up getting into food fights and refused to eat much at all. For example, the mother of a very young client was actually referred to child protective services by the psychiatrist involved in the treatment. This mother had had a sister who had died in a starved state from anorexia nervosa. Because of this, she associated being underweight with death and became terrified that her child would be underweight. As a result, she stuffed her little boy with enormous amounts of food. This was seen as emotional child abuse.

The most fundamental step in ensuring that a child retains all of his innate ability around hunger and fullness is trust. Ellyn Satter, in her groundbreaking book, *Child of Mine: Feeding with Love and Common Sense* (2000), aptly states that it's the parents' job to provide the food, and the child's job to eat as much or as little as he needs. In infancy, it's not often that a parent deviates from this give and take, but as children move out of the "milk only" phase, parents have a more difficult time staying tuned in to a child's eating signals. Parents believe that there are so many "legitimate" reasons for them to try to take control of the child's eating. In this era of the epidemic of childhood obesity, the fear of a child gaining too much weight often leads well-meaning pediatricians to give parents the advice to monitor what and how much a child is eating. The opposite situation can also be present, if there is a fear that the child is not gaining enough weight. In addition, many parents who want to help their children be as healthy as they can, allow them to eat only nutritionally dense foods and restrict them from play food. Although this attempt to control the amount and type of food children are eating is often born from good intentions, it also brings the potential for the child's mistrust of his signals. Not only are his hunger and fullness signals missed, but also his innate understanding of his food preferences and how his body feels after eating different amounts and types of foods. Instead of listening to and respecting her own physical reactions to the eating experience, the child reacts to the parent's external message, rather than her own internal knowledge. This reaction can run the gamut of being the "good little girl" and doing everything that Mommy wants, to acting out as the rebellious child, who refuses to eat most everything.

FAMILY EXPERIENCES

We have worked with many parents and children whose stories have spoken of some of the difficulties that arise in knowing how to handle the feeding arena with children. In future sections of this chapter, you will read about our tips and guidelines for protecting your child's inborn intuitive signals and for healing some of the problems that may have already arisen. Some families are able to transcend these difficulties by adopting an Intuitive Eating approach, and some have a harder time making this shift. This process of prevention and healing will be illustrated by vignettes of some real-life clients.

As you've been reading so far, you may have been thinking, "How can I trust that my child will be an Intuitive Eater? How can I allow my child to make these decisions on her own—all she'll want to eat is candy?!" Before learning how to heal existing problems, let's first explore the stories of some children who have been able to grow up with all of their Intuitive Eating signals intact. Fortunately, we have the great honor to hear about many children who have been born to and raised by parents who have sought our help to return to their own Intuitive Eating. As a result, these parents are committed to raising their children with the same philosophy. And how incredible it is to watch the fruit of their labors!

Jeannie and Jimmy

Jeannie has been a client for many years. She now has a two-and-a-half-year-old son, who continues to amaze her with how intuitive his eating is. Jimmy's favorite play food is chocolate-covered blueberries. At every meal, his mom puts a bowl of these blueberries on the table, along with all of the other foods she has prepared. She mentioned that, sometimes, all that Jimmy eats are the blueberries. Sometimes, he eats a few of them, and at other times, he eats all of his other food and eats none of the blueberries. Sometimes, he just likes to take the blueberries out of the bowl and then put them back. His mom has no agenda about Jimmy's eating. She sees that over a week's time, he eats a well-balanced array of foods, is growing beautifully, and is full of health and energy.

Jeannie's sister has a different approach for her children. Her daughter had loved M&Ms since she first saw them as a small toddler. This little one's mother was so afraid that she would eat too many, that she began to ration them out whenever they were around. This little girl has become obsessed with M&Ms, and cannot get enough of them. Her cousin, Jimmy, on the other hand, occasionally asks for a lollipop or two. Sometimes, he wants to hold one in each hand or open several of them. He takes one lick and is more fascinated with the wrapping than he is with the actual candy!

Andrea and Allie

Andrea was referred for counseling by her pediatrician when her baby, Allie, was seven months old. Andrea had told her doctor that she had no idea how to feed her child, having suffered with anorexia, bulimia, and compulsive overeating throughout her teens and twenties. Allie was more than ready to eat solid food, but Andrea not only didn't know how to proceed, she was terrified to create an eating disorder in her own child. She arrived in the office on that first session and offered a big hug in hope and gratitude, and said, "Please teach me how to feed my daughter." In those first few months of counseling, Andrea was not only taught how to introduce vegetables and fruits and grains and meats, etc. to Allie, but she was also introduced to Intuitive Eating to help heal her own disordered eating.

Through Allie's toddler years, she had the advantage of being offered every possible nutritious food that her mother would prepare and would sit at the table with her parents while eating. She wasn't introduced to play food in her home as a tiny child, but when she was at other's homes, no restriction was put on her exploration of foods that were offered. Carrots and ice cream and spinach and candy were all treated equally. Andrea made no comments and gave no judgmental glances at Allie's choices. As a result of this freedom, Allie, at seven years old, has only a moderate interest in play food and a true desire for a wide range of more nutritious food. A couple of years ago, she woke up one morning and asked Andrea for tofu and hearts of palm for breakfast! When it was her turn to bring a snack to nursery school, she wanted to bring bok choy. At a friend's house, where all of the visiting children were eating ice cream, she asked for carrots. When asked at school to draw a picture of her favorite food, Allie drew brussels sprouts! But don't get the wrong impression—Allie also loves candy and cookies. She simply has no need to fill up on these foods, because they're never restricted and never judged.

Allie is also a very active little girl and loves her dance classes with a passion. There are no food fights between her and her parents. Instead, there is a healthy relationship with food, which is acutely attuned to her hunger, fullness, and food preferences. It was recently Allie's seventh birthday. She decided that she wanted to have crab legs at her birthday dinner and chose sides of carrots and potatoes. When she had had enough of her dinner, the server asked what she wanted for dessert, and she told him she was full and didn't feel like dessert. He was stunned and kept pressing her about it being her birthday and needing to celebrate with cake. Allie politely explained: "I'm very full and don't want more to eat. But you can sing me happy birthday!" Her mother is regularly taken by Allie's comments about how poorly other children eat. She just doesn't understand why they're stuck on one type of food or are begging for dessert. The only unfortunate experience that Andrea can report involves a dance teacher who saw Allie eating little cubes of tofu. The teacher said something like, "Ick, I don't like tofu." As this teacher was deeply admired by Allie, it's not surprising that Allie has refused tofu since having had this experience. What power we adults have on these impressionable children!

ROLE MODELING

The tofu experience, just described, brings up an extremely important aspect of the relationship between a child's eating and the eating of adults who influence the child. Parents tend to serve as the primary role models in the realm of eating. There is great power in setting an example of eating when hungry, stopping when full, and eating a large variety of foods. This is a case of "do what I do," rather than "do what I say." The more talk there is about food, whether it's positive encouragement to try foods or negative strivings to reduce a child's quantity of food, the more the opportunity for a child's resistance or rebellion toward the "authority" figure. The less talk and the more role modeling, the more likely it is that the child will try new foods, find vegetables interesting, and have more balance in the entire eating experience.

Jill and Billy

Jill is a client who first sought nutrition counseling after a lifetime of eating-disordered behavior and body image problems. Her mother was always on a diet throughout Jill's childhood, and Jill began attempting to control her weight in her late teens, through diets and restrictive eating. Her restrictive eating ultimately led to a diagnosis of anorexia nervosa and a mind that could think of nothing else but food and body. At the time she sought counseling, she was married and thinking about having children. She was very worried that if she didn't heal her own problems, she would eventually transmit them to her future children. She was finally ready to make some changes!

Jill worked very hard to let go of diet thinking and to start feeding herself according to her body's hunger and fullness signals. She eventually became pregnant, and, to this day, she credits her improved eating for her ability to become pregnant. She also credits her Intuitive Eating work for the profound effect it has had on the raising of her first son, and later her second son. She recently told a story that exemplified this. Her oldest son, Billy, who is four, was sitting at dinner with the family. He turned to his father, and said, "Daddy, you need to eat your vegetables—they're good for you!" Jill has cooked and served her children a wide range of nutritious foods since each was able to eat solid food. She also keeps play food in the house, attempting to buy foods that offer some nutritional value. Her children love Fig Newtons, graham crackers, dark chocolate almonds, and ice cream. When they're at other children's homes, they are never restricted from any foods that they may find there. Jill has also never commented on how much or how little food the children eat or classified foods as good foods or bad foods. Above all, she has never told Billy that vegetables are healthy and that he should eat them. She has no idea how he got the thought to tell his father to eat his vegetables and that they're healthy!

Jill is raising her boys with the trust that they will get a sufficient variety of food and nutrients, if they are allowed to make their own decisions about what they eat and how much. One evening, Billy was eating ice cream and said he was full, after having finished half of it. He asked his mom to put the other half in the freezer and save it. The next morning, when Jill asked Billy what he would like to have for breakfast, he said that he'd like to eat ice cream and grapes for breakfast, and that's what he ate! Some mornings, he wants eggs; some mornings he wants oatmeal. He's never told that he can have ice cream only if he finishes other foods first. Both boys are growing appropriately and are getting the full spectrum of foods that they need to be healthy.

SUPPORTING YOUR CHILD'S INNATE RELATIONSHIP TO FOOD AND EATING

It's important for parents to know some of the basic concepts of a child's relationship with food. Below, you'll find some of these concepts, along with some practical tips for protecting your child's inborn Intuitive Eater:

Children Are Self-Regulating. For the most part, children are self-regulating in terms of how much food they need. Some children have a lower growth rate and some a faster growth rate, and this varies from time to time. They'll eat exactly what they need in order to follow their own path.

- Children grow in spurts. Sometimes they eat as much as an adult and sometimes as little as an ant. If left alone and not nudged, they'll get everything that they need.
- If they are physically active, they will be hungrier than if they are sedentary.
- Children's food preferences vary regularly. Don't worry if your child only wants peanut butter and jelly for many weeks and then won't look at it for months afterward. If no issue is made (such as, "you've always loved this—why aren't you eating it now?"), the child is quite likely to go back to this food sometime in the future.
- Conversely, if you serve the same food every day, the child might become disinterested in it. As in the concept of habituation, too much of a good thing can become boring and rejected. Alternate foods every few days to maintain children's interest in different foods.
- Look at the whole week, instead of a particular meal or day of eating, and you will see that your child will get everything that he needs.

Children Seek Autonomy. An important developmental task of childhood is the quest for autonomy. This can show up as early as two years old or even before, and continues throughout childhood, peaking in adolescence. In adulthood, a sense of autonomy is one of the signs of a psychologically healthy person. If we help our children to feel empowered, whenever safe and appropriate, this developmental task will take root.

- Allow your children to serve themselves, as soon as they are developmentally able to do so. If you serve them, you are presuming how much they need to satisfy their hunger. They will take what they need, without feeling pressured to "clean the plate."
- Saying "no" to eating is often a way for a toddler to show his independence, especially if he's not hungry. Don't worry, when he's hungry, he'll eat!
- If you have raised your children as Intuitive Eaters, you can feel safe allowing them to order for themselves in a restaurant. If not, they may need more guidance from you.
- Involve children in food shopping and meal preparation—they'll be more interested in eating the foods they pick and prepare.

Introducing New Foods Is an Art. Parents often expect their children to try a new food when offered, even if it's only a bite. The first moment of feeding conflict can begin at this point, if foods are not introduced without understanding how children can react to this new experience.

- Allow children to experiment with food, especially if introducing a new food or an already accepted food prepared in a new way. A child might put it in his mouth, take it out, play with it, and then try it once again. Or he might not be ready to eat it at all at that time. Let children be a little messy—this sensory experimentation phase is part of normal development.
- It can sometimes take fifteen exposures or more for a child to accept a new food. Just because you introduce something new once or twice, and the child refuses it, don't give up. Keep serving it from time to time, without any pressure. At some point, the child might try it.
- When offering a new food, offer it with some familiar foods. Don't put out several new foods at once. This can be overwhelming for the child, and he might refuse everything.
- At around age two, children often become fearful of new things, including new foods. Again, don't worry—if the child isn't pushed, he'll eventually be willing to try new things, when he's ready.

• There are going to be some foods that your child simply doesn't like, just as adults have particular food preferences and dislikes.

Your Role as the Parent Is Powerful. Parenting is an awesome task. In the realm of feeding your children, following some basic guidelines will smooth the way to a positive outcome.

• Stay neutral when serving food, instead of pushy. If you're invested in what or how much your child eats, your child will react to you, instead of to his inner signals.
• Eat a variety of foods yourself, and enjoy and appreciate food together as a family. Remember, children love to mimic their parents, even in the realm of eating.
• Above all, do not bribe, reward, or attempt to comfort with food. Food is for hunger, satisfaction, and nourishment. Help your children learn how to endure feelings. Let them know that their feelings are real and valued and that there are ways to be comforted without using food.

THE POWER OF RESTRICTION AND DEPRIVATION

Mary, Denise, and Molly

The examples above illustrate the best outcome of raising children with respect for their intuitive signals. These children were provided an early eating experience that involved an orientation to a wide variety of food, which was also served to the whole family. There were no messages of food-type restriction or comments about food amounts. Other clients, especially those who are still struggling with their own disordered eating, have a bit more trouble giving the same message.

Mary has four-and-a-half-year-old fraternal twin girls. Molly is naturally lean and extremely active. Denise is more sedentary and softer in build. From early on, Mary worried about Denise's weight and, after the girls learned that play food existed, marveled at what limited interest Molly had in these foods.

Mary had done a wonderful job of cooking nutritious food and serving it to the girls at family meals. The problems began, however, when the parents began to set limits on how much play food Denise could eat. Mary recently reported a story that had a troubling outcome. Molly rarely was interested in play food, so she was left alone. Denise, on the other hand, loved it. One day, Denise had found two bags of M&Ms and offered one of them to Molly. Molly wasn't interested, so Denise took the second bag and brought it to her room. At first, this appeared to have a happy message. Denise was willing to share with her sister and did not need to eat both bags at the same time. Mary has been working on liberalizing her message about play food to her daughters, and she thought that this example showed that she had made some progress. A little later that day, Mary noticed that Denise had shut herself up in a room and was secretly eating her stash of candy. Mary walked in and seeing a guilty look on Denise's face, asked her if she thought she had to sneak candy. Denise said, "Yes, I thought you would be mad." Mary said, "Denise, you can have as much candy as you want. I won't get mad. I just want to make sure you eat enough nutritious food too (which she definitely does). But I understand that some days you want eight pieces of candy, and some days you don't care about candy at all (also true). As long as you eat other foods too, you can have as much candy as you want." Denise then asked, "Will Daddy be mad?" Mary answered, "I'll talk to Daddy," to which Denise replied, "Sometimes I just want spinach and corn and rice." She followed that by saying, "I want to do the candy dance," and she sang a very happy song and dance about how much she loves candy!

Mary expressed concern to her husband Danny about the message he was conveying to Denise and told him about the sneaking story. She convinced him that if they continued to put limits on Denise, they would basically be telling her that she could not trust her body. In addition, she warned him that Denise would end up like Danny's mother, who is constantly on diets and beating herself up for "blowing her diet." She told him that if he wanted to inflict that kind of pain on his daughter, then he should keep telling her that it's bad to want to eat candy.

This poignant story shows what can happen when parents have anxiety about their child's weight and believe that they must control the amount of play food a child can have. Molly never got this message, as they weren't worried about her weight, and she self-regulated her play food intake. Fortunately, Mary was wise enough to see what the future could hold, if they continued to give the message that there were good foods and bad foods. For Mary, who had grown up with extreme food restriction, the outcome of this childhood environment was a serious eating disorder. Fortunately, she continues to receive counseling for herself and for the whole family. With hope, both parents will learn to treat their daughters equally and eliminate diet mentality messages.

There are numerous studies that support the concept that dietary restriction can have serious consequences for children. These include the potential for increased weight gain, eating that is not connected to hunger, preoccupation with food, and, eventually, lowered self-esteem (Eneli, Crum, and Tylka 2008). Putting pressure on children to eat when they refuse food, misinterpreting normal weight as overweight, restricting certain foods, and soothing children with food all interfere with children's trust in their inner signals about eating. Ellyn Satter believes that "overcontrol" and "undersupport" are at the basis of many childhood weight problems (Satter 2005).

Nancy

The foundation for Intuitive Eating is based on a number of psychological and physiological factors. The power of deprivation can be a profound psychological factor, leading a child (as well as an adult, of course) to make some very dysfunctional food choices. This point is well illustrated by a frightening story that I was recently told by a client of mine (ER), who is an early childhood educator. She told me about a little girl who was in the preschool class that she taught. Little Nancy was a beautiful child with graceful hands and fingers. Nancy's mother believed that sugar was a dangerous food and forbade Nancy from eating anything that had sugar as one of the ingredients. She even went so far as to inform the teachers that Nancy was never to be given any food that contained sugar. One day, my client noticed that Nancy had not gone onto the playground to play with the other children. Instead, she stayed back in the classroom and was found picking up the crumbs from the floor that were left behind from the snacks that the other children had eaten. Those dainty little fingers not only picked up crumbs but also picked up pieces of dirty raw rice and dried beans, which the children used for play. This child was so desperate to taste what she couldn't have, that she went to this extreme to fix her feelings of deprivation. After seeing this behavior continue, the teachers went to Nancy's house to confront her mother and ask her to stop restricting Nancy from eating what the other children were eating. Even after being told what Nancy had done, her mother remained vehement that Nancy was never allowed to have sugar!

HEALING DEPRIVATION

Pamela and Eric

Fortunately, many parents are more receptive. Pamela is a mother of a healthy, average weight five-year-old, who was referred to work on her lifelong history of restrictive eating. In the early part of her treatment, she mentioned that her son Eric was hyper-focused on dessert. After each bite of dinner, he would beg for the dessert, while not appreciating the tastes of the other foods served to him. Pamela's husband was very adamant that Eric finish his dinner before he could have dessert, and the dinner table became a battleground. Pamela and her husband came in for counseling together one day and were astonished to hear the recommendation of putting all of the foods on the table at once—yes, including the cookies, along with the chicken and the broccoli and the bread. Although Pamela and her husband were skeptical, they were open-minded about this new approach.

It didn't take very long before Eric stopped seeking the desserts over all other foods. Did he still eat the cookies? Of course! But instead of eating them first, for fear that this new way of eating would disappear (along with the cookies), he began to eat all of the nutritious foods along with the cookies. Fear of deprivation is a powerful force in the seeking and overeating of restricted foods. The surest way to get a child to be disinterested in the foods the parent wants him to eat is to tell him that he can't have his dessert until he finishes his dinner. Quickly, "dinner" becomes the enemy and the barrier to getting what he really wants. The limited access, conditional availability, and the measured serving size of the dessert create an overvalued treasure. In addition, the child's need to express his autonomy is displayed through fighting about how much he "has to eat" before he gets the prize or whether, in a defiant nature, he'll eat anything at all.

Once the parents stop being so invested in controlling what goes into the mouths of their children and stop metering out the amount of disapproved foods, an amazingly rapid "cease fire" emerges and calm falls upon the feeding experience.

STEPS FOR PROTECTING AND REINFORCING YOUR CHILD'S INTUITIVE EATING EXPERIENCE

Introduce Foods According to Your Pediatrician's Guidelines. Introduce a variety of nutritious foods to your baby as soon as your pediatrician recommends that solid foods are appropriate. Begin with grains or vegetables, depending on what your pediatrician tells you. If you begin with grains, offer as many whole grains as possible, so your child gets used to the flavor of the whole grain. When instructed, introduce vegetables. Start with mild green vegetables, and after the child is accustomed to them, introduce the orange, sweeter vegetables. Again, when instructed, add fruits, and then all other foods.

If Your Child Is Thirsty, Offer Water, Rather than Juice. Juice was only introduced into the food supply during the early 1900s. Before juice was invented, people mainly ate fruit and drank water (*Los Angeles Times* 2009). Juice can fill up a child's stomach and distract from true hunger signals. Filling up with juice within an hour before a meal will lead the child to feel too full at the next meal.

Prepare Balanced Meals. When children are able to eat all foods, prepare balanced meals that include protein, complex carbohydrates (especially whole grains), fats, fruits and vegetables, and high calcium foods (dairy products provide the most reliable source of calcium).

Postpone Introducing Play Food to Very Young Children. There is no need to introduce play food to very young children. They'll have plenty of opportunities to experience these foods. If, however, someone offers a play food to a toddler who is at an age to be able to eat it, don't forbid it. Allow the child to experience this food without comment (either negative or encouraging). How many times have you seen a parent try to urge the one-year-old to try his birthday cake! And how many more times have you seen a parent tell a child that she can't eat what the other children are eating? If your child has been oriented to a wide variety of foods when he or she begins to eat solid foods, the play food will not become overvalued. It will take its place in the child's healthy and unself-conscious relationship with food.

Share the Power of Nutrition Early on. Teach your children that food can have the power to give them energy, make their bones and muscles strong, help them grow, help them avoid getting sick frequently, help them think well at school, and help them heal their wounds. Some people call these foods "nutritious foods." Others call them "growing foods." One person even named them "vital foods." Pick a word that works for you.

Talk about Foods in Non-Moralistic Terms, Rather than "Good" or "Bad." Telling children that a food is a bad food can instill a feeling of guilt. Instead, tell children that there are some foods that don't necessarily help the body, but exist, just to taste good. You can call these foods "play foods." Don't call them "junk food," because that implies that they serve no purpose and could elicit shame for eating something of no value. Tell them that just as they don't go to school all year round, without weekends or breaks, they also don't play all year round without going to school. Their minds need school to help them learn, just as their bodies need nutritious foods, for the purposes mentioned above. Tell them that they also might want some play foods just for fun, just as they have some playtime, along with their learning time. In this way, they'll have a reason to eat healthy foods and not overvalue the play foods. Balanced eating is the result of this kind of thinking. It will also reduce the risk of your child gravitating toward the play food at another child's home because it has been restricted in your home.

Put a Variety of Foods on the Table. Prepare balanced meals for your children, and try to eat with them whenever possible. When the children have become aware of play food, occasionally put some on the table, along with all of the nutritious food. Make no comments about which foods or how much food a child should eat. Some days he may only want the play food, but most days he'll eat an array of most everything that is served. Refrain from telling your children to eat a certain amount of the nutritious food, before eating dessert. Otherwise your child will likely start a negotiation process that can only lead to tension and bad energy at the meal. Remember, your child's food choices may change from meal to meal or day to day. In the big picture, he'll get all the nutrients that he needs.

Pack Lunches That Have a Variety of Choices, Including a Little Play Food. If your child never gets a cookie in her lunch, you can be sure that she'll trade something with another child to get what she wants.

Make Healthy Snacks Available for Your Children. Have healthy snacks readily available for when your child gets hungry between meals. These snacks might include cut-up fresh fruit and vegetables, nuts, cheese, hummus, whole grain crackers, etc. If these foods are ready to eat and visible in the refrigerator or on the counter when your child gets home from school or is home during the day, there's a good chance that she'll go for them when she's hungry.

Do Not Be a Short-Order Cook! Make one meal for the whole family, but be sure to have a number of choices of side dishes, so that each child has something to eat, even if he doesn't like the main course. Tell them that you will be preparing meals that are well balanced, because you believe that well-balanced meals will help them grow tall and strong and will help to keep them healthy. Let them know that you won't be making several dinners for the family, but assure them that you will be serving some foods that you know they each like. Reassure them that you will not be monitoring which of the foods or how much of the foods they are eating. That will be their job.

Trust Your Child's Innate Abilities. Children know how much to eat to match hunger needs and to stop eating when full. In the big picture, your child will get everything needed for growth and health and will maintain a flowing and positive relationship with food.

HEALING A BATTERED RELATIONSHIP WITH EATING FOR YOUR CHILD

Parents often seek nutrition counseling for their young children, hoping that the children will either learn to eat a wider variety of foods or will lose weight. Often, it's unnecessary to actually work with the child. Instead, the parents are taught about the Intuitive Eating philosophy and are given practical guidelines. Sometimes, it is still necessary to directly help a child to change eating habits and feelings about food.

Five Tips for Parents for Making Changes at Home

Here are some of the steps that can help you make changes. These tips can apply to children as young as the age of five and even through the teens.

This is especially geared toward children who are known to be aware of the household "eating rules." For younger children, changes can be initiated without actually talking about them. Explain the following:

1. Tell your child that you have read a book or talked to a professional who has given you some very different ideas about eating than what happens in your house. Acknowledge that parents can learn new things and change and that you are eager to make some of these changes. This will intrigue your child and get the soil ready for implanting the new ideas.

2. Kids have the ability to know how much to eat—but it gets confusing when parents take over the job of making these decisions. Tell him that from now on, he will get to choose how much he wants to eat at mealtime and that you will be providing a variety of foods at meals, which includes previously forbidden foods. It will be up to him to decide which foods he wants to eat of the foods offered to him and how much or how little of these foods his body tells him he needs.

3. Make sure to state that you are not a "short-order" cook, but assure him that you will be serving some foods that you know he likes (See p. 233).

4. Ask him if there are any foods that he would like to have in the house that are not usually present. You'll see a great deal of excitement and disbelief in the child's face at this point.

5. Most importantly—stick to your promise. Your child will test you to see if this is too good to be true. He might wait for you to slip and say that he doesn't need more food, or that "he should eat some vegetables," or that he has to eat a certain amount of nutritious food before he can have any dessert. It will take time before your child believes that you really aren't going to interfere with his eating.

This advice can be scary for many parents. Fears stem from worrying that others will think that they're not good parents because they're not enforcing strict eating rules, to worrying that the child will never stop eating, will only eat desserts, or won't eat enough food.

For some parents, it is helpful to seek counseling with a nutrition therapist or a psychotherapist who is supportive of Intuitive Eating. With counseling, the concerns can be vented to the professional instead of to the child. It is also very important that both parents are aligned. Just as in any parenting issue, a united front allows the child to feel safe and not confused.

In addition to the guidelines, it is critical that each parent examine his or her own beliefs about food, eating, and the body. If there is any form of disordered eating in the family, it can be difficult to heal a dysfunctional eating experience in a child. Remember, parents are important role models, which is critical in helping a child return to his Intuitive Eating roots. Eating family meals together, and regularly, is important. This provides an opportunity for your child to witness parents or siblings eating nutritious foods, even when your child is not ready to try them. When this is layered upon a neutral atmosphere about what and how much the child is eating, your child will eventually eat balanced meals.

WHEN YOUR CHILD IS OVERWEIGHT

Over 30 percent of kids in the United States are overweight. Doctors and parents are naturally concerned and worried that if "something isn't done about it," these children will be at risk for many health issues. Unfortunately, well-meaning attempts to manage this problem often yield dismal results.

Placing eating restrictions on children who are overweight can have a powerful influence on future disordered eating and body image. Leann L. Birch, a professor of Human Development at Pennsylvania State University, and her research group have extensively evaluated these issues. Their studies show that parents using restrictive feeding practices backfire and create bigger problems, which lead children to eat when they aren't hungry, often resulting in greater weight gain.

In a study of five-year-old-girls—some overweight and some at normal weight, the girls whose mothers used restrictive feeding patterns were shown to have the greatest level of overeating behavior by age nine (Birch, Fisher, and Davison 2003).

Parental restriction is only one side of the coin. The other side is parental pressure to eat more healthy foods. In yet another study of five-year-old girls, when they simply perceived parental pressure and control about food, it resulted in them pulling away from their internal signals of hunger and fullness. Instead, some began to restrict certain foods, to eat emotionally, and to eat with abandon (Carper, Fisher, and Birch 2000).

It can be very difficult and even terrifying for parents to let go of monitoring their children's eating patterns, especially if a child is overweight. But, as in any behavior, the more a person is pushed to change a habit, the less likely that the habit will change.

In the case of a child who has been overeating and/or is overweight, limiting the amount or the type of food that the child eats can only lead to feelings of deprivation and rebellion, just as diets do for adults. The child who is told that he must limit his eating, will have a deepened sense of mistrust of ever having enough. This child is likely to sneak food, eat as much as he can at a friend's house, or, eventually, develop a serious eating disorder. Feelings of shame can emerge in a child who breaks the rules in an over-controlling eating environment. It can also ultimately affect the health of the child's relationship with his or her parents.

The solution, once again, is to help the child listen and respond to his own hunger and fullness cues. The child's job involves first healing the fear of deprivation or the rebellion that has emerged in response to being told what to do. When this healing takes place, the child can then begin to learn to trust his hunger and fullness signals.

This might feel like taking an impossible leap of faith—to give up the attempt to control your child's eating, especially if he or she is overweight. Perhaps Michele's story will help reassure you that it can be done.

Michele

About ten years ago, a call came in from the parents of an eight-year-old girl seeking help for her overeating. They were concerned about her weight and worried about potential health issues. The parents reported that they were both dieters but knew that a diet was the wrong approach for their daughter. They didn't think that they were ready to change their own habits but said that despite this, they would do anything they could for their daughter. After a few sessions with the parents, it became clear that this child would benefit from counseling.

The first time that Michele came into the office, she said that she wanted to have her parents present during her session. In subsequent sessions, one or the other of the parents and sometimes an aunt accompanied Michele in her session. Their presence was wonderful, as not only did Michele feel that her parents would be supporting her in the changes that were suggested, but also that she would have an arena to speak up to her parents about her feelings. The first session with Michele was remarkable for her. She was excited to hear that her parents were willing to make changes, and that because of these changes, she was going to start to feel better. During that session, Michele revealed that she often ate too many desserts at parties. She'd eat so much, especially chocolate, that she would end up having "a very bad tummy ache" and would have to leave the party. When asked why she thought that she ate enough dessert to make her feel sick when she was at her friends' houses, she said that her parents wouldn't allow any desserts at home, unless they were low in calories. She didn't like the diet desserts, so, in order to get what she liked, she felt the need to eat as much as she could at her friends' homes.

In these sessions that Michele attended, there was never a word spoken about weight. No scale was ever used, and the emphasis was always on how Michele felt, both physically and mentally. Any focus on a child's weight, either by her parents or by any professional, whether doctor or dietitian, runs the risk of giving some very damaging messages to the child.

Michele was a very intelligent, perceptive, and healthy little girl, with good self-esteem. The chief concern was to maintain this self-esteem, by avoiding giving her the impression that she wasn't good enough at her present weight. By emphasizing the hope that she wouldn't have to overeat and get the resulting stomachaches, she had a concrete reason to make changes.

Almost any child who is overeating will have the ability to say that he or she feels too full and uncomfortable, even if it doesn't result in stomach pain.

Talking to a child about future health issues is also not the correct course. First of all, it can scare the child and make her have excessive worry about herself. Unfortunately, we hear parents tell their children that they will get diabetes or have heart problems if they don't lose weight. Secondly, the concept of future heart problems is too abstract, even for an adult, let alone a child. Worry about future health issues does not have the power to motivate behavior change. Feeling physically better in the moment has far more impact.

After Michele talked about eating too much at parties, she was asked to list the foods that she would like to regularly have in her house. (Of course, chocolate was one of them!) She gave her parents a list, with the promise that they would take her shopping to buy them. When asked how she felt about that change, she was elated but also skeptical that her parents would follow through.

In the nutrition counseling session, Michele was taught that her body would give her a message about when she was hungry and when she was full. She said that she knew when she was hungry, and she usually knew when she was full. Then she asked a provocative question, "How can I stop eating when I know that I'm full?" Rather than provide a pat answer,

Michele was asked: "If your tummy is full, does your body need more food?" She replied, "Well, no." Michele was then asked, "So, if your body doesn't need any more food, then what do you really need?" This eight-year-old child got it, right there, and responded, "I need to know that I'll be able to get the sweets I want at my own house."

Michele added, "Sometimes I need to eat when I'm feeling bored or sad or lonely or scared." Many adults can't make that connection! After it was explained that some people think they need food to help soothe their feelings, Michelle was asked if she could think of anything else she could do to help her when she feels bad. Michele proposed that she could color in a coloring book, play with her dog, or talk with her mom. This was the beginning of helping Michele heal her feelings of deprivation about food, and start to separate her physical cues from her emotional cues for eating.

Michele's parents followed up on their promise to bring previously restricted foods into the house. Over time, Michele started trusting that she would have sweets at home when and if she wanted. As a result, her feelings of deprivation vanished, and she found that she only needed moderate amounts to satisfy her. She stopped overeating at parties, talked about balancing her nutritious foods with her play foods, and grew into a tall, athletic young woman.

Michele continued to come in for sessions, from time to time, until she was fourteen. Not only did her disordered eating stop, but, more importantly, she was no longer at risk for developing an eating disorder. The success of this story rests on her parents' willingness to change the way they handled food for the family, their support of her and her needs, and their wisdom to not draw any attention to her weight. Eventually, they were even willing to give up dieting themselves and to strive to reconnect with their own intuitive signals.

Preventing Overeating Problems

To learn about preventing eating problems, reference the earlier sections, "Supporting Your Child's Innate Relationship to Food and Eating" and "Steps for Protecting and Reinforcing Your Child's Intuitive Eating Experience." It is also extremely important to work on your own eating issues, if they exist. Get help for disordered eating, and, above all, make no negative comments about food or body to your child. Remember, children want to be like their parents. Pay attention to what you think and say about your body or your eating, because your child will absorb your comments and will imitate what you say and how you eat.

Ten Steps for Working with Your Child Who Is an Overeater

With the previously mentioned guidelines, you'll have a much better chance of preventing eating problems for your child. If a child is already in the throes of overeating, you may be able to solve the problem utilizing the ten steps listed below. If you feel uncomfortable doing this on your own and need more help, don't hesitate to seek the counsel of a nutrition therapist who is trained in Intuitive Eating. (See the link to the list of Intuitive Eating Counselors listed in the Intuitive Eating Resource section at the end of the book.)

1. Ask your child if he knows what hunger feels like and where in his body he feels hunger. Tell him that most of the time, he'll feel it in his stomach, but sometimes he might feel it in his throat. If he's not paying attention, he might even feel it in his head! Tell him that, sometimes, people get headaches from not eating soon enough when they need fuel.
2. If your child is too young to get food on his own, teach him to make sure he tells an adult when he's hungry, so he can get the food he needs.
3. Ask him if he knows what fullness feels like. Tell him that his stomach is like a balloon filled with air. The balloon can be filled a little bit, leaving lots of space to fill it with more air, just as his stomach can be filled a little bit, leaving room for more food. The balloon can be filled with a little more air to make it bigger, just as his stomach can be filled with a little more food to make him fuller. Or either of them can be filled with so much air/food that it seems as if either could pop!
4. Explain that filling his stomach with enough food will give him plenty of energy to run and play, but filling it with too much food could give him a stomachache. You can illustrate that just as the car needs gas/fuel so that it can drive, his body also needs fuel to be active. If the car gets filled with too much gas, the extra gas will run over the side of the car. But for him, unlike the gas tank, too much fuel/food can make him feel uncomfortable or even sick.
5. Ask him if, after he feels comfortably full, he thinks that his body needs any more food. If he says "no," present a question about what

he really needs, since his body doesn't need the food. If he doesn't know, tell him that sometimes people eat too much food because they're bored, or because they want something to make them feel better when they're sad or scared. Help your child come up with some alternatives to eating if he's feeling an emotion that's leading him to avoid the feeling or soothe it with food.

6. Above all, never talk to your child about weight, and never put her on the scale. Talk about the immediate benefit of feeling more comfortable in her body if she eats according to her hunger and fullness signals. Do not talk to her about future health problems.

7. Ask her if there are foods that she'd like to have in the house, which have previously been forbidden. Tell her that you will buy those foods and keep them in the house.

8. Tell your child that you are going to back off from telling him what to eat, what not to eat, and how much to eat. Tell him that you will provide him with a variety of foods at a meal—some nutritious and some play foods. It will be up to him to have what he wants in a meal and how much he needs to take care of his hunger.

9. Let him know that you trust that he will eventually be guided by his own internal voice about hunger, fullness, and food preference. Tell him that you know that his body will help him know how to get balance in his eating. The more that your child knows that you trust his inner wisdom, the more he will eat in an attuned way, and the less he will eat in reaction to you.

10. Ask her if there is any kind of help that she would like from you. You don't want her to feel abandoned by you. You simply want her to know that you will no longer attempt to control her eating. She may say that she would like you to remind her to pay attention to her hunger signals, or to remind her to eat slowly, so that she can notice her comfortable fullness. Or, she may ask you to stay out of it. Honor her wishes!

WHEN YOUR CHILD IS UNDERWEIGHT OR RESISTING FOOD

Addressing the early stages of food resistance can greatly reduce the risk that your child will end up with a full-blown eating disorder in the future. (See Chapter 16 for more information on treating eating disorders.)

We frequently receive calls from parents who report that their children are not eating enough or that they can't get them to eat anything but "white carbs." They tell us that the dinner table (and usually all other meals) has become the battleground between the parents and the child. These food fights are preventable, and once they have become established, they are treatable.

But what happens if there has been a disconnect between the child's innate signals and the parents' agenda for eating? How do you take the eating experience out of the "boxing ring"?

Five Steps for Reestablishing Peace Between You and Your Food-Resistant Child

Your child's need to exert his or her autonomy, by rebelling against eating enough or eating nutritious foods, can often take precedence in the child's psyche. These needs can include the need to either please the parent or the need to eat enough to meet biological and/or nutritional needs.

1. If you back off on pressuring your child to eat more or to "eat better," it is likely that his rebellion will diminish and eventually vanish. Hunger is a very powerful motivator for seeking food, if the more potent psychological need to rebel isn't present. Trust that your child's relationship with food will heal, and he will begin, once again, to meet his hunger needs. It might take quite a while for your child to trust that you mean it, when you say you're backing off and leaving the food decisions in his hands. Seek help, if necessary, to support you during this stressful time.

2. Use the same strategy that was discussed above, in regard to beginning a dialogue with your child about the change that is about to take place. Let him know that you love him and truly believed that you were doing the right thing by trying to direct his eating. Tell him that because you have been worried that he wasn't eating enough nutritious food, you have stepped in to guide him but have found that your suggestions have only led to tension between the two of you.

3. Explain that one of the exciting things that you have learned is that he has all of the innate knowledge he needs to guide him to eat healthfully. Because of this new knowledge, you're going to leave the decisions about what he eats and how much to him, while preparing

and serving an array of foods. His job will be to listen to the signals that his body gives him about how much he needs to eat, and to check in with his body to see how he feels physically after making his food choices.

4. Assure him that you're not going to worry about his eating anymore, because you truly believe all of the new information that you have learned.

5. Once again, be prepared for the child's disbelief, excitement about the lifting of the pressure, and then distrust about whether you will really stick to your word. The more time that goes by without your comments, the more your child will trust that the match is over, and you will see a remarkable transformation take place before your eyes. Your child's food intake will increase, and the ratio of play food to nutritious food will begin to decrease.

Parents who have been engaged in food fights with their children have very challenging work cut out for them. They are worried about what others will think of them, if they see that their children are underweight or not eating healthfully. They are worried that people will think that they're neglectful parents, if they are no longer making comments to their children about eating. They think that it is their job to continue to push them to eat "correctly." But once they surrender and accept that what they're doing isn't working, they begin to take the first steps to healing their relationship with their children in the realm of eating, and helping their children heal their relationship with food.

As a caveat, there are some situations that require adjunct work with a psychotherapist, specializing in children's behavior and/or eating disorders. Unfortunately, we're hearing more and more about very young children who are being diagnosed with anorexia nervosa. If you feel that your child's eating refusal is deeper than a rebellion against being pushed to eat, then please seek psychological help. Also, if you suspect that there may be sensory integration problems (neurological problems with organizing bodily and environmental sensations—for example, a child having extreme reactions to different textures of food), then you may need to seek the help of an occupational therapist specializing in sensory processing dysfunction.

ADOLESCENTS

Adolescents are filled with contradictions. One day they can be delightful and almost childlike in the their openness and trust. On other days, they can be sullen and barely talk. Understanding the developmental tasks of adolescence is tantamount to helping teenagers heal their relationship with food.

In order to find their own identity, teens need a sense that they are emotionally independent from the adults in their lives. They attempt to achieve independence in many arenas—some that can be healthy, such as developing their own political viewpoint, finding hobbies or interests that are different than those of their families, or playing music that their parents hate. They may experiment with behaviors that are unhealthy—using alcohol and drugs, having sexual experiences before they're emotionally mature, and eating in a way that they know will anger and frustrate their parents.

Having fed my son (ER) a large variety of healthy foods throughout his childhood, I admired how well he ate in comparison to some of his friends. When he became a teenager, however, I was astonished to see how often he would stick a soda or some other example of play food under my nose, just to taunt me! I later learned, of course, that this was one of the ways he could exert his independence from his nutritionist mother!

We frequently receive calls from the parents of adolescents who are worried that their teens are eating too much, gaining too much weight, or are eating unhealthily. Some of the concerns that we hear range from parents hoping to help their teens avoid the unhappiness that they had experienced as adolescents, to parents who have been told by the doctor to monitor their teens' eating, in order to help them lose weight to avoid medical problems. We also work with many adolescents who have put themselves on diets.

Whether the diet comes from the doctor, the parent, or is self-imposed—it will inevitably have unfortunate results. Put simply, teens who dieted were more likely to gain weight in the future than those who didn't diet as adolescents.

- A 1999 study of teen girls who were followed for four years showed that the girls who labeled themselves as dieters at the beginning of the study were about three times more likely to become overweight than girls who were non-dieters (Stice et al. 1999).
- In 2003, it was found that binge eating was associated with dieting for both preadolescent and adolescent girls and the boys. In a

follow-up of three years, there was more weight gain in the dieters than in the non-dieters (Field et al. 2003).

• In yet another study of adolescents in 2007, it was also found that dieting predicted future weight gain. This study found an increase in binge eating and a decrease in breakfast eating for teen girls who dieted. Teen boys were also found to have an increase in binge eating, as well as a decrease in physical activity (Neumark-Sztainer et al. 2007).

Since dieting is not the answer, how can we help our teens to maintain their innate Intuitive Eating or help them get back on the right track to rediscover their intuitive signals?

Ten Steps for Promoting Intuitive Eating During Adolescence

Remember, that just as in the "terrible twos," adolescents are fighting for their autonomy. They are likely to rebel against anything that is forced upon them.

1. Provide easily available, balanced food for your teens. Keep a variety of nutritious foods in the house, as well as the play foods that your teen enjoys.
2. Ask your teens how you can help them. They may appreciate your help in making breakfast or lunch and by providing snacks that can be taken with them.
3. Involve teens in food shopping and in the preparation of meals. Many teens love to cook and are happy to be included in this experience.
4. Don't fall into the trap of telling your teen that he can watch television after school, only while he's having his afternoon snack. Pairing these activities can give a dangerous message. Teens need time to "chill" before beginning their homework. If you connect relaxation with snacking, they might learn to overeat as a procrastination technique. Some teens have reported that the roots of their overeating behavior began here. As long as they were having their snack, they were allowed to watch TV. In order to get more down time, they would continue to eat (and eat and eat). Let them know that you understand that they need to relax after their long day at school. Encourage them to eat a snack if they're hungry after school, and then suggest that

they do a relaxing activity before starting their homework. In this way, you are separating eating the snack for hunger from watching TV for relaxation.

5. Maintain family mealtime as often as possible. This can be a challenge when teens are involved in many activities that take them away from mealtime. It will still be beneficial if only a few meals in a week are eaten as a family.

6. Do not make mealtime the time to reprimand or ask too many questions. It is best for mealtime to be a calm and peaceful time to allow for optimal satisfaction and recognition of fullness signals. The best way to get a teen to overeat or to refuse to eat is to begin a fight at dinner!

7. Make no comments about what or how much your teen is eating. Also be aware of your own body language or body scanning of your teen. No "eye rolling"! Adolescents are highly sensitive to criticism and judgment. Even the slightest perception that his or her weight is unacceptable can lead to shame, attempts at dieting, rebellion, or even eating disorders.

8. If you notice that your teen is overeating, bingeing, or gaining weight rapidly, recognize that this may be a sign of emotional distress or unmet needs. Instead, spend quality time with him or her. Be patient, and let it be known that feelings are appropriate and may be expressed as much and as long as needed.

9. Rule out any medical problems by having regular checkups. If there is no medical problem, and it becomes clear that your teen needs more help, seek the help of a counselor, psychotherapist, and/or nutrition therapist who is trained in Intuitive Eating. Be extremely careful to speak with the professional first. Explain what you're noticing, and also ask about this person's belief about dieting vs. Intuitive Eating. Many teens have reported the onset of an eating disorder coinciding with seeing a professional who has prescribed a diet or a meal plan.

10. Be highly aware of your own relationship with food and your body. Never make disparaging comments about your body or spend time talking negatively about what you've eaten or about how much or how little you've eaten.

To illustrate the process of helping a teen move from resistance to making changes in his eating to becoming an Intuitive Eater, take a look at Bobby's story.

Bobby

Bobby was fifteen when he first walked through the door for nutrition counseling. He was a teen who had been referred by his doctor, with the prescription to lower his cholesterol and lose weight.

It was clear that he was a super smart teenager, with a fair share of skepticism. When he was asked what his goals were, he said that he was only there because the doctor had sent him, but he guessed that he would like to be healthier. Similar to many teens, Bobby exhibited a high level of sophistication and appeared to be capable of understanding the tenets of Intuitive Eating. As sophisticated as he was, however, when he heard that no foods were going to be forbidden, the grin that came across his face was priceless.

When the psychological concepts of deprivation and drive for autonomy were explained to him, he relaxed and was eager to share his story. His history included a report about parents who were overly focused on healthy food and exercise, countless attempts by these parents to get him to lose weight, and poignant tales of emotional eating that felt uncontrollable to him.

In the beginning, Bobby's treatment was centered on helping him find satisfaction in his eating. This meant paying attention to eating when he was moderately hungry, so that he wasn't in primal hunger when he started a meal. Additionally, he was guided to find foods that he truly enjoyed, and to eat more slowly, so he could appreciate the taste of the food. He set his own goals, so that his need for independence was honored. Bobby reported that he was eating unhealthy foods, which he was buying at school and not really enjoying them. One of the first goals that he set was to find more enjoyable foods, which would replace the foods that were not giving him satisfaction.

It was remarkable to see a young man suddenly take interest in eating more healthfully, after he had been told that all foods were fair game and that nothing would be forbidden. This was a boy who would regularly buy play food at school, as his parents didn't know what he was buying. There is that adolescent rebellion at work! He soon decided that he wanted to focus on throwing away food after he noticed that he was full. He had recognized that the food wasn't as satisfying after he was full, and he was committed to work on ending his meal at this point.

After several months of treatment, Bobby saw his urgency to eat foods lessen, because there was no forbidden food. He now trusted that he would always be free to eat them, if that was his choice.

Sifting out the eating triggered by defiance and rebellion freed him to look at the times at which he was eating for deeper emotional reasons. He saw that the anxiety that came with striving for excellence in school was the hardest emotion to handle. Now that he had a license to eat whatever he wanted, whenever he wanted, he found that he could deal with most other emotions, without using food.

Bobby identified ways in which he could find joy in life and realized that these were the things that soothed him more than food had. He also got more support for his schoolwork, which reduced his anxiety in that area.

When certain foods are forbidden, people often look for a justification to eat them, based on emotional distress. Once they have made peace with food, this justification is no longer needed, and they can explore other coping mechanisms.

Soon after this point, Bobby shared that his blood cholesterol was down to a normal level. It is important to note that weight loss was not the focus of Bobby's nutrition counseling. The focus was on helping him respond to his inner cues about eating and to help him separate his physical cues for eating from his emotional cues. (The psychotherapist with whom Bobby was working at the time was in support of his Intuitive Eating work.)

After about a year and a half of working toward reclaiming his Intuitive Eater, Bobby arrived at the office wearing a new sweater. He casually mentioned that he had to buy some new clothes, because all of his clothes were now two sizes too big. When asked how he felt about this, he talked about how great he felt that he was healthier and that is cholesterol had dropped. He knew that this had happened as a result of his own motivation to do his Intuitive Eating work. He said that it was the first time in his life that he wasn't being pushed to diet. He also proudly said that his cardiologist was so impressed by his progress, that he had asked Bobby if he would talk to his other patients and teach them what he had done. He then began a diatribe of his experience, including:

- "No one was pushing me to do this. There were no high stakes. I wasn't trying to please the doctor. It was me! It was my choice."
- "This wasn't a competition. There was no pressure to lose weight or get on a scale. There was no concrete number that I was trying to achieve, so there were no expectations. I haven't fulfilled or surpassed a goal. No one was focused on weight loss or was saying that I wasn't doing enough."

- "I never felt any deprivation." In fact, when talking about what he had eaten that day, he mentioned that he had ice cream.
- "I never felt guilty about what I ate."
- "This was a lifestyle change, not a diet."
- "Before this work, my mother told me that I would have to watch what I eat for the rest of my life."
- "People don't want to be ambushed in order to scare them. People don't respond to fear."
- "Instead of being told to lose weight, people need to be given the tools to know what to do and how to stop eating, when enough is enough!"
- "When people overeat, they're doing it for a reason. They don't want to be told that they're a bad person. It doesn't help. It hurts and makes them feel bad and have shame. Then they eat to push down that feeling."
- "People don't want to be pushed to do it all at once. The best thing is to start slow."
- "When people say a food is bad and you shouldn't eat it, you don't get the good taste of the food—you get the feeling of rebellion when you eat that food. That feeling of rebellion feels good!"

Out of the mouth of an adolescent babe! Bobby's explanation of his process said it all. He spoke to the concepts of deprivation, independence vs. rebellion, fear, anger, shame, etc.

MOVEMENT

There is an entire chapter in this book about exercise, or as we often prefer calling it, movement. Most newborns can be seen flailing their arms and legs. They're most likely attempting to stretch out, after their long stay inside the crowded boundaries of the mother's body. As infancy progresses, babies learn to turn over in their cribs, sit up, and eventually, crawl. They're eager to move around and explore all of the new and exciting things in their environment. Eventually they're walking and running, and they can barely be kept out of trouble. No one who has been around a small child can deny this natural desire to move. There are many explanations as to why so many children ultimately become inactive, but we won't reiterate them here. Suffice to say that an active family helps children to maintain their innate desire to move. Just like sitting with your children when they eat in order to model eating a variety of foods, playing outside games with the family or dancing together inside the house can do the same job for movement. Even as teenagers or, especially as teenagers, kids need to see their parents being active, as role models for movement.

If there were less focus on trying to control children's eating and more focus on families being active together, we might see far fewer sedentary children and teens and fewer weight problems. Just as eating is intuitive, the intuitive desire to move, with which we are born, needs to be treasured and nurtured!

The Intuitive Eating Approach to Physical Activity for Your Children and Teens

By following these five guidelines, you will ensure that your children establish a lifelong appreciation for movement in their lives.

1. Infants and toddlers have an intuitive sense about movement. As the years go by, build on this inner signal to move, in order to promote and maintain health for your teens. When possible, engage in family activities, such as taking walks, hiking, basketball, family camp, tennis, rollerblading, biking, skiing, swimming, etc.
2. Encourage your children to be involved in group sports, dance, martial arts, or other forms of movement, as early as possible. For example, the American Youth Soccer Organization starts kids as early as age four. Help your child find an activity that gives him a sense of identity and self-esteem, without promoting competitiveness.
3. Again, just as with eating, role modeling is imperative. You can't sit surfing the Internet or watching television all day. Find an activity that you enjoy, so your children will know that you practice what you preach. On the other hand, be sure that you're not engaged in compulsive exercise. Watching a parent who overexercises can be a surefire way to turn a child off from exercising altogether.
4. Be aware of the effect of extended screen time on children. Whether they're watching too much television, playing excessive video games, or even working too many hours on the computer, these activities will affect their chances for optimal health. The American Academy of Pediatrics (AAP) recommends that children under two not watch

any TV and that those older than two watch no more than one to two hours a day of quality programming.

5. Finally, physical activity should not be promoted as a weight loss device. If a child recognizes a parent's anxiety about the child's weight, any talk about movement being for purposes of health will be interpreted as movement for weight loss (and is sure to be resented and rejected).

PULLING IT ALL TOGETHER

Whether you have a brand new infant who arrived intact with an inborn set of intuitive signals, or a child or adolescent who has strayed from these signals, the happiness and peace of the child, as well as the entire family, resides in a commitment to Intuitive Eating. Give your child the confidence to know that you have trust in his or her innate ability to eat and move. Base your own relationship with food on Intuitive Eating. Parents are the primary role models for their children. Providing a wide array of healthy foods, when the children are very small, will ensure that they will have the opportunity to know that most foods can be delicious. Avoiding the labels of "good food" and "bad food" will help children make neutral food choices and prevent the sense of shame that comes with doing something they feel is wrong. Eating together as a family, whenever possible, and engaging in an active life together will put your children on the path to a happy, healthy, and well-balanced life. All you have to do is trust!

Chapter 16

The Ultimate Path Toward Healing from Eating Disorders

Eating disorders are not just a fad or a phase. They are serious, potentially life-threatening conditions that affect a person's emotional and physical health.

—National Eating Disorders Association

As you have explored this book, you may have noticed a number of references to eating disorders, especially comments about how dieting has been found to be one of the most provocative and powerful catalysts in the development of an eating disorder.

We have yet to meet a patient who declares, "I wanted to have bulimia, anorexia, or a binge-eating disorder." It usually starts off with, "I just wanted to lose a few pounds," which evolves into dieting, disordered eating, and finally, to a full-syndrome eating disorder. In fact, 35 percent of so-called normal dieters progress to pathological dieting. Of those, 20 to 25 percent will progress to partial or full-blown eating disorders. In the United States alone, it is estimated that there are five to ten million girls and women struggling with some type of eating disorder. In *addition,* there are one million boys and men with an eating disorder. These are conservative estimates from the National Eating Disorders Association.

But let's not focus on statistics in this chapter. Instead, let's get into the real lives and painful experiences of some of our patients who have plunged into the world of dieting. As a result, they then catapulted into a full-fledged, diagnosable eating disorder and have ultimately come to work with us in their paths to recovery. Before we begin their stories, however, let's look at how and when Intuitive Eating can be introduced and incorporated into the treatment of various eating disorders.

THE INCORPORATION OF INTUITIVE EATING IN THE TREATMENT OF EATING DISORDERS

Most patients in the throes of anorexia nervosa, bulimia nervosa, or binge-eating disorder have lost touch with their innate signals of hunger, fullness, and taste preference. For some patients who are medically compromised, residential treatment may be the only appropriate setting to begin the healing process. For others, outpatient day treatment may be the solution that is prescribed. For those who are deemed healthy enough to work with a registered dietitian/nutrition therapist in private practice, clients must be given the clear message that attempting to follow the principles of Intuitive Eating in a literal sense will lead to negative results. This is true, especially for those who are suffering from anorexia nervosa. The physical starvation associated with anorexia is often so grave, that an attempt to rely on certain intuitive signals can only lead to confusion and maintenance of the underfed state. Some patients love to say to us: "I'm only eating when I'm hungry, because that's what the book says (and I'm hardly ever hungry!)" or "I'm full after a few bites, so I don't need to eat more." We reassure them that they will someday be able to trust their hunger and fullness, but at the moment, their starved bodies are not able to give them accurate signals. One of the symptoms of starvation is slowed stomach emptying. As a result, ingesting even the smallest amount of food can create a false sense of fullness and push away signs of hunger. At this point in their healing process, we consistently emphasize the unreliability of waiting for the hunger signal as a cue to eat.

In the early treatment of anorexia, we attempt to feed patients in a very slow, deliberate fashion, so as not to physically overstress the body. We also don't want to overstress a patient's emotional state and create excessive fear. We teach them about the body's physiology and drive toward homeo-balance, the role of brain chemistry, fundamentals of nutrition, the mechanism of metabolism, and the potential dangers of undernourishment.

Along with our role as teachers, we strive to help patients feel empowered by becoming part of the "nutrition team." They are encouraged to give their input about food likes and dislikes, uncover what is a feared food rather than a disliked food, and plan the eating risks that they're willing to take. They can talk freely about their food fears and body image struggles and can reveal their eating "secrets," knowing that they will never be judged. They feel free to reveal the outcome of undereating vs. eating enough, as not eating enough is often the constant theme. In other words, the members of the "team" bounce the ball back and forth, as they move forward to the common goal. Conversely, if we were to give them a prescribed meal plan, written authoritatively by us, without their input, it would reinforce their anguish of having all of the control taken away from them. This feeling can lead to rebellion, anger, and a lack of cooperation. It also creates the risk that this meal plan will become cemented in their minds as the only "correct" way to eat. We guide them, advise them, and steer them toward finding a flexible way to eat. As time goes on, their eating choices increasingly originate from their inner desire.

Our patients are taught to take each setback as a learning experience, rather than a failure. They are consistently reminded that the healthier they become, the more they will be able to trust their signals of hunger and fullness and finally reclaim their ability to eat without anxiety.

The treatment for binge-eating disorder and bulimia begins in a slightly different way. If patients with these disorders are at a normal weight and not in a starved state, they will more rapidly be able to tune in to their intuitive signals of hunger and fullness than patients healing from anorexia. With bingeing disorders, patients have become accustomed to eating quantities of food that are larger than their normal needs. As a result, their interpretation of fullness is initially highly skewed. As they rarely feel hungry, asking them to listen to hunger signals can feel alien and frustrating. They so often have ignored hunger and fullness and are eating for many other reasons. These reasons can include boredom, loneliness, anger, etc., and often, guilt about what they're eating.

We also help our patients by putting on our nutritionist caps. We give them scientific information, in order to challenge their cognitive distortions and myths about food and their body.

For anyone with an eating disorder, Intuitive Eating can be presented as the model of eating that will ultimately become one's own. The vision of a future, free of obsessive thinking and compulsive behaviors, is very powerful. This hope can facilitate the patience it will take to get through the period of time that is needed for healing. The body must heal physically, and the mind must heal emotionally. We must emphasize the importance of working with a treatment team, which will require a commitment to working with a psychotherapist who has been trained in the treatment of eating disorders. A medical doctor who can monitor the physiological state of a patient is also critical in many cases, and, for some, a psychiatrist may be involved to evaluate medication need. In our work, we, as nutritionists, are a part of a well-oiled and communicative treatment team.

Now let's get into the lives of Carrie, Skylar, Lila, Dana, Laurel, Trevor, and a few other of our patients to see how their experiences with dieting led them down the path to their eating disorders. We'll then see how making Intuitive Eating their own has freed them completely from their fear of eating and of unnatural weight gain. Ultimately, this philosophy has led them to a happier and fuller life experience.

Carrie

One Friday afternoon the telephone rang, and the answering machine began to record a powerful plea from Carrie, who apologized for calling so late. She became filled with emotion, as she said that she knew that the only way that she would ever be able to fully heal from her anorexia nervosa was to learn how to become an Intuitive Eater. She had heard about *Intuitive Eating* on a Web site and, after reading it, was convinced that this was her last chance.

Carrie was almost twenty-two years old at the time and reported that she had been hospitalized eleven times in the past four years. Each time, she was kept in the hospital until she reached a normalized goal weight, yet upon release, she would immediately lose all the weight she had gained, only to be rehospitalized once again. At the point that she made this call, she had returned to a very low weight (not her lowest) and was dropping weight by the day. She was determined to never allow herself to go back in the hospital again, and that it was time to finally get well. She also knew that she could not keep doing the same things and expect different results. Carrie explained that each time that she had committed to regaining weight, she was haunted by the fear that she would return to a normal weight, without feeling the freedom to eat and trust that her body wouldn't betray her. A lightbulb had turned on in her head when she read *Intuitive Eating*. For the first time, she had hope that there was a solution!

During her first session, Carrie described her understanding that her eating disorder served her as a method of control, distraction, tension release, and running away from life. She believed that a big factor in the development of her eating disorder was a fear of growing up, getting married, and leaving her parents' home. In her words, "Contrary to the common belief about eating disorders, I had a very secure childhood and did not come from a dysfunctional family. I grew up in a loving family and had a very happy childhood."

Carrie was confident, easygoing, and liked herself and felt that she had never had any big eating and body-image issues. She reported being a picky eater but ate enough of the foods she liked to grow and be healthy. She tried dieting on several occasions, "just because it was what people around me were doing, and it was kind of an activity." The majority of the women talked about needing to lose weight and about which foods were "fattening" and needed to be restricted. Dieting was just part of her culture!

In the midst of high school, she was prescribed some medication for a medical condition that had to be taken with food. To avoid side effects, she forced herself to eat a large amount of food and drink a lot of juice, late at night. At this point, she also began to do some emotional eating to calm her fears. Soon she started gaining weight, and eventually gained a significant amount of weight. She then decided that she needed to go on a diet.

It's not difficult to predict the outcome of this story. The longer that Carrie dieted and lost weight, the more she liked having the feeling she got from controlling her food and her body. Her fears about growing up were pushed down by the achievement she felt by losing weight and by the false sense of control that this gave her. At first, her weight loss was admired by those around her. It soon, however, became evident that it had gone too far and that she was in a serious health crisis. She also went from being a popular, lovable girl who loved school, to one who was irritable, moody, and grumpy. She had become someone who now only cared about what she did or didn't eat and what the scale said each morning. Eventually, she was diagnosed with anorexia nervosa and was hospitalized for the first time.

In some of Carrie's early hospitalizations, she had no desire to get better. As a result of some beneficial psychotherapy, Carrie eventually felt ready to get better, and went into one of her hospitalizations with that goal. But it didn't work out as she had hoped. In her own words, she said, "Hospitals are not the answer. It's all a quick fix. I did not get to work on my mind long enough and did not maintain my eating and weight long enough for it to have any lasting outcome." One problem was that, just as the thought of going on a diet had led her family and friends to last supper eating, the thought of having to gain weight in the hospital led Carrie to "last supper restricting" before each readmittance. But, mostly, she said that she never really learned how to eat in the hospital. All she knew how to do was to gain weight when she was in and how to subsequently lose it when she was out. After each discharge, she would restrict food, overexercise, compulsively weigh herself and lose weight—all the things she was not allowed to do in the hospital. It was as if she were on a tightrope and could fall off on either side of the weight continuum. Go into the hospital and gain—come out and lose! She knew that if she didn't learn how to trust her body, she would always be afraid of eating and gaining too much weight.

So, where does one begin, in helping a young woman with a serious history of anorexia nervosa, who wants to learn to become an Intuitive Eater? The first step was to capitalize on what motivated her, and this was the freedom that she hoped she could achieve by trusting her body. Here are some of the guidelines that formed the foundation for how the principles of *Intuitive Eating* were used in Carrie's treatment:

1. **Honor Your Hunger**—Carrie could always trust that if she felt hunger, then her body was giving her a message that she needed to eat. This did not, however, mean that if she didn't feel hunger, she was getting an accurate message that she didn't need to eat. If this guideline was not emphasized, reemphasized over time, and believed—then the "contract" would be broken.

2. **Feel Your Fullness**—Carrie needed to accept that until she was at a healthy weight, her fullness signals were not reliable! With anorexia, there is slowed stomach emptying, which can lead to getting full very quickly and feeling full most of the time. She would have to accept that this principle couldn't be implemented until she returned to a normal weight.

3. **Make Peace with Food**—A commitment to taking risks and eating the foods that she had been restricting for years was something she could practice, even at her low weight. (When she began, Carrie was eating only a limited variety of safe foods each day.)

4. **Discover the Satisfaction Factor**—Eating foods that she wanted to eat and that were satisfying her palette would empower her and remove the rebellion that came from having been told what to eat. Rather than a rigid meal plan, there would be guidance in helping her figure out what she liked and encouragement to take risks incorporating these foods into her eating life. She would also be supported in

gradually increasing the amounts of satisfying foods she needed, in order to normalize her weight.

5. Cope with Your Emotions without Using Food—In Carrie's case, this would shift to learning to cope with her emotions without restricting food or getting on the scale. She would learn that pushing down her feelings by counting calories, cutting out foods, or getting on the scale could only give her a false sense of control and no solution to her problems. She would learn to talk with her therapist, nurse practitioner, religious leader, family members, and, of course, her nutrition therapist, instead.

6. Respect Your Body—Carrie needed to accept that starving her body was the antithesis of respecting her body. In order to honor her body, she needed enough food to nourish her and help her gain weight. Respecting her body would also mean accepting her normal, healthy size and not trying to change it. She also needed to throw away her "anorexic" clothes and make peace with the fact that they would never again fit her. She needed to buy comfortable clothes that would fit a healthy body.

7. Reject the Diet Mentality—Carrie had seen the ill effects of dieting on her family members, and she especially saw how dieting was one of the factors that led her to her eating disorder. All of the people she knew who were dieting were overweight. As a result, she knew that diets didn't work and that she never wanted to diet in order to manage her weight, but she had never had another alternative.

8. Challenge the Food Police—Oh, and there were many Food Police in Carrie's head. The Food Police spoke from the voice of her anorexia. She would have to challenge her distorted thoughts and replace them with thoughts that came from the logical, emerging Intuitive Eater within. She would have to let go of valuing perfectionism. She would learn to get right back on track toward her goal, every time she would revert to a restrictive behavior—this was a process, not a perfect, straight line to recovery!

9. Exercise: Feel the Difference—Carrie would have to learn that any exercise beyond her normal walking would be counterproductive to her healing process. She would learn to look forward to the time when she could trust her body to tell her how much movement was just right for her and to feel the positive effects that movement would offer her.

10. Honor Your Health: Gentle Nutrition—The healthier that Carrie's
body would become, the more she had cravings for healthier foods.
Ironically, Carrie had no problem eating play food. At first, it was
mainly play food that she craved. Eventually she would want to add
more protein and fruits and vegetables.

During her treatment, Carrie was repeatedly reminded that she could
not trust her fullness until her body was at a normal weight, but she was
also told that her hunger could always be honored. In her process toward
this goal she used every experience as a learning opportunity, rather than as
a failure. In this way, she stopped beating herself up for not "doing it" perfectly. When she would get extremely hungry very late at night, she would
take that as a message that she had not eaten enough during the day. When
she would get on the scale after being advised to abandon that practice,
Carrie learned that she would suffer for days with an increase in obsessive
thoughts about her weight. Carrie also learned that her meals did not sustain her if she wouldn't eat enough protein, or, at other times, enough fat or
enough carbohydrates at a meal. And, most importantly, when she had intermittent instances of losing weight, the message became very clear—eat
more! Carrie directed her own recovery. She was counseled about what
would make up a sustaining and balanced meal, but she was never told
what to eat or how much to eat.

Carrie didn't have the need to feel rebellious, because she was always
led to evaluate her own decisions and decide whether they worked for her.
In other words, with the goal of freedom ahead of her, she was motivated
to stay on her journey to becoming an Intuitive Eater. Having reached her
goal, Carrie has recently become a happily married woman, maintaining
a healthy weight, and hoping to become pregnant very soon. She wants to
shout her relief and excitement to the world. She is convinced that the gift
of being an Intuitive Eater and the freedom it brings surpasses any benefit
she ever gained from anorexia!

Skylar

Skylar was referred for treatment of her "anorexia" by her psychotherapist
at the age of fifty-seven. To look at Skylar at that time, one would see a
striking, well-dressed woman who did not look emaciated. Even though
she looked somewhat listless and had no sparkle in her eyes, she certainly

did not give the image of someone with anorexia nervosa. Yet, the thoughts and behaviors of this woman mimicked those that had imprisoned her from the age of fifteen. They had followed her through a hospitalization for anorexia at an extremely low weight, through gradual weight gain over the years, and finally to a normal weight for her height. This weight was reached with very little increase in caloric intake. Instead, as a result of inadequate calorie input to compensate for her caloric output, her metabolism had slowed down over the forty-plus years of her eating disorder. Her continual starved state signaled her brain to send the message to her body to slow everything down, especially her ability to burn calories. At her weight at that time, she certainly did not meet the weight loss criterion of anorexia nervosa. But her pattern of restriction, with its lack of sufficient energy intake, and her obsessive thinking and fear of food and eating, certainly qualified her as having an eating disorder.

Skylar's story began, as it does for so many of our patients who develop anorexia nervosa, with a history of being overweight as a child and then being delivered into the world of dieting as a way to "rescue" her from the fate of obesity. She reported being aware of a sense of being overweight at age ten. At twelve to thirteen she was counting calories with her mother. (As an aside, many well-intentioned, but ill-informed parents believe that restricting calorie intake or certain types of food will help their children lose weight and feel better about themselves. Unfortunately, in most cases, just the opposite occurs. Children end up feeling different, deprived, and frequently rebellious. And, as a result of these feelings, they are often led right into the trap of an eating disorder.)

At about the same age that Skylar began counting calories, her family went on a summer visit to her grandfather's home. Two other families, with whom her family was very close, joined them on this vacation. Within this group were three very thin girls of Skylar's age. Of course, the comparisons began, not only in Skylar's mind but also by her mother. Her mother was very focused on weight and told Skylar that she was eating too much. When the family got home at the end of this trip, Skylar was taken to the doctor, who put her on a regimented diet to lose weight.

In subsequent years, Skylar's food intake was carefully watched, except when she went to summer camp. At camp, she would eat freely but would naturally lose weight from all of the activity. There was no focus on weight at camp, and she never felt overweight. The summer she turned fifteen, she became very excited to go back to camp. It had been a very tough year in school and looking forward to the inevitable weight loss was a relief for her. After the summer, Skylar decided to take an active part in continuing her weight loss. She ate no breakfast or lunch, would only eat Jell-O during the day, and at dinner said that she was on a diet. In her home, dieting was praised, so there was no objection to her small food intake. Anguish and fear always accompanied the food she actually ate. Her solution to these feelings was found in spitting as much of her food as she could into her napkin when no one was watching and then flushing the food down the toilet.

Skylar's fear and obsessive thinking became so intense that she began not using water when brushing her teeth, as she was sure that anything that went into her mouth, even water, would "make her fat." She never used salt, as she was afraid that the salt would "get into her body" and cause her to retain water and become fat. Ultimately, all that she would allow into her body was one apple a day. Now, ironically, her mother was angry with her and would try to get her to eat, but Skylar would refuse. Finally, while visiting a friend who was in the hospital, Skylar passed out from malnutrition. She was admitted to the hospital for three to four days and was then discharged to the care of "Dr. Smith," who weighed her and told her she looked like a concentration camp victim and that she would never have children.

Little by little, Skylar began to eat moderately. She gradually gained weight but was getting on the scale two to three times a day. Ultimately, she stopped weighing herself and began bingeing on ice cream—the main food that she ate. In her twenties, Skylar began using diet pills and diuretics in her frantic attempt to control her weight.

At age thirty-two, and at a very low weight, Skylar moved to California. She resumed weighing herself, and as the scale kept creeping up, the powerful force of her anorexia grabbed her once again. She stopped eating and, subsequently, lost a good deal of weight. In her late thirties and early forties, she began to eat again, subsisting mainly on frozen yogurt. She finally began her nutrition therapy in her fifties. She was still in an extreme state of food restriction, had gained weight without increasing her caloric intake or variety of food, and was living with an enormous fear of food and further weight gain.

Skylar spent two years healing her anorexic experience. During those years, she searched for and eventually was able to rediscover her Intuitive Eating signals. Today, ten years later, Skylar continues to appreciate her normal relationship with food. She eats three meals and two snacks a day and regularly eats in restaurants—something that had previously gripped her with terror. She eats a wide variety of foods and restricts nothing. She has said that she actually prefers to eat a normal meal, finding it far more satisfying than her two pints of frozen yogurt. She exercises consistently, but not excessively and takes in enough food to sustain her during exercise. Sufficient food and exercise have helped her build healthy muscle. Honoring her body's need for proper nourishment has also sped up her metabolism. Skylar has maintained a healthy athletic body and has been an Intuitive Eater ever since. The years of being afraid to eat are gone forever!

(It is important at this point to restate that weighing oneself is contraindicated in the Intuitive Eating process. The procedure of weighing clients in the doctor's office or dietitian's office is used for medical necessity, especially in the case of anorexia nervosa, to assure that patients are progressing toward health. Patients are usually weighed backward, so that the numbers do not become the focus. Eventually, being an Intuitive Eater means that one trusts the body to give the accurate signals to know how much and what to eat—not the scale!)

Lila

Anorexia is only one serious outcome that can emerge from the world of dieting. Bulimia nervosa, or the pursuit of the elimination of calories after they have been consumed, often becomes the desperate solution to failed dieting. As you have seen throughout this book, there is an inevitable rebound of overeating that occurs after someone has restricted either a particular food, or quantity of food. In fact, nearly half of those with anorexia will develop bulimia, with binge-eating behavior. This rebound can be physiologically/neurochemically triggered, as a result of the secretion of brain chemicals, such as neuropeptide Y and others. Or it can be psychologically triggered, due to the rebound from deprivation that results from restrictive thoughts or behaviors. More often, we see both physiological and psychological rebound. Once overeating takes hold, subsequent to dieting, patients feel out of control and terrified that all of the weight that was lost will return. Or, even worse in their minds, they fear that they'll end up *yep* at a higher weight than before they had begun dieting. In this desperation, they will look for ways to rid themselves of the calories consumed from overeating or from a binge. Purging attempts include excessive, compulsive exercise, vomiting, the use of laxatives, diuretics, or diet pills, or starving for a period of time after overeating. (As a note, laxatives and diuretics mainly remove water from the body, not calories. The resultant dehydration gives someone with bulimia a false sense that she/he has lost weight. This dehydration is inevitably followed by rebound water retention. This then leads to a recurring cycle of dehydration, followed by bloating, followed by further use of these drugs to rid the body of bloat—and on, and on, and on. There are extremely serious medical consequences accompanying the over-use of these drugs, as there are with diet pills, purging, and even compulsive exercise.)

For Lila, dieting began when she was a senior in high school, as she and her girlfriends were preparing for the prom. Prior to this time, Lila always felt that she was a "bigger" girl, with bigger legs than those of her friends, but she wasn't overly concerned about this. Lila describes this time as one in which she was enjoying the "bonding" experience of going on a diet together with her girlfriends, so that they would "look good" for the prom. The daily meal plan for the girls included an apple for breakfast, salad with vinegar for lunch, and chicken and vegetables for dinner. They decided that they would do this for one week before the prom to "see what would happen." Lila remembered seeing an immediate weight loss in the week—for which she was elated.

Graduation came after the prom, with a subsequent trip to the Caribbean for three and a half weeks. For the first time in her life, she felt completely free and independent. It was a time for partying and eating and losing her virginity. She drank many piña coladas and ate excessive amounts of French bread and desserts—foods that she had previously been restricting. When she got home, she saw that she had gained back all the weight she had lost and more.

Rebounding from her diet experience, she continued her overeating during the summer before college. At the same time, she was navigating a multitude of emotions—anxiety about her newly found independence and sexuality and her impending move away from home. As a result, Lila continued to eat emotionally and to gain further weight.

Immediately after arriving at college, Lila became involved in a relationship with a boy that was to last throughout her college years. She also found herself going from a very active, athletic high school student who wasn't worried about life, to an inactive college freshman. She continued overeating, began actual bingeing, and had episodes of secret eating. She found herself thinking, "I can't believe I've eaten so much!" and began purging her food as a way to undo her out-of-control behavior. Since Lila did not lose any weight as a result of her bulimia, she never thought of bulimia as a weight control mechanism. She saw it purely as a means of erasing the results of her bingeing. (Note, quite a significant amount of calories are still absorbed, even if one vomits after a binge.)

Frequently, the experience of feeling out of control and consuming an enormous amount of extra food can become horrifying to a person. As a result, the impulse to eradicate any remnant of the behavior can become as compulsive as the behavior itself. As one makes purging a regular part of life, the sense of responsibility for one's actions disappears. As we have seen, coping with feelings without using food can be a very difficult challenge for many people. Bulimia, once discovered, sometimes begins as a seemingly exciting alternative to either dealing with feelings or overeating. Patients report feeling as if they're "getting away with murder." Of course, as bulimia progresses, with its mental and physical side effects (most seriously, its potential for death) and its influence on one's normal pattern of eating, this "solution" ultimately becomes one's nemesis. Very quickly, shame emerges. Hiding the food wrappers, isolating in order to find time for the bingeing, or stealing away to the bathroom when eating in public, becomes a daily ritual.

By Thanksgiving, Lila's bingeing and purging led her to her all-time-high weight. Although still involved with her boyfriend, she felt insecure about herself and about her weight. She began a hard workout program, once or twice a week and was alternating periods of starving with binge/purge incidents. By the end of freshman year, Lila's normal exercise turned into compulsive overexercising. Before going back to school, she sought the help of a nutritionist who helped her to curb her bulimia. During sophomore year, she joined a sorority and began a crusade to save her sorority sisters from the dangers of developing an eating disorder.

For the rest of her time in college, Lila was able to manage her eating and her exercise, was free of bulimia, and was maintaining normal weight. Unfortunately, after graduation, she moved into an apartment with two roommates, one of whom was an overeater and the other, a restrictor. It was a highly emotional year, as she broke up with her college boyfriend and was facing the stress of postgraduate life. With the influence of living with roommates who had eating disorders combined with the problems in her life, she felt depressed and went back to some of her old behaviors of restricting, then bingeing and purging.

In the healing of a serious eating disorder, we often see periods of time when the symptoms of the eating disorder return. These times are associated with periods of increased stress. This stress can be greater than the person's ability to cope with it. When this happens, one needs to see the return of symptoms as a red flag, which is not to be ignored. It represents a need to seek help in order to get back on the path of healing. And Lila did just that. She sought a psychologist at an eating disorder clinic who helped her to stop purging. Directly afterward, she began doing the work required to help her find her way back into Intuitive Eating.

Although she had had a respite from her eating disorder during her last three years of college, she had not truly made peace with food. She had become a careful eater, and a diligent exerciser. As her stress levels increased dramatically, she again sought the behavior of controlling her food as a way of giving her a false sense of control of her life. She also began overeating again, as a way of comforting herself and numbing her pain. And, once again, the bulimia had returned. At this point, Lila began to follow the guidelines of Intuitive Eating. These included a commitment to never diet or restrict again. As a result, Lila was able to discover that eating primarily for hunger, and respecting her body's signal of fullness, gave her an inner sense of empowerment. Choosing to eat what was appealing to her allowed her to receive satisfaction from her meals. She began to spend time with her feelings, rather than pushing them down. She found that by developing her "emotional muscle," she was far better able to cope with life than she had ever been while practicing bulimic behavior.

Today, Lila is a happily married woman with three children. She eats intuitively, includes healthy exercise in her life, doesn't weigh herself, and maintains a normal weight.

Dana

There are many influences that can become the catalyst for the entry into the world of an eating disorder. With Skylar, we saw that being an overweight child and counting calories with her mother led her down the path to anorexia. In Lila's case, dieting, as a bonding experience with friends, coinciding with dramatic life changes, was a powerful precursor to bulimia. Dana's story begins with comparing herself to others. Dana began to feel somewhat self-conscious about her body at about age twelve and began to compare herself to her classmates. In this comparison, she assessed herself as bigger than the others girls. By the time she was fifteen and in the beginning of ninth grade, or her first year of high school, she decided that she had to "do something to make a difference." This thinking coincided with several emotional traumas. Her parents had gotten divorced, her mother subsequently remarried, and then suffered a heart attack (from which she recovered). All of these events set the stage for eating and body image problems for Dana.

To complicate matters further, when Dana was at her dad's house, he regularly made comments about portion sizes and often told her that she had "had enough," even though she usually still felt hungry. Dana's mom had a natural interest in nutrition and regularly bought what she thought were healthier foods. As a result of her mom's focus on healthy food and her dad's investment in the amount of food she ate, Dana developed an excessive consciousness about food.

Dana had regularly enjoyed ice-blended chocolate drinks from the local coffee bar. Her first attempt at "making a difference" began by cutting out these drinks and was followed by cutting out one small item after another. As a result of these restrictions, she soon found that her clothes were beginning to fit looser. Concerned about her behavior, Dana's mother took her to see a nutritionist, who, unfortunately, turned out to be unqualified. Concluding that Dana carried a little extra "fluff" around her middle, the nutritionist inappropriately and incorrectly told her that her body couldn't handle carbohydrates. When she told her to cut down on her starch intake, Dana was eager to agree to the restriction. Dana complied even further, by believing that she should also restrict fruits, and even some vegetables, such as carrots! (Note: In many states, there are no legal requirements to call oneself a "nutritionist." Be sure that your nutritionist is, at minimum, a registered dietitian (R.D.).) Dietitians must have at least a bachelor's degree, postgraduate training, pass a national exam, and maintain continuing education.)

As anyone reading this might now predict, Dana continued restricting what she ate and how much she ate and began to feel fearful of many foods. Being fueled by her sense of accomplishment, her search for identity, and a false sense of control, she continued to restrict. She went on to cut out lunches at school, allowed herself to have only half a bagel at breakfast, and barely ate anything at dinner. While Dana had at first felt larger than her friends and was observed by the nutritionist to have "fluff" around her middle, she was actually at a rather low weight for her height! Not too many months later, her weight dropped to a worrisome level. By the time she reached nutrition therapy, her weight had reached a critical level. She was very weak, and her thinking was blurred by malnutrition. It was decided that she needed more help than she could get in weekly nutrition sessions and that she would need to be admitted to an intensive day-treatment program for eating disorders.

(As a note, a journey into the Intuitive Eating process must begin, not just with a motivation to heal, but also with a mind that is clear enough to understand what is taught and retain the information. Dana, at this point, was far beyond this ability.)

By the time the arrangements were made for admittance, Dana had lost even more weight. Unfortunately, day treatment was not enough to help, as she continued to starve herself on weekends, when not at the program. Eventually, she was admitted to inpatient treatment at a hospital that had an adolescent eating disorder program. After six months, she was able to leave the hospital, greatly improved. With more sufficient nutrition, Dana began to grow again, and grew two or three inches. She also saw a return of her menstrual cycle.

But, unfortunately, this was not the end of Dana's story. Although Dana's weight was restored to a normal range, she still held the fear of eating certain foods and of eating early in the day. Undereating during the day led to excessive overeating at night, accompanied by excessive weight gain. It's not hard to understand why she felt a total lack of control of her body and her life. Dana was now dealing with all of her previous emotional issues. In addition, being back in school, she experienced all of the normal issues of being a sixteen-year-old in high school. With this emotional angst, Dana continued to distract herself from these feelings by focusing on her battle with food and body.

Dana's overeating at night finally scared her so much that she began once again to restrict her total caloric intake. Fortunately, she was unable to maintain this serious restrictive behavior for more than three weeks. She then returned to her pattern of daytime under eating, followed by the inevitable nighttime overeating.

At this point, extremely frustrated and frightened, Dana was open to returning to nutrition therapy. Unhappy with her excessive hunger during the day and the discomfort that resulted from overeating at night, she was finally ready to make peace with food and eating. Since she was at a healthy weight, she very quickly began practicing the principles of Intuitive Eating and was overjoyed by the results. She learned that by not eating enough for her body's needs during the day, she had quickly fallen into primal hunger and was inevitably set up to overeat at night. As soon as she committed to eating sufficient amounts during the day, the nighttime overeating diminished. Added to this, once she embraced the belief that no food was her enemy and allowed herself free access to foods she had been avoiding, she found that those foods took a normal balanced place in her eating life. While working on Intuitive Eating principles, she also continued in her psychotherapy with her psychologist. In this setting, she was able to deepen her ability to cope with her feelings, instead of using food for this purpose.

By the time she was a high school sophomore, Dana became a stable Intuitive Eater. Dana's path began with a dangerous and frightening slope to climb. Because she was far too malnourished, her initial introduction to appropriate nutrition therapy expectedly suffered a quick demise. She required restoration of weight in an inpatient hospital setting in order to be ready for this journey. For the many patients we've seen—both female and male—the willingness to change entrenched habits and let go of old coping mechanisms could only begin with trust.

The office of the nutrition therapist must provide an atmosphere of safety and hope. Trust can only be developed when one believes that everything that he or she shares will be heard, absorbed, and not be judged. He or she needs to know that the nutrition therapist understands that any behaviors that are revealed, no matter how dangerous or even life threatening, were developed as a way to cope with a private world that was very scary or lonely or sad. Letting go of these coping mechanisms requires patience, a leap of faith, and a learning of new ways to think about food, body, and life. All of this is possible—these patients are just a few of the many who have healed their eating disorders with this work.

An eating disorder can potentially have a short course and be resolved without permanent physical and/or psychological damage, if it is treated with both psychotherapy and nutrition therapy in the early days of its inception. Unfortunately, there can be lifelong suffering and anguish, and even death for those who go without proper treatment. This can also be the case for those who drop out of treatment before they are fully able to embrace the Intuitive Eating philosophy. But, on the bright side, let's look at a few cases of patients who were able to catch their eating disorder early enough, with appropriate treatment, and come away more rapidly healed.

Laurel

In the previous case histories, we've seen many influences that triggered the development of an eating disorder. Comments by family members frequently have a powerful effect on a young person's body image. School pressures, transitions into new phases of development, and other life experiences often create anxieties that are calmed or even numbed by the overuse of food. Dealing with these emotional issues can also be avoided by putting the focus on under eating and obsessive thinking about food and body. In Laurel's case, a combination of illness and personal trauma set off her eating disorder.

Laurel was a healthy girl and a normal eater until she was almost seventeen years old. Just before her seventeenth birthday, she became very ill with tonsillitis, which decreased her normal appetite. Losing a few pounds led to positive comments by her friends. Liking this attention, Laurel found herself dieting for the first time in her life. She would tell herself that she didn't need "that cookie" or "that bag of chips." One month later, she got sick again, this time with the flu. Once again, she lost more weight and was given even more attention.

Soon after this, Laurel discovered that her boyfriend was cheating on her with her best friend—news that understandably devastated her. Feeling betrayed, she completely stopped eating and began to isolate from her friends. In the first week, she felt no hunger and lost even more weight. After that, even though her hunger returned, feeling so unhappy, she chose not to eat. She also began using laxatives, thinking that they would help to lose more weight. Laurel was trying to feel some semblance of control in her now out-of-control life.

Deeply concerned about her well-being, her parents sent her to treatment with a psychotherapist, with whom she had a wonderful relationship. She was also sent to a nutritionist, with whom she did not connect. She was given a high-calorie meal plan by the nutritionist, was told to weigh and measure her food, and to keep a food log. Unfortunately, this excessive amount of food caused rapid weight gain, with its accompanying "refeeding edema" (water retention that occurs when eating begins again after a period of starvation). In order to get some relief from her physical discomfort, Laurel began purging her food. Ultimately, she stopped seeing the nutritionist, stopped her bulimic behaviors, and stopped any kind of healthy eating. Instead, all she began to eat was candy!

At this point, Laurel was referred to nutrition therapy by her psycho-therapist. As in other cases previously mentioned, the safety that Laurel felt in this new experience led to a strong feeling of trust. With this trust, she became willing to absorb information that would help her change her thinking about eating and begin the journey to rebuilding a healthy relationship with food. Laurel was treated as part of the team in her recovery. She was told that, ultimately, her body was hers to protect and that a decision to get healthy again had to come from within. Clearly, it hadn't worked for her to follow an authoritarian recommendation. In her new treatment, she felt respected as an individual who was intelligent and capable of making healthy decisions. She also appreciated hearing that all of the behaviors she had attempted in her eating disorder were created as coping mechanisms to deal with emotional and physical feelings.

Laurel was taught about starvation's effect on her energy levels, immune system, sleep patterns, cognitive functioning, and metabolism. She was taught the many advantages of eating in a balanced way that would be respectful to her body but still include the play foods that she had come to love. If she chose to eat this way, she would prevent large blood sugar fluctuations, and she would be providing her body with the nutritional building blocks for making hormones, strong bones, immunoglobulins, muscle tissue, neurotransmitters, and more. She soon began to examine the trade-off between what she would be getting by maintaining her disordered eating and what she would be giving up.

Part of Laurel's disordered behavior included isolating, out of a fear of eating in public. Soon, she was able to see that this emotionally damaging isolation, along with her potentially physically dangerous current patterns, were far more frightening than actually learning to eat again. This time around, however, she began by taking tiny baby steps, rather than giant leaps. Adding a bit of protein to her day, such as a string cheese in the morning or some cottage cheese or yogurt at lunch was acceptable to her. It was not too much food to encourage excessive bloating, but it was a step in a healthy direction. Little by little, she added new foods, always working toward a balance of protein, carbohydrates, and fats. She began to include fruits and vegetables, waffles and brown rice and pizza, nuts and beans, beef jerky, and avocado. She also came to trust that she could include play food in the day, without tipping the balance. Little by little, she began gaining weight, with very little physical discomfort.

She practiced and rehearsed what it would be like to go to dinner with friends. Although feeling scared, she took the risk and got through the initial experience, feeling triumphant. Her friendships were renewed, and she accomplished the task of college applications, the joy of the senior prom, and graduation. Eventually, Laurel left for her first year at college, where she was preparing and providing food for herself, as well as eating out with friends. She was able to again experience normal hunger signals, regained a healthy amount of weight, and began, once again, to regularly get her period.

At college, as was to be expected, Laurel experienced a few emotionally uncomfortable situations. These experiences led her to an initial loss of appetite and a fleeting thought that controlling her eating might give her a sense of emotional control. But she very quickly remembered the conversations she'd had in the early days of her psychotherapy and nutrition therapy and was able to get right back on track. She stayed in touch by weekly calls and felt that this support was an important part of her transition into independence.

All of the stories we've told so far were those of girls and women. But eating disorders are not absent from the world of men. Let's now look at one case history of a young man whose eating disorder was not only triggered by some of the same factors as seen before, but was also influenced by the media.

Trevor

Trevor was a thirty-one-year-old man, whose weight was normal until the age of twelve. Problems in school and living with a dysfunctional family triggered emotional discomfort and overeating. Although his sister teased him mercilessly and called him disparaging names, he blocked this out and remained in denial of his compulsive eating problem. By the time he was eighteen, Trevor realized that his overeating had let him to an uncomfortably large size.

At this point, Trevor decided that he was going to tackle his weight problem. His solution was to begin taking laxatives, which he mistakenly thought would produce true weight loss. He knew that both his sister and her friend were taking laxatives, with this purpose in mind. He also knew that his mother was regularly taking suppositories. As expected, Trevor lost no weight from this dangerous practice and decided to join a health club to see if that would help. Unfortunately, he was lonely and depressed and was eating most of the time, again precluding any weight loss. At that point, he read a story in a magazine that said that a particular celebrity was only consuming orange juice as a weight control method. Impressionable, Trevor decided to try starving himself in the same way. (As a note, many people, especially those suffering from low self-esteem and eating disorders, often worship celebrities and project onto them a great deal of power and wisdom. They often admire their looks and copy their styles of dress and behaviors—a potentially dangerous act!)

At twenty, Trevor moved to California, bringing his starving behavior along with him. He began taking college classes in the mornings and would go to the market afterward to make a salad with nonfat dressing from the salad bar—his only allotted food choice for the day. As time went on, he changed his routine and began to allow himself only one bag of rice cakes per day. He began taking sedatives, so that he could sleep all day in order to avoid feelings of hunger, but his hunger became so intense that it would awaken him. Regardless of what Trevor ate, he continued taking laxatives and began to purge.

Soon, friends were telling Trevor that he was looking skinny and pale. This attention, no matter how negative, pleased him deeply. Eventually, the rice cakes were eliminated, and Trevor was in a complete state of starvation. Finding himself in such primal hunger, Trevor one day consumed an entire bottle of ketchup. At this point, realizing how sick he had become, he entered treatment with a psychotherapist, who referred him for nutrition therapy.

Although emaciated, Trevor still saw himself as the "fat boy" he had been in high school. He didn't believe that he deserved to eat and felt that food was like poison for him. Developing a healthy therapeutic relationship, Trevor slowly took the steps toward becoming an Intuitive Eater. In fact, he even felt so much trust during the first session, that he actually bought and ate a bran muffin directly after the session—the first of many steps on his path.

With continued treatment, Trevor became an Intuitive Eater. He came a long way from believing that the simple suggestion to eat was a ridiculous thought and that starving, laxatives, and purging were the only method of weight control for him. He accepted that throwing up what he ate didn't work for him. Instead, he saw that consuming balanced meals and eating regularly throughout the day sped his metabolism and allowed him to maintain a normal weight. In his psychotherapy sessions, he learned new coping skills to deal with his emotional problems. Trevor regularly reflected on his prior dysfunctional eating behaviors and never stopped being in awe of this transformation!

DEFINING MOMENTS

It is immaterial whether an eating disorder happens to a female or a male or whether it begins as a result of dieting to prepare for a prom or as an answer to avoiding painful feelings. What is most important is the ability to connect with a psychotherapist and a nutrition therapist. These professionals should be trained to understand the psychology of eating disorders and be able to offer a safe arena for the exploration of the thoughts and feelings that form the basis of a patient's relationship with food. Sometimes, during the treatment, there can be one defining moment that can affect the healing process profoundly. The following two vignettes illustrate defining moments:

Kelly was a college senior whose anorexia and bulimia were so severe that she had, at one point, reached a dangerously low weight and was purging anything that she ate. Under the threat of hospitalization, she had managed to increase her weight somewhat before she was first seen for nutrition therapy. She was, however, still firmly entrenched in her eating disorder and was still seriously underweight.

Although Kelly was extremely resistant to changing her habits, she was open to answering a question that became critical to her recovery. She was asked to explain what was her greatest fear in the realm of her nutrition therapy treatment. It was expected that she would say that she was afraid of never being able to stop gaining weight. Surprisingly, she answered that she was afraid of giving up her bulimia, because she used the act of purging as a way to reduce anxiety.

Kelly was stunned by the relief that she felt, when she reflected on two main facts: 1) She came from a normal weight family, and 2) She had never worried about her weight prior to the development of her eating disorder. Kelly was able to acknowledge that she didn't believe that her body could gain an unreasonable amount of weight. This realization became the defining moment that catapulted her recovery in leaps and bounds. As a result of her malnutrition, she was in an extremely depleted physical state. She was well aware that her energy levels were very low, that she was isolating from her friends, and that she was having difficulty focusing in school. If her poor health continued, she would be at imminent risk of being hospitalized, which would make continuing in school impossible. But, for the first time, she realized that she didn't have to be afraid of excessive weight gain! At that moment, Kelly became willing to eat again. She decided that she could focus on reversing starvation, even if it might take a long time to resolve her bulimia.

This shift did not occur as a result of being externally forced. Instead she decided that she truly wanted to get well and be able to maintain normalcy in her life. This new resolve was born from the epiphany she had had about her genetics. She had now become a teammate in her own recovery!

Kelly was now ready to take in more food. Her weight restoration and the return of her menstrual cycle were rapid. Along with this came an ability to feel appropriate hunger and fullness again—sensations she hadn't recognized for a very long time.

At this point, the time had come to work on refining Kelly's sense of satisfaction in eating. When asked if there was any one thing that particularly helped her during this period, Kelly's face lit up, and she said, "Yes, it was your story about eating a chocolate truffle during the movie, *Chocolat*"— one more defining moment! She loved hearing about the sensual experience of slowly tasting and savoring a delicious piece of chocolate, while watching a film about a chocolate shop in Paris. She had also seen the film, wishing that she could enjoy the chocolate—a food she had forbidden herself. With a commitment to make peace with food, as well as trust in her nutrition therapist as a role model, Kelly began an exploration of all the foods which she had restricted for years—especially chocolate!

After a year and a half, Kelly continues to maintain the weight that she had regained and eats with a freedom that she hadn't felt since before her anorexia began. In addition, her bulimic episodes drastically decreased. A large percentage of her bulimic behavior had been triggered by primal hunger and by the rebound from restricting the foods that she loved. Kelly's remarkable progress was attributed to challenging her destructive thoughts, honoring her hunger, and making peace with food. Kelly's ultimate goal of completely letting go of the bulimia also required continued work with her psychiatrist to find ways of coping with her anxiety, without using food.

Della, a beautiful and striking six-foot-tall twenty-three-year-old, had been in a battle with food all of her life. Taking after her father's side of the family, Della tended toward a stocky build. She always felt self-conscious about her body, in comparison with her ultrathin sister and also her mother, who was hyper-focused on maintaining her slimness. Della began dieting at age fourteen, beginning a roller-coaster ride of drastic weight fluctuations, diet pills, food restriction, compulsive overeating, laxative abuse, and purging, which lasted until she began nutrition therapy at the age of twenty-two.

In her first session, Della was asked about her favorite foods. She mentioned many nutritious foods, such as beans and soups and vegetables and meat, and then, guiltily, acknowledged that she liked candy, but could only eat it in excess. As the Intuitive Eating process was explained to Della, she heard that she would always be able to eat any food that she desired, even candy. At first, she had a sense of disbelief, which was soon followed by a sense of calm. Della has since said that this moment of hope was one that has changed her life forever. She knew that all of her attempts at weight loss had not worked and decided to give up the battle of weight loss and focus on "just feeling good."

She left the office with a resolve to quit dieting once and for all. Immediately, she experienced a quieting of her mind and a feeling of peace, which she had never remembered feeling in relationship to eating.

Although past experiences with losing weight gave her a temporary feeling of well-being, this couldn't compare with what she ultimately felt as an Intuitive Eater. After a year and a half of this work, Della still loved candy, but she no longer needed to eat the whole box—in fact, she never even thought about doing that again. Eating became a pleasurable experience. As she followed her hunger and fullness and taste preferences, she received satisfaction from her meals, enjoyed the small amount of play food that she desired, and never felt stuffed. All remained quiet on the front of Della's war with food and body, and her concerns about her weight disappeared—what a surprise!

As we have seen in hundreds of people, becoming an Intuitive Eater can have a powerful effect on many aspects of one's life. Many people, whom we've seen, have spent the majority of their waking moments thinking about what they've eaten and about their physical inadequacies. Some have used these obsessions as a way to distract themselves from difficult thoughts and feelings. Others have literally numbed themselves from traumatic experiences. Many feel shame about aspects of their eating disorders or about a body that doesn't meet society's current standards. For some people, the only emotion that triggers overeating is one that is associated with a feeling of guilt about eating itself. To their disbelief, once they are able to release this guilt, by making peace with food, their overeating vanishes.

Regardless of the source of overeating, under eating, or other behaviors associated with eating disorders, an unhealthy or uncomfortable relationship with food can impede one from moving forward in life. Through their journey on the path of Intuitive Eating, we have seen people change jobs, leave abusive relationships, mend bad feelings with friends or family, and simply regain or achieve, for the first time in their lives, peace and joy and contentment. Just ask Della, or any of the others mentioned in this chapter—each would tell you, without a moment's hesitation, that the trade-off is worth far more than anything they could have ever imagined!

READINESS FOR INTUITIVE EATING

Eating disorders can take from a few months to many years for healing to take place. This depends on how long you've had the eating disorder, when you're ready to seek help, and other mitigating factors. It's important to be patient with yourself. It's unlikely that anyone with an eating disorder can fully dive straight into Intuitive Eating. If you start too soon, without professional help, you may end up feeling scared, frustrated, and overwhelmed.

Here are some of the indicators of when you are ready to move into work on Intuitive Eating. Remember, this should be done in conjunction with your health-care team:

- **Biological Restoration and Balance.** If you have anorexia, this means weight restoration. It's not realistic to expect yourself to be able to regularly hear hunger signals, let alone honor hunger and fullness. If you have bulimia or a binge-eating disorder, this means moving from a pattern of chaotic eating to regular meals. Regardless of the eating disorder, it will usually take some sort of nutrition counseling with a nutrition therapist to get you back into balance.
- **Recognition that the eating disorder is not about weight or food, but rather something deeper.** Once you begin to accept this, eating will move into the realm of self-care, rather than a staunch attempt at defending its existence.
- **Ability to recognize and willingness to deal with feelings.** As you are able to identify and appropriately cope with your feelings, the need to turn to eating disorder behaviors will decrease.
- **Ability to identify your wants and needs.** As you are able to identify your wants and needs, the less you will need your eating disorder behaviors to fill that unmet void.
- **Ability to risk.** As your body begins to heal, both physically and psychologically, you will be ready to take and tolerate risks with your eating. For someone with anorexia, it may simply be eating a food without knowing its exact calorie content. For someone with bulimia, it might be savoring chocolate for the first time.

INTUITIVE EATING CHART
How Intuitive Eating Principles Apply to Eating Disorders

Core Principle	Anorexia Nervosa	Bulimia Nervosa/ Binge-Eating Disorder
1. Reject the Diet Mentality	Restricting is a core issue and can be deadly.	Restricting does not work and triggers primal hunger, which can lead to binge eating.
2. Honor Your Hunger	Weight restoration is essential. The mind cannot function and think properly. You are likely caught in an obsessive cycle of thinking and worrying about food, and have difficulty making a decision. Your body and brain need calories to function. Your nutrition therapist will work with you to create a way of eating that feels safe to you.	Eat regularly—this means three meals and two to three snacks. Eating regularly will help you get in touch with gentle hunger, rather than the extremes that often occur with chaotic eating. Ultimately, you will trust your own hunger signals, even if they deviate slightly from this routine.
3. Make Peace with Food	Take risks; add new foods, when ready. Do this gradually with baby steps.	Take risks, try "fear" foods, when ready and not vulnerable. (Vulnerability includes being overhungry, overstressed, or experiencing some other feeling state.)
4. Challenge the Food Police	Challenge the thoughts and beliefs about food. Take the morality, judgment, and rigidity out of eating.	Challenge the thoughts and beliefs about food. Take the morality and judgment out of eating.

INTUITIVE EATING CHART
How Intuitive Eating Principles Apply to Eating Disorders

Core Principle	Anorexia Nervosa	Bulimia Nervosa/ Binge-Eating Disorder
5. Feel Your Fullness	You can't rely on your fullness signals during the beginning phases of recovery, as your body likely feels prematurely full, as a result of slowed digestion and stomach emptying. There is also a feeling of being bloated from "refeeding edema."	A transition away from experiencing the extreme fullness that is associated with binge eating. Once regular eating is established, gentle fullness will begin to resonate. Note: If you are withdrawing from purging, especially from laxatives, the feeling of fullness may temporarily be distorted by feeling bloated from water retention.
6. Discover the Satisfaction Factor	Frequently, there are fears or resistance to experiencing the pleasure from eating (as well as other pleasures of life).	If satisfying foods and eating experiences are included regularly, there will be less impetus to binge.
7. Cope with Emotions Without Using Food	Often emotionally shut down. Food restriction, food rituals, and obsessive thinking are the coping tools of life. With renourishment, you will be more prepared to deal with feelings that emerge.	Binge eating, purging, and excessive exercise are used as coping mechanisms. Can begin to take a time-out from these behaviors to start experiencing and dealing with feelings.
8. Respect Your Body	Heal the body-image distortion.	Respect the here and now body.
9. Exercise	Will likely need to stop exercising, or might include gentle movement.	Overexercising can be a purging behavior. Moderate exercise can help manage stress and anxiety.

INTUITIVE EATING CHART How Intuitive Eating Principles Apply to Eating Disorders		
Core Principle	Anorexia Nervosa	Bulimia Nervosa/ Binge-Eating Disorder
10. Honor Your Health	Learning to remove the rigidity of nutrition— where there is a strict adherence to "nutritional principles," regardless of their source. Recognize that the body needs: Essential fat Carbohydrates Protein Variety of foods	Learning to remove the rigidity of nutrition. There is a strict belief as to what constitutes healthy eating, and if this belief is violated, purging consequences can ensue (if bulimic). Recognize that the body needs: Essential fat Carbohydrates Protein Variety of foods

Eating Disorders Resources

ORGANIZATIONS

National Association of Anorexia Nervosa & Associated Disorders (ANAD)
P.O. Box 7
Highland Park, IL 60035
Crisis Hotline: (847) 831-3438
Web site: www.ANAD.org
   An association of lay and professional people dedicated to alleviate the problems of eating disorders through advocacy, education, and prevention. One particular benefit of this group is that it offers over three hundred *free* regional support groups throughout the country.

National Eating Disorders Association (NEDA)
603 Stewart St., Suite 803
Seattle, WA 98101
Hotline: 1-800-931-2237
Web site: www.nationaleatingdisorders.org

Helpful Web site includes referral sources, links to other eating disorder organizations, and basic facts about eating disorders. A good place to start when trying to get information on eating disorders.

Professional Organizations

Academy for Eating Disorders (AED)
6728 Old McLean Village Drive
McLean, VA 22101
Phone: (703) 556-9222
Web site: www.aedweb.org

The Academy for Eating Disorders is a multidisciplinary association of academic and clinical professionals with expertise in the field of eating disorders. Their official peer-reviewed publication is the *International Journal of Eating Disorders*. AED's objectives include advancing research, advocacy, and prevention of eating disorders; and promoting effective treatment and care of patients with eating disorders and associated disorders. AED has some limited public information on their Web site.

International Association of Eating Disorders Professionals (IAEDP)
P.O. Box 1295
Pekin, IL 61555-1295
Phone: (309) 346-3341
Membership: 1-800-800-8126
Web site: www.iaedp.com

IAEDP offers education, training, and certification for professionals treating eating disorders. The organization also promotes public awareness of eating disorders and assists in prevention efforts.

Other Web Sites

Anorexia Survival Guide
www.anorexiasurvivalguide.com

Offers a very helpful (and *free*) monthly e-newsletter, *Eating Disorder Survival Guide for Parents*. Archives of past newsletters are available on the Web site. Especially valuable for parents with a child with an eating disorder.

Eating Disorder Referral and Information Center
www.edreferral.com
An easy-to-navigate site with many helpful topics on eating disorders. This site is free to the public, but professionals pay a fee to get listed on the referral list.

Families Empowered and Supporting Treatment of Eating Disorders (FEAST)
http://www.feast-ed.org/
FEAST is an international organization of and for parents and caregivers to help loved ones recover from eating disorders by providing information and mutual support, promoting evidence-based treatment, and advocating for research and education.

Gurze Books
www.bulimia.com
Run by a small publishing company that specializes in eating-disorders publications including newsletters, books, and workbooks. Free catalog upon request.

Something Fishy Web site on Eating Disorders
www. eating-disorders.net
A comprehensive Web site that includes online support and is often cited as one of the most helpful Web sites by our patients.

Chapter 17

The Science Behind Intuitive Eating

Based on the research to date, it can be argued that Intuitive Eating is a measurable eating style that may be beneficially associated with health indicators . . .

—Steven Hawks

When we cultivated the premise of Intuitive Eating, we reviewed evidence from hundreds of studies, which, in addition to our clinical experience, ultimately formed the basis for the ten Intuitive Eating principles. Although our original concept was evidenced-based (or more accurate to say, evidenced-inspired), it's really not the same thing as saying, "studies show that Intuitive Eating works." Until recently, that is.

To date there are over twenty-five studies on Intuitive Eating, with several more currently underway. In this chapter, we highlight some of the studies validating the process and characteristics of Intuitive Eating. For a complete list and summary of the studies, see Summary of Intuitive Eating Studies, located at the end of this chapter.

MEDIA IGNITES PUBLIC AND SCIENTIFIC INTEREST

Although our book was originally published in 1995, the tipping point for both research and public interest in our work occurred ten years later, triggered by the publication of two different studies on Intuitive Eating, which sparked global media attention.

In 2005, a professor of health science at Brigham Young University, Steven Hawks, and his colleagues published one of the first studies exploring

Intuitive Eating and health in college students (Hawks et al. 2005). It was a small study, in which women scoring high on an Intuitive Eating scale developed by Hawks and colleagues (2004a) were shown to have a lower body mass index, lower levels of fat in the blood, and a reduction in the overall risk for heart disease, compared with participants who scored low. In other words, Intuitive Eaters were associated with better health indicators.

In an Associated Press interview about his study, Hawks disclosed his personal weight battle, and that, despite his knowledge and advanced degrees, he could not keep his weight off until Intuitive Eating—which was instrumental in his fifty-pound sustained weight loss. The headline from that interview was, PROFESSOR LOSES WEIGHT KEEPS IT OFF BY EATING WHATEVER HE WANTS (Vergakis 2005), which ignited media frenzy. Very soon afterward, Dr. Hawks and I (ET) appeared on the *Today* show, discussing Intuitive Eating. Dr. Hawks also gave several more national interviews, including CNN, MSBNC, and the *Washington Post*.

SCIENTIFICALLY DEFINING AND MEASURING INTUITIVE EATING

In 2006, Dr. Tracy Tylka of Ohio State University published a large study on nearly thirteen hundred college women, which validated three key features of Intuitive Eating (Tylka 2006):

1. Unconditional permission to eat when hungry and what food is desired.
2. Eating for physical rather than emotional reasons.
3. Reliance on internal hunger and satiety cues to determine when and how much to eat.

Tylka's research was a big undertaking, because in order to assess and validate the key components of Intuitive Eating, a series of four studies were conducted. In the first part of the study, Tylka created and validated the Intuitive Eating Scale (IES) to measure and indentify Intuitive Eaters. Our quiz in Chapter 2, "Are You an Intuitive Eater?" is based on the results from this study.

Next, the college women completed the Intuitive Eating Scale, along with a series of other tests, in order to evaluate the relationship between Intuitive Eating and several indicators reflecting mental health, body awareness, and eating disorder symptoms.

Women scoring high on the Intuitive Eating Scale were identified as Intuitive Eaters. Compared to women scoring low on this scale, Intuitive Eaters were found to have higher body satisfaction, without internalizing the thin ideal, which indicates that Intuitive Eaters are less likely to base their self-worth on being thin. Intuitive Eating Scale total scores were also positively associated with self-esteem, satisfaction with life, optimism, and proactive coping.

Intuitive Eaters also had better body awareness, or *interoceptive awareness,* a process in which your brain perceives physical sensations originating from within your body, such as fast heartbeat, heavy breathing, hunger, and fullness. Interoceptive awareness also includes the physical sensations triggered by emotions. Every emotion has a physical sensation. For example, when you experience feeling scared, you may perceive a pounding and rapid heartbeat, or perhaps you experience an overall physical tightness in your body or chest. This emotional-physical connection is so profound (and accessible) that psychiatrist Daniel Siegel, M.D., helps his patients get connected with their emotions by first having them identify the physical sensations they are experiencing in their bodies. (Dr. Siegel describes this process in his book, *Mindsight.*)

Next, Tylka evaluated the relationship between body mass index (BMI) and Intuitive Eating scores. She predicted that individuals who eat intuitively are less likely to engage in behaviors that may lead to weight gain (such as eating in the absence of hunger, eating in response to emotional fluctuations, and situational factors) compared to people engaged in dieting behaviors. As expected, women with higher IES scores were negatively related to BMI, which suggests that listening to body signals in determining what, when, and how much to eat is associated with a lower body mass index. (Recall that several studies show that dieting predicts increased weight gain. So, this finding is not surprising, but it is validating.)

Notably, Tylka and Hawks, each independently, created and validated different tools to assess Intuitive Eating characteristics. Hawks's Intuitive Eating scale (2004a) has four components:

1. Intrinsic Eating (eating is based on inner cues).
2. Extrinsic Eating (eating is based on external influences such as mood, social, and food availability).
3. Anti-Dieting (eating is not based on diets, counting calories, or desire for weight loss).
4. Self-Care (body acceptance, taking care of body regardless of size).

The development of these assessment scales has opened up possibilities for other researchers to explore even more issues related to Intuitive Eating. These studies are described in the next section.

STUDIES INDICATE BENEFITS AND CHARACTERISTICS OF INTUITIVE EATING

Adolescents

Sally Dockendorff and colleagues (2011) adapted Tylka's Intuitive Eating Scale (2006) for adolescents and presented her findings at the 119th annual American Psychological Association conference. Dockendorff identified an additional key component of Intuitive Eating—trust; as in the ability to trust the body's innate hunger and satiety cues. In other words, it wasn't enough to be aware of hunger and satiety cues, Intuitive Eaters in this age group also trusted their bodies to tell them when and how much to eat. Given the growing food and fat phobia, trust may be a significant feature of all Intuitive Eaters, regardless of age.

Dockendorff reported beneficial findings of Intuitive Eating for this group of over five hundred middle school adolescents, which are consistent with Tylka's results on college women (2006). Adolescents who scored high on Dockendorff's Intuitive Eating Scale had lower: a) body mass index levels, without internalizing culturally thin ideals, b) lower body dissatisfaction, and c) less mood problems. Intuitive Eaters had better life satisfaction scores and experienced a greater positive mood. This is a noteworthy finding, as adolescents are particularly vulnerable to hormone fluctuations and peer pressure to fit in, which can influence mood and life satisfaction.

Health Properties of Intuitive Eater's Food Choices

Some critics express concern about one of the key components of Intuitive Eating—*unconditional permission to eat when hungry and what food is desired*. They assert that if people were "allowed" to eat whatever they wanted, it would result in unhealthy diets and weight gain. To address this contention, Smith and Hawks (2006) designed a study involving nearly 350 male and female college students and evaluated the health-related properties of the food choices made by Intuitive Eaters. Contrary to the expectation of critics, students scoring high on the Hawks Intuitive Eating scale

(2004a) ate a more diverse diet and had a lower body mass index. Furthermore, there was no association between Intuitive Eating and the amount of "junk food" eaten in the diet. In other words, Intuitive Eaters were not eating an unhealthy diet. Intuitive Eaters also reported taking more pleasure in their eating. Interestingly, more men than women were rated as Intuitive Eaters (173 and 124 students, respectively).

Health and Well-Being

Positive health psychology represents the pleasant end of emotional states, which include feeling upbeat, happy, appreciative, and has been shown by several studies to predict future levels of health and well-being. Moreover, these effects accumulate and compound over time, making people healthier, more socially integrated, effective, and resilient. Also, there are documented physical health benefits of such states, which include lower levels of the stress chemical cortisol and less inflammation. A study by Tylka and Wilcox (2006) on 340 college women showed that two core constructs of Intuitive Eating, (1) eating for physical rather than emotional reasons and (2) reliance on internal hunger and satiety cues to determine when and how much to eat, uniquely contributes to the psychological well-being including: optimism, psychological hardiness (an indicator of resilience, or the ability to recover from adversity), unconditional self-regard, positive affect, proactive coping, and social problem-solving.

The study's findings highlight the importance of a person's ability to detect and attend to their emotions and their biological cues of hunger and satiety, as detection and awareness of these states are uniquely connected to well-being. These findings validate many of the Intuitive Eating principles (*Honor Your Hunger, Respect Your Fullness, Coping with Feelings without Using Food, Reject the Diet Mentality*).

Intuitive Eating Holds Promise for U.S. Military

The U.S. Army conducted a promising pilot study on the merits of Intuitive Eating for its troops (Heilson and Cole 2011). Researchers from the U.S. Army–Baylor graduate program in nutrition evaluated both motivation for eating and the Intuitive Eating characteristics of one hundred active duty military service members aged eighteen to sixty-five years old. The results indicated that military service members with a normal body mass index scored the highest on the Intuitive Eating Scale, were more likely to eat for physical reasons, and relied upon their internal hunger satiety cues, whereas participants with above normal body mass index levels were inclined to eat for nonintuitive or nonphysical reasons. Because of these promising results, a larger study is underway, which will evaluate the effectiveness of an Intuitive Eating program to help break the emotional, environmental, and social connection with eating in the military service.

FACTORS THAT PROMOTE OR INTERFERE WITH INTUITIVE EATING

Studies show that there are many factors that influence Intuitive Eating, such as comments and feeding practices by parents and other caregivers, self-silencing of thoughts and feelings, body acceptance and appreciation, and cultural westernization. These studies are described in the following section.

Parent/Caregiver Feeding Practices and Eating Messages

Parental Feeding Practices. Galloway and colleagues (2010) evaluated the impact of parental feeding practices on Intuitive Eating and body mass index with a novel study design. Nearly one hundred college-aged students *and* their parents completed retrospective questionnaires of parental feeding practices regarding the college students' childhood. Examples of the questions included, "Did your parent keep track of_____:

- The sweets (candy, ice cream, cake, pies, and pastries) that you ate?
- The snack foods (such as potato chips) that you ate?
- The high-fat foods that you ate?

Next, the researchers measured the students' current body mass index and assessed their Intuitive Eating levels using Tylka's Intuitive Eating Scale. The results showed that parental monitoring and restriction of food intake had a significant impact on their college student's body mass index, emotional eating, and Intuitive Eating Scale scores.

Parents that monitored and restricted their daughters' eating had daughters who: a) reported significantly more emotional eating, b) had a higher body mass index, and c) were less inclined to eat for physical reasons of hunger and satiety. The association was different for the male college students. Parents who recollected restriction of their son's food intake had sons with significantly heavier body mass index levels, but they did not report higher emotional eating.

Once again, another study shows that Intuitive Eating is associated with a lower body mass index. The researchers concluded that controlling feeding practices by parents have potentially long-term consequences, and may contribute to the development of emotional eating.

Impact of Parent and Caregiver Eating Messages. Kroon Van Diest and Tylka (2010) report similar findings from a study on college-aged men and women. They created and validated a questionnaire, which asked students to rate the degree to which their parents/caregivers emphasized the following types of behaviors while growing up:

- Told you that you shouldn't eat certain foods because they will "make you fat."
- Talked about dieting or restricting certain high-calorie foods.
- Commented that you are eating too much.

They found high levels of critical and restrictive eating messages from caregivers were associated with low Intuitive Eating scores and higher body mass index scores.

These Intuitive Eating studies on parental feeding practices add to the body of research by L.L. Birch, which shows that when parents attempt to restrict children's eating, it backfires by disconnecting them from their natural hunger and satiety cues, ultimately creating the very problem they were trying to circumvent. These studies also support many principles of Intuitive Eating, including *Reject the Food Police, Make Peace with Food, Honor Your Hunger, Feel Your Fullness,* and *Make Peace with Food.*

Self-Silencing

Self-silencing is the suppression of one's thoughts, feelings, or needs and it is a gender phenomenon influencing women's mental health. The process of self-silencing is thought to begin in adolescence, a vulnerable time when body dissatisfaction and social pressures emerge. When silencing their voices, young women may begin to ignore or suppress physiological or hunger cues that are inconsistent with societal ideas of thinness. Expression of thoughts, feelings, or needs appear to be a critical aspect of healthy eating behaviors. Shouse and Nilsson (2011) evaluated the relationship between disordered eating, Intuitive Eating, and self-silencing and found that Intuitive Eating is maximized when a woman has high levels of emotional awareness, combined with low levels of self-silencing. However, when high emotional awareness was coupled with more self-silencing, participants had more disordered eating and less Intuitive Eating. The researchers believe that when women have clarity about their thoughts and feelings, but silence their voices, hunger signals may become confused, which may decrease trust of internal signals of hunger and satiation. The most intuitive and least disordered eaters in the study displayed high emotional awareness and low self-silencing.

The results of this study validate the principles: *Challenge the Food Police* and *Cope with Your Emotions without Using Food*.

ACCEPTANCE AND BODY APPRECIATION

While the ability to eat intuitively is inborn, the likelihood of remaining an Intuitive Eater is influenced by the environment, which includes family, friends, and culture. Intuitive Eating can be thwarted by an environment that lacks acceptance and/or imposes rigid rules for eating that ignore a person's inner experience (such as hunger or satisfaction). Furthermore, when people encourage others to be critical of their bodies, they (women especially) learn to eat in a disconnected manner in an attempt to regulate their appearance, instead of listening to their bodies. Additionally, pressure to lose weight by family members, friends, and culture (in lieu of body acceptance) contributes to focusing on appearance-related eating. Many people are surprised to learn that body compliments can be a form of judging a person by their appearance, such as "You look great—how much weight did you lose?" or "I wish I had a body like yours."

Acceptance Model of Intuitive Eating. A series of studies by Tracy Tylka and colleagues (Avalos and Tylka 2006, Augustus-Horvath and Tylka 2011), on nearly six hundred college women and eight hundred women ages eighteen to sixty-five years old, respectively, found that placing emphasis on body function and body appreciation are key ways to translate body acceptance into Intuitive Eating behaviors.

When women emphasize the functionality of their bodies over appearance, they are more inclined to eat according to their body's biological cues. Furthermore, they found that adopting an attitude of body appreciation predicted Intuitive Eating, because favorable body attitudes are associated with greater awareness of body signals, combined with a greater tendency to honor these signals. Their research indicates that it is important to promote a positive body orientation, which focuses on body appreciation and body functionality, rather than appearance, which in turn, facilitates Intuitive Eating.

Tylka and colleagues found that body appreciation was uniquely and positively related to Intuitive Eating in a wide variety of age groups for women. They identified four hallmarks of body appreciation:

1. Possessing a favorable opinion of the body despite size and perceived imperfections.
2. Being aware of and attentive to the body's needs.
3. Engaging in healthy behaviors to take care of the body.
4. Protecting the body by rejecting unrealistic media body ideals.

Tylka and colleagues believe that it is important to challenge Western promulgation of the thin ideal stereotype and promote acceptance of a diversity of body sizes.

Cultural Acceptance. A fascinating series of multicultural studies by Hawks and colleagues indicate that prior to and during the early stages of westernization, individuals from their native countries are *natural Intuitive Eaters,* but this process of eating is sacrificed at the expense of the westernized thin ideal (Hawks et al. 2004b, Madanat and Hawks 2004). During acculturation, the westernized standard of beauty becomes internalized, via the bombardment of unrealistic media images of thinness, and indigenous Intuitive Eating styles erode away, toward external cues of eating, both of which can lead to obesity and eating disorders.

These acceptance studies support and validate Principle 7—*Respect Your Body.*

What about Men? Many of the Intuitive Eating studies have been conducted on women, or on mixed groups of men and women, but not men only.

There are studies underway exploring Intuitive Eating issues in men. A preliminary study on 181 college men by Gast and colleagues (in press) found that men scoring high on the Hawks's Intuitive Eating Scale were associated with a lower body mass index, compared to men with low Intuitive Eating scores. The men also placed more value on being physically fit and healthy, rather than on an ideal weight. The researchers suggested that Intuitive Eating seems ideally suited for men because it builds on men's anti-dieting views (men often perceive dieting behaviors as feminine), and builds on self-care fitness beliefs that appear to be more likely held by men.

Together the results from these studies show that Intuitive Eaters have many attributes associated with both physical and mental health, as summarized below.

INTUITIVE EATING CHARACTERISTICS	
This chart summarizes the research findings of characteristics associated with Intuitive Eating.	
Intuitive Eaters have lower	Intuitive Eaters have higher
• Body Mass Index • Internalized culturally thin ideal • Triglycerides • Disordered eating • Emotional eating • Self-silencing (suppressing one's thoughts, feelings, and needs)	• Self-esteem • Well-being and optimism • Variety of foods eaten • Body appreciation and acceptance • HDL (good cholesterol) • Interoceptive awareness • Pleasure from eating • Proactive coping • Psychological hardiness • Unconditional self-regard

STUDIES ON BINGE-EATING TREATMENT AND EATING DISORDER PREVENTION

Up until recently, research on eating disorders has been pathology and symptom-based, without considering positive eating behaviors. But in 2006, Tylka and Wilcox evaluated the constructs of Intuitive Eating and concluded that they were distinct and contributed uniquely to psychological well-being—and that Intuitive Eating is more than the absence of eating disorder symptoms. Furthermore, they recommended that Intuitive Eating be part of the educational process for treating eating disorders, as it could contribute to the patient's ability to flourish and thrive in recovery.

A recent study (Young 2011) found that the Intuitive Eating model is a promising approach for eating disorder prevention on college campuses. Intuitive Eating was found to have more appeal because it did not have the perceived stigma of "eating disorders," which is less threatening for voluntary student participation.

Binge-Eating Treatment

A promising study by Laura Smitham from the University of Notre Dame used an eight-week Intuitive Eating program (based on our book) for treating thirty-one women diagnosed with binge-eating disorder (Smitham 2008). The results of this study showed a significant reduction in binge eating, so much so, that the women no longer met the diagnostic criteria for binge-eating disorder. A caveat of this study was that there was no control comparison group.

However, there were control comparison groups for two larger studies on binge eaters, using an approach similar to an Intuitive Eating process, which also resulted in a significant reduction in binge eating (Kristeller and Wolever 2011). The treatment process used was Mindfulness Based-Eating Awareness Training (MB-EAT), which was developed by Jean Kristeller, Ph.D., and it shares a significant number of features with Intuitive Eating, as shown in the table on page 292. Although the MB-EAT training program does not have a specific "Reject the Diet" component, Kristeller agrees that dieting interferes with mind-body attunement, and this hazard is reinforced many times throughout her program.

Intuitive Eating—the Solution for Prevention of Eating Disorders and Obesity

Because of the growing body of research, indicating that Intuitive Eaters eat diverse foods, have better self-esteem, healthier weights, better psychological hardiness, and reduced eating disorder symptomatology—we believe that Intuitive Eating can be the unifying solution to prevent both eating disorders and obesity.

We are afraid that the well-meaning public health policies fighting the "war on obesity" may create unintended problems, from perpetuating

SIMILARITIES BETWEEN MB-EAT AND INTUITIVE EATING PRINCIPLES	
Mindfulness Based-Eating Awareness Training Components	Intuitive Eating Principles
Hunger Awareness Training	Honor Your Hunger
Taste and Enjoyment of Eating	Discover the Satisfaction Factor
Awareness of Fullness	Respect Your Fullness
Food Choices Based on Liking and Health	Satisfaction, Make Peace with Food, Honor Health with Gentle Nutrition
Nonjudgmental Awareness of Eating	Challenge the Food Police
Meet Emotional Needs in Healthy Way	Cope with Your Feelings without Using Food
Acceptance and Nonjudgment of Body	Respect Your Body
Gentle Exercise	Exercise—Feel the Difference

greater weight gain to increasing the risk of eating disorders, the hazards of which are documented in a position statement by the Academy for Eating Disorders. Public health policies promote external solutions, rather than attunement of food, mind, and body. They also tend to promote weight stigma and body dissatisfaction, both of which are risk factors for eating disorders and obesity.

SUMMARY OF INTUITIVE EATING STUDIES

There are more than twenty-five studies on Intuitive Eating, with research currently underway. These annotated studies are listed alphabetically, by the first author.

Augustus-Horvath, C. L., and Tylka, T. L. (2011). The acceptance model of intuitive eating: A comparison of women in emerging adulthood, early adulthood, and middle adulthood. *Journal of Counseling Psychology,* 58, 110–125.

Body acceptance by others was found to help women appreciate their own body and resist adopting an observer's perspective of their body, which contributes to eating intuitively.

Avalos, L., and Tylka, T. L. (2006). Exploring a model of intuitive eating with college women. *Journal of Counseling Psychology*, 53, 486–497.
Unconditional acceptance with an emphasis on body function and body appreciation predicted Intuitive Eating.

Bacon, L. et al. (2005). Size acceptance and intuitive eating improves health for obese, female chronic dieters. *Journal of the American Dietetic Association*, 105, 929–936.
Two-year study demonstrates non-dieting methods improves health for obese chronic dieters.

Cole, R. E., and Horacek, T. (2010). Effectiveness of the "my body knows when" intuitive-eating pilot program. *American Journal Health of Behavior*, 34(3), 286–297.
This study evaluated the effectiveness of an Intuitive Eating program tailored to assist military spouses in rejecting the dieting mentality. The program was able to significantly transition participants away from a dieting mentality toward Intuitive Eating lifestyle behaviors.

Dockendorff, S. A. et al. (Aug. 2011). *Intuitive Eating Scale for Adolescents: Factorial and Construct Validity*. Paper presented at the 119th annual American Psychological Association conference, Washington, DC.
Tylka's Intuitive Eating scale was adopted for adolescents, and Intuitive Eating was associated with health benefits including lower body mass index, without internalizing the thin ideal, positive mood, and greater life satisfaction.

Galloway A. T., Farrow, C. V., and Martz D. M. (2010). Retrospective reports of child feeding practices, current eating behaviors, and BMI in college students. *Behavior and Psychology* (formerly *Obesity*), 18(7), 1330–1335.
Nearly one hundred college-aged students and their parents completed retrospective questionnaires of parental feeding practices regarding the college students' childhood. The results showed that parental monitoring and restriction of food intake had a significant impact on their

college student's body mass index, emotional eating, and Intuitive Eating scale scores.

Gast, J., Madanat H., and Nielson A. (in press). Are men more intuitive when it comes to eating and physical activity? *American Journal of Men's Health.*
Men scoring high on Hawks's Intuitive Eating scale was associated with lower body mass index. Men placed value on being physically fit and healthy, rather than on an ideal weight.

Hahn, K. O., Wiseman M. C., Hendrickson J., Phillips J. C. and Hayden E. W. (2012). Intuitive eating and college female athletes. *Psychology of Women Quarterly*
Preliminary data indicate favorable results between Intuitive Eating and collegiate female athletes. [Personal communication with J. Phillips, March 10, 2011.]

Hawks, S. R., Madanat, H., Hawks, J., and Harris, A. (2005). The relationship between intuitive eating and health indicators among college women. *American Journal of Health Education,* 36, 331–336.
Intuitive Eating was associated with reduced body mass index, lower serum triglyceride levels, and with reduced risk for overall risk for heart disease.

Hawks, S. R., Merrill, R. M., and Madanat, H. N. (2004a). The intuitive eating validation scale: preliminary validation. *American Journal of Health Education,* 35, 90–98.
This study developed a scale to define and operationalize Intuitive Eating. Intuitive Eating is a valid orientation that can help individuals regain a normal relationship with food and achieve a healthy body size, when dieting so far has been ineffective or even harmful.

Hawks, S. R., Merrill, R. M., Miyagawa, T., Suwanteerangkul, J., Guarin, C. M., and Shaofang, C (2004b). Intuitive eating and the nutrition transition in Asia. *Asia Pacific Journal of Clinical Nutrition,* 13, 194–203.
The Intuitive Eating scale (IES), a measure of food consumption that is primarily characterized by the satisfaction of physical hunger, was used to evaluate agreement with Intuitive Eating principles in the U.S. and four Asian countries.

Heileson, J. L., and Cole, R. (2011). Assessing motivation for eating and intuitive eating in military service members. *Journal of the American Dietetic Association*, 111 (9 Supplement), page A26.

Intuitive Eating was associated with lower body mass index levels in one hundred active military troops.

Kroon Van Diest, A. M., and Tylka, T. (2010). The caregiver eating messages scale: development and psychometric investigation. *Body Image,* 7, 317–326.
Critical and restrictive caregiver messages were negatively associated with Intuitive Eating.

MacDougall, E. C. (2010). An Examination of a Culturally Relevant Model of Intuitive Eating with African-American College Women. University of Akron. Dissertation, 218 pages.
The present study explores the model Intuitive Eating with African-American college women. Results of the present show that Intuitive Eating may extend and generalize to more diverse cultures.

Madanat, H. N., and Hawks, S. R. (2004). Validation of the arabic version of the intuitive eating scale. *Global Health Promotion* (formerly *Promotion and Education),* 11, 152–157.
The Hawks Intuitive Eating Scale was validated for a completely different culture, and may be an appropriate tool to assess Intuitive Eating status among Arabs.

Madden, C. E., et al. (2012) Eating in response to hunger and satiety signals is related to BMI in a nationwide sample of 1601 mid-age New Zealand women. *Public Health Nutrition*, Mar 23:1–8.
Women with high Intuitive Eating Scale (IES) scores had significantly lower body mass index, which suggests that people who eat in response to hunger and satiety cues, have unconditional permission to eat, and cope with feelings without food, are less likely to engage in eating behaviors that lead to weight gain.

Mensinger, J. (2009, November) Intuitive eating: A novel health promotion strategy for obese women. Paper presented at the American Public Health annual conference in Philadelphia.
Intuitive Eating is a novel health improvement strategy that considers the temporality of dieting and negative consequence of weight cycling.

Sarah, H., Shouse S. J., and Nilsson, J. (2011). Self-silencing, emotional awareness, and eating behaviors in college women. *Psychology of Women Quarterly,* 35, 451–457.

Expression of thoughts, feelings, or needs seems to be a critical aspect of healthy eating behaviors. The suppression of voice, combined with high levels of emotional awareness, may decrease trust of internal signals of hunger and satiation and disrupt Intuitive Eating. Intuitive Eating is maximized when a woman has high levels of emotional awareness and low levels of self-silencing. Conversely, Intuitive Eating is disrupted.

Smith M. H., et al. (2010, May). Validation of Two Intuitive Eating Scales Among Females Receiving Inpatient Eating Disorder Treatment. Paper presented at the 2010 annual ICED conference, Salzburg, Austria.

Validation of Intuitive Eating scales in a clinical population provides strong foundation for further examination of the role of Intuitive Eating in prevention and intervention of eating disorders, as well as highlights the rationale for the inclusion of Intuitive Eating principles in inpatient, residential, and outpatient eating disorder treatment.

Smith, T. S., and Hawks, S. R. (2006). Intuitive eating, diet composition, and the meaning of food in healthy weight promotion. *American Journal of Health Education,* 37, 130–136.

Higher intuitive Eating scores were associated with an increase in the enjoyment and pleasure of eating, lower BMI, less dieting, and reduced anxiety over food.

Smitham, L. (2008). Evaluating an Intuitive Eating Program for Binge Eating Disorder: A Benchmarking Study. University of Notre Dame. Dissertation, November 26, 2008.

An eight-week Intuitive Eating intervention program was used on thirty-one women meeting the DSM-IV criteria for Binge Eating Disorder (BED). Overall, the women experienced significant improvement, with a significant reduction in binge eating.

Tylka, T. L. (2006). Development and psychometric evaluation of a measure of intuitive eating. *Journal of Counseling Psychology,* 53, 226–240.

Seminal study identified the three key components of Intuitive Eaters and associated health benefits. Intuitive Eaters were found to be more optimistic, had better self-esteem, a lower body mass index (BMI), and were less likely to internalize the culture's unrealistic thin ideal.

Tylka, T. L., and Wilcox, J. A. (2006). Are intuitive eating and eating disorder symptomatology opposite poles of the same construct? *Journal of Counseling Psychology,* 53, 474–485.

Intuitive Eating and trust in responding to hunger and satiety cues predicts psychological health above and beyond disordered eating.

Tylka, T. L. (in press). A psychometric evaluation of the Intuitive Eating
scale with college men.
Two preliminary studies on men and Intuitive Eating and on the Intuitive Eating Scale indicate promising effectiveness.

Tylka, T. L., and Wei, M. (in press). Do perceived social support and self-
esteem mediate the relationship between attachment and Intuitive Eating?
Wei, M., and Tylka, T. L. (in press). Do perceived body acceptance by
others and body appreciation mediate the relationship between attachment and Intuitive Eating?

Weigensberg, M. J. (2009). Intuitive Eating Is Associated with Decreased
Adiposity (Abstract). http://professional.diabetes.org/Abstracts_Display.
aspx?TYP=1&CID=72812 [accessed 12-30-2011].
Intuitive Eating was associated with lower adiposity and less insulin resistance, especially for girls who valued general health more highly
than physical appearance.

Young, S. (2011). Promoting healthy eating among college women:
Effectiveness of an intuitive eating intervention. Iowa State University.
147 pages. Dissertation. AAT 3418683.
This is the first study to evaluate the effectiveness of an Intuitive Eating
program designed to increase normative eating behaviors and reduce
eating disorder risk factors. Overall, these results indicate that the Intuitive Eating model can be a promising approach for disordered eating
prevention on college campuses.

Epilogue

This may be the end of the book, but if you choose to become an Intuitive Eater, it becomes a new beginning.

Take the journey to becoming an Intuitive Eater, and you will go through a process that is bound to challenge some of your most entrenched thoughts, and perhaps stir up some deeply hidden feelings and fears. You know that living in a world of dieting chaos with its self-blame and failure doesn't work. It doesn't work metabolically or emotionally, and it certainly doesn't work spiritually. Clients talk over and over about feeling beaten down, defeated—as if their souls are actually hurting. By the time they come to this process, many have given up hope of ever being a normal eater.

Intuitive Eating is an empowering process, which not only promotes health, but is also your gateway to freedom. When you are freed from the tyranny of food and body anxiety, you have the space and renewed energy to pursue your dreams and discover your purpose in life. But becoming an Intuitive Eater requires a highly conscious decision and commitment. It means letting go of the old way of surviving and opening up to a new way of viewing life. It might take soul searching and introspective work to decide whether dieting has been keeping you from your deepest appreciation of life. Making this viewpoint change can be difficult to accomplish initially, but can ultimately become a way of living that knows no return.

To begin this paradigm shift, you'll need to consider that there are many trade-offs in the eating world. Having the "willpower" to stay on a diet can give you a temporary sense of power and control, while being an Intuitive Eater can give you a lifelong sense of self-empowerment. The acts of dieting and rebound bingeing can offer excitement. So does eating forbidden foods. But when excitement no longer comes from food or dieting, other aspects of life are freed to be experienced. When you are using food or the obsession that dieting creates to numb yourself or to distract yourself from your feelings the majority of time, you might feel calmer and less stressed, but your life can seem like a blurred, out-of-focus home movie. You know you're alive and racing through life, but you rarely experience its highs, lows, and nuances of sensation. Once you peel off the layers of dieting and overeating numbness, you'll discover a richness in life that for some has been buried for decades.

When you become an Intuitive Eater who responds to those innate biological and food preference signals, you become acutely in touch with your body, thoughts, and feelings. Ultimately, this sensitivity can transcend to the rest of your life.

You also learn to operate from a framework of curiosity rather than judgment. When dieting, every digression from the food plan becomes an opportunity to become critical of yourself. And criticism can become deadly and infectious. It's not unusual for this critical viewpoint to spill over into other behaviors or even to family members and friends. As an Intuitive Eater you see the food experience as an opportunity to learn more about your thoughts and feelings. You may find that this curiosity triggers other explorations in your life. You may even decide to make serious changes in other parts of your life that have been making you stressed or unhappy. Some clients have decided to change jobs or remove themselves from abusive relationships as a result of going deeper into the meaning of life. Others decide to get into counseling with a psychotherapist.

One of our clients aptly suggested that Intuitive Eating is about *waiting* and learning to be patient. She finds herself *waiting* to eat until she is hungry. Then she describes *waiting* during a time-out in the midst of her meal to see if she is full. When she is experiencing a difficult feeling that she used to cover up with overeating, she now sits with the feeling and *waits* it out until she feels better. And in the bigger picture, she is *waiting* for her eating to normalize so that she feels the freedom and peace in her life that she has so badly craved. She says that this process has taught her to be more patient than she has ever been in her life. She has decided that patience is golden, that what she has learned about herself as she "patiently *waits*" is more valuable than all the pounds she has lost (and, of course, regained) and all the money she has spent on her failed diets. Learning to *wait* has freed her from the burden of dieting and from a life in which she felt locked and trapped, with no escape.

We deeply hope that you will be able to free yourself from dieting by reclaiming the Intuitive Eating ability with which you were born.

Common Questions and Answers About Intuitive Eating

We have compiled some of the most frequently asked questions by our clients as they go through the process of Intuitive Eating. We hope that these answers will also be answers to some of your questions.

Question #1: How long will this process take?
Answer: Unfortunately, this question has no pat answer. It depends on how long you've been dieting and how entrenched the voices of the Food Police are. It also depends on how willing you are to put weight loss off and concentrate on changing your relationship with food. We have seen some people connect quite rapidly with the concept and take only a month or two to be eating in a new way. For others, it's taken two or three or even five years to accept the principles and make serious changes.

Question #2: If I let myself eat whatever I want, won't I eat uncontrollably and gain lots of weight?
Answer: When you have made complete peace with food and know that what you like will always be available to you, you'll be able to stop after a moderate amount. If you're only giving yourself pseudo-permission, it won't work, because you don't really believe you'll always have access to this food. So check out how genuine your permission-giving is. Remember, guilt is what tends to make people eat uncontrollably. Intuitive Eating means having no guilt in your eating. When you first begin the healing process, you may find that you're eating more of the foods that you had previously restricted. This restriction has led to deprivation, and you may end up eating more of these foods for a while. Once the deprivation has healed, these foods will take a balanced place in your eating life.

Question #3: Won't my friends be judgmental and question my eating?
Answer: You may find that many people won't understand what you're doing. Most of our society is conditioned to dieting as a way of living. In fact, some people are perpetually talking about being on diets or saying that they should be on diets. So, yes, some people will be judgmental. You may find that it's hard to explain what you are doing. Remember, this is an intuitive process. Some of the time, you'll just be feeling your way through it and knowing that it feels right to you.

Question #4: Should I try to explain what I'm doing?
Answer: You can try, but it might be frustrating. Key phrases to give out would be:

- Dieting leads to deprivation, deprivation leads to craving, and craving can lead to out-of-control behavior.
- I eat whatever I want when I'm hungry and find that I'm more easily able to stop when I'm full.
- When I feel satisfied with what I eat, I eat less.
- I'm learning to cope with my emotions without using food.

Question #5: Will I ever lose weight doing this?
Answer: The most important statement that we can make is that *weight loss must be put on the back burner*, as you go through the Intuitive Eating process. If you focus on losing weight, it will affect your decisions about eating and sabotage the process. If you have been eating without attention to your intuitive signals and have been eating for emotional reasons, it's likely that you're not presently at your *natural healthy weight*. As you heal from the diet mentality, it is likely that your weight will normalize. If, on the other hand, you have an unrealistic view of what normal weight is and are trying to be thinner than your natural healthy weight, you won't lose weight.

Question #6: What if I can't lose weight? What's this all worth?
Answer: If you are someone who is genetically destined to weigh more than society's standards or your own unrealistic standards, and, therefore, cannot lose weight, you will derive a great deal of peace and contentment with this process. You will get off the "treadmill" of deprivation and guilt. You will eat in a way that's pleasurable and satisfying. You will stop feeling guilty about your eating and stop blaming yourself for being overweight.

You will stop overeating and with it stop feeling uncomfortable and bloated. You'll stop intermittently under eating and, with that, stop feeling starved and uncomfortable. All in all, achieving an Intuitive Eating style will free your time for more enriching thoughts and feelings (rather than food-worry and guilt). For many people, that means ultimately feeling happier.

Question #7: What if I never feel hungry?
Answer: Some people report that they don't feel hunger in their stomachs, but ultimately get raging headaches or some other symptom of not having eaten. For some people, they've dieted and/or binged for so long that they've lost complete touch with hunger. If this is the case for you, you can give yourself a period of time where you purposely eat every three to four hours to try to reestablish your hunger signals. Your body needs food in these intervals, and you may find that after awhile your body trusts that it's going to get fed and will respond by expressing hunger.

Question #8: How will I know when I'm full?
Answer: When you have learned to *honor your hunger,* you'll find that your fullness signals are much more apparent to you. If you eat all of the time and don't feel hunger, it's hard to experience fullness. You'll have no base with which to start to judge the difference. It's helpful to take a time-out in the midst of your meal to test your fullness.

Question #9: Can I ever eat something if it just looks good, but I'm not hungry?
Answer: The Intuitive Eating process is not another diet with a set of absolute rules. Although *honoring your hunger* is one of the first principles, there will be many times when you'll choose to eat something just for its taste or sensual pleasure, without being hungry. We call this taste hunger. If you give yourself permission for occasional responses to taste hunger, you'll feel more satisfied with your entire eating experience and find that you end up eating smaller quantities of food in general.

Question #10: What about sweets? Should I eat them when I'm hungry?
Answer: In general, if you wait until you're hungry to eat sweets, you'll find that you may end up eating a larger quantity than you might need to satisfy your sweet tooth, because you'll be trying to satisfy your biological hunger. Most cultures offer sweets after the meal to please the palate and to punctuate

the end of the meal. Having something sweet, then, is usually in response to taste hunger.

Question #11: What if I want to eat when I can't handle my feelings?
Answer: Generally, the quickest route to resolving emotional conflict is to allow yourself to experience your feelings to their utmost. But sometimes this can be overwhelming. Some people need to be with a friend or a therapist to feel safe enough to let their feelings come out. Others are able to tolerate their feelings for some period of time, but then need an escape for awhile until they feel able to deal with them again. If that is where you find yourself, then search for healthy ways to comfort and distract yourself from the feelings so that you don't end up diving into food as a way of coping.

Question #12: What about good nutrition? If I eat whatever I like, I won't be healthy.
Answer: We have found, in case after case, that giving yourself permission to eat whatever you like ultimately results in a balance of food choice. You'll find, after you have finally made peace with food, that the majority of your food choices will be nutritionally healthy and a smaller portion will be play food. The nutritionally healthy foods take care of your body while the play food takes care of your soul! After all, if you never have to be deprived of a favorite food again, you won't have a great urge to overdo it. You'll want to feel good, and feeling good comes from eating according to your hunger and fullness signals, without stuffing yourself.

Question #13: Do I have to exercise to make this work?
Answer: We have put our chapter on exercise toward the end of the book, because we find that too much emphasis on exercise in the beginning of this process can make some people feel as if they're on another diet. Exercise is something that you'll probably want to do because it makes you feel good. If you disconnect your eating from your exercise, you'll find that you don't get into the old trap of feeling that exercise is for the purpose of weight loss. Exercise is a benefit for all people, young or old, regardless of weight. It's part of a healthy existence. Look for opportunities to move that are fun and enjoyable. If, on the other hand, you are someone who is adamant about not exercising, this process will still be of benefit to you, because it frees you from the world of dieting. But wait and see, you may find yourself moving despite yourself!

Question #14: Should I tell others that they should try this process?
Answer: Most people don't like being told what to do. It usually makes them feel rebellious. You're probably better off just living this new lifestyle. If people ask you why you seem so calm and not obsessed about food or why you look so radiant, you can tell them what you're doing. They might then ask about doing it themselves.

Question #15: What do I do if a host or hostess tries to push more food on me when I don't want any more?
Answer: This person is not respecting your boundaries and does not have a right to pressure you. Say "No, thank you," firmly. Say that you're full and don't want to feel uncomfortable. Remember, your intuitive signals are what count, and you need to honor them.

Appendix B

Step-by-Step Guidelines

If you're someone who cooks, you'll know that before you learned how to cook, just pulling out a recipe card might have caused you to feel anxious about whether the finished concoction would ever resemble any cooked dish you'd ever before seen. In order to gain a comfort level in your kitchen, you probably needed to understand some of the basic concepts of cooking. If the recipe said "simmer," you wouldn't have known the difference between boiling, simmering, or sautéing. The following guidelines are similar to your recipe card. If you look at them before you read the rest of the book, you might get confused and misunderstand the purpose of each. Once you've become comfortable with the Intuitive Eating philosophy, however, these guidelines can become a quick and easy reference when you need to reconnect with the process.

STEP 1 — PRINCIPLE ONE:
REJECT THE DIET MENTALITY

Throw out the diet books and magazine articles that offer you false hope of losing weight quickly, easily, and permanently. Get angry at the lies that have led you to feel as if you were a failure every time a new diet stopped working and you gained back all of the weight. If you allow even one small hope to linger that a new and better diet might be lurking around the corner, it will prevent you from being free to rediscover Intuitive Eating.

1. Make a firm commitment to give up dieting for the rest of your life. As long as you hold on to even the slightest thought, promise, or hope that

dieting is in your future, you will sabotage your ability to become an In-tuitive Eater.

2. Throw out all of your calorie counters and old diet books and articles.

3. When friends talk about the newest fad diet, or you see a TV com-mercial or magazine article on dieting—avoid getting drawn into the ex-citement that might arise. Instead, take a deep breath and gently assure yourself that you are committed to a new way of thinking and feeling about food and eating, and that dieting is not a part of this new process.

4. Protect your food boundaries by refusing to allow others to tell you what to eat, when to eat, or how much to eat. Protect your body boundaries by refusing to allow others to make comments about your weight and body.

5. If you notice that you're feeling rebellious or beginning to eat uncon-sciously, check in with yourself to see if you're still holding on to diet thinking and diet rules that are triggering this reaction or if you're being bombarded by any outside boundary invaders.

STEP 2 — PRINCIPLE TWO:
HONOR YOUR HUNGER

Keep your body biologically fed with adequate energy and carbohydrates. Otherwise you can trigger a primal drive to overeat. Once you reach the moment of excessive hunger, all intentions of moderate, conscious eating are fleeting and irrelevant. Learning to honor this first biological signal sets the stage for rebuilding trust with yourself and food.

1. Begin to listen to the smallest noise or feeling that indicates that you are experiencing hunger, such as a growling or grumbling stomach, a slight headache, a lack of mental focus, grouchiness, lack of energy, etc.

2. As soon as you recognize your biological hunger, make the time to eat.

3. If you neglect this most basic signal and get overhungry, it will be very hard to identify what you really want to eat or when you've had enough. Experiment with beginning to eat at around a "3" or "4" on the "Hunger Discovery Scale."

4. If you don't seem to experience hunger signals over long periods of time, you might want to try eating every three to four hours. Eventually, your body will get used to being fed regularly and will begin to provide you with dependable hunger signals.

5. Keep in mind that if you are sick or stressed, hunger signals may be blunted. It's important to feed your body on those days, too, even if you don't feel the hunger.

6. Be prepared—be sure to make time for shopping for food, cooking or picking up premade food, and for gathering snacks or even meals to put in a lunch bag or to carry in the car. In this way, you show respect for your body's signals and can provide for your needs.

STEP 3 — PRINCIPLE THREE: MAKE PEACE WITH FOOD

Call a truce, stop the food fight! Give yourself unconditional permission to eat. If you tell yourself that you can't or shouldn't have a particular food, it can lead to intense feelings of deprivation that build into uncontrollable cravings and, often, bingeing. When you finally "give in" to your forbidden food, eating will be experienced with such intensity, it usually results in Last Supper overeating, and overwhelming guilt.

1. Give yourself unconditional permission to eat whatever you really like. Make avocado emotionally equivalent to lettuce and peach pie equivalent to a peach.

2. Beware of giving yourself "pseudo-permission" by telling yourself that you can eat what you like, but continuing to hold guilty thoughts about your food choices. It won't work!

3. Do not deprive yourself of any food that sounds appealing to you.

4. Observe how your body feels when eating this food and how satisfying it is to your tongue. Make a mental note of these experiences for your memory bank.

5. Keep an ample supply of all the foods that you think you might like to eat. (Restock the supply when it gets low.)

STEP 4 — PRINCIPLE FOUR: CHALLENGE THE FOOD POLICE

Scream a loud "NO" to thoughts in your head that declare you're "good" for eating minimal calories or "bad" because you ate a piece of chocolate cake. The Food Police monitor the unreasonable rules that dieting has created. The police station is housed deep in your psyche, and its loudspeaker shouts negative barbs, hopeless phrases, and guilt-provoking indictments. Chasing the Food Police away is a critical step in returning to Intuitive Eating.

1. Identify your distorted food, dieting, and eating thoughts and beliefs. Throw them out and replace them with the truth.

2. Listen for the destructive voices which can speak harmful thoughts:

- **The Food Police** voice is harsh and critical and is driven by the dieting mentality. It can be stimulated by listening to the media, parents, and peers. It keeps you at war with your relationship with food and your body.
- **The Nutrition Informant** voice is judgmental and colludes with the Food Police. It gives you nutrition facts to help justify your dieting.
- **The Diet Rebel** voice is angry and is born in response to boundary invaders who cross over the line into the private space that holds your Intuitive Eating signals and feelings about your body. It protects your autonomy while also causing some destructive eating behavior.

3. Develop the helpful voices that can get you through hard times and make your eating relationship more comfortable:

- **The Food Anthropologist** voice describes neutral observations. It notes your thoughts and actions with respect to your food world to help you make choices about what you want to eat, when you want to eat, and how much you need to eat. It can also record these thoughts in your memory bank, so they will be easily accessible when needed in the future to help you make eating decisions.
- **The Nurturer** voice is soft and gentle and provides soothing and reassuring statements that support you through this process.
- **The Rebel Ally** voice evolves from the Diet Rebel voice and helps you protect your boundaries against anyone who invades your eating space.
- **The Nutrition Ally** voice replaces the Nutrition Informant voice when the Food Police are exiled. It is interested in healthy eating with no hidden dieting agenda.

- **The Intuitive Eater** voice speaks to your gut reactions. You were born with this voice, and it gives you messages and answers about your eating that only you can know. It also helps you make decisions that only you have the right to make.

4. Watch out for negative self-talk based on the following irrational beliefs and distorted thinking:

- Dichotomous thinking—thinking in an all-or-nothing, black-and-white fashion.
- Absolutist thinking—magical thinking that believes that one behavior will absolutely affect and control a second behavior.
- Catastrophic thinking—thinking in exaggerated ways.
- Pessimistic thinking or "The Cup Is Half Empty"—where a given situation is seen in its worst-case scenario.
- Linear thinking—thinking in a straight line, allowing for no variables, focusing on the end results.

5. Replace negative self-talk with positive self-talk based on rational thinking. Some examples of rational thinking include:

- Living in the gray—moderate thoughts, not black and white.
- Permissive thoughts and statements.
- Accurate, nonexaggerated thoughts.
- "The Cup Is Half Full" thoughts—creating the best-case scenario.
- Process thinking—focus on continual change and learning, prioritizing the means rather than the end.

STEP 5 — PRINCIPLE FIVE:
FEEL YOUR FULLNESS

Listen for the body signals that tell you that you are no longer hungry. Observe the signs that show that you're comfortably full. Pause in the middle of a meal or food and ask yourself how the food tastes, and what your current fullness level is.

1. Pay attention to your fullness signals. But, remember, the only way that you can do this is to give yourself unconditional permission to eat. You

must firmly believe that you will be able to eat again when you get hungry in order to be able to stop when you're full.

2. Be sure to honor your hunger. If you're overhungry, your urgency to eat will create great difficulty in recognizing your fullness signals. Equally, if you begin eating before true hunger arises, your fullness signals will be muted—you're likely to be guided by your tongue instead of your stomach.

3. Discard the notion that you must finish everything on your plate because you fear wasting food. Far more damage can be done to your body and your psyche by eating extra food than by discarding it.

4. Increase your consciousness in order to help you identify satiety.

- Try eating without distraction so that you can be fully present during your meal.
- Pause in the middle of a meal or snack and take a time-out to check your fullness level. This is not a commitment to stop eating but a commitment to check in with your body and taste buds.
   —Take a taste check. Ask, "How does the food taste? Does it meet your expectations? Is it satisfying your taste buds? Or are you continuing to eat just because it's there?"
   —Take a satiety check. Pay attention to the signals that your stomach gives you to indicate that you're becoming comfortably full. Ask, "What's my hunger or fullness level? Am I still hungry? Is hunger going away? Do I feel insatiable? Am I beginning to feel satisfied?"
   —Practice stopping at a level "6" or "7" on the "Fullness Discovery Scale."
- Identify the *Last Bite Threshold*. This is the endpoint. You know that the bite of food in your mouth is the last. Don't worry if you can't do this at first—it will ultimately become intuitive. If you feel disappointed that you have to stop at this point, remember, you can eat this food or another food again, when your hunger returns. Eating is actually more satisfying when you're comfortably hungry, rather than already full. You're giving yourself a gift by stopping now.
- Make a concrete statement to yourself that you've reached the threshold bite by putting your fork and knife on your plate or by moving your plate forward a little bit.

• Give your leftovers to the server to wrap up if you're at a restaurant or put them in the refrigerator if you're at home.
• Say, "No, thank you" firmly to your host or hostess if more food is being thrust upon you. You have a right to say "no."

5. Make sure that you have plenty of food available for your meals. If you give yourself too little to eat, you'll never feel satisfied or full. You don't need "too much" food, but "too little" food will sabotage this process.

6. Select foods that have some substance. If you only choose "air foods" such as rice cakes and raw vegetables, you'll get a false sense of satiety, only to get hungry again much too quickly. Feed yourself "real food."

STEP 6 — PRINCIPLE SIX:
DISCOVER THE SATISFACTION FACTOR

The Japanese have the wisdom to promote pleasure as one of their goals of healthy living. In our fury to be thin and healthy, we often overlook one of the most basic gifts of existence—the pleasure and satisfaction that can be found in the eating experience. When you eat what you really want, in an environment that is inviting and conducive, the pleasure you derive will be a powerful force in helping you feel satisfied and content. By providing this experience for yourself, you will find that it takes much less food to decide you've had "enough."

1. Give yourself permission to seek pleasure in your eating. The more pleasurable your food is, the more satisfaction you'll derive from your eating experience. (The more satisfied you feel, the less you'll need to eat—especially if you know that this food will never be forbidden.)

2. Figure out what you *really* want to eat by paying attention to the following sensations associated with eating:

• taste—sweet, savory, salty, sour, or bitter
• texture—hard, crunchy, smooth, creamy, etc.
• aroma—sweet, acrid, mild, etc.
• appearance—color, shape, eye appeal, etc.
• temperature—hot, cold, icy, temperate
• volume or filling capacity—airy, light, dense

3. Think about how your body might feel when you finish eating:

- Will you be physically satisfied by your choice?
- Will a dense food make you feel uncomfortably full later or an airy food leave you feeling empty?
- Will an overly rich meal give you stomach distress?
- Will a primarily sweet meal send your blood sugar on a roller coaster ride?

4. Make your eating environment enjoyable:

- Eat when gently hungry rather than overhungry.
- Make time to appreciate your food.
- Create an aesthetic environment—try pretty placemats, candles, colorful dishes, classical music. Keep the noise level down.
- Sit down to eat.
- Take several deep breaths before you eat.
- Savor your food.
- Pay attention to eating as slowly as you can.
- Taste each bite of food that you put in your mouth.
- Provide variety in your meal.
- Avoid tension while eating.

5. Don't settle. Eliminate the unenjoyable—*if you don't love it, don't eat it, and if you love it, savor it!*

6. Check in with your taste buds in the midst of your meal to see if the food still tastes as good as it did when you began.

7. Remember, it doesn't always have to be perfect—sometimes meals are not in your control. There are many more opportunities ahead for satisfying meals.

STEP 7 — PRINCIPLE SEVEN: COPE WITH YOUR EMOTIONS WITHOUT USING FOOD

Find ways to comfort, nurture, distract, and resolve your issues without using food. Anxiety, loneliness, boredom, and anger are emotions we all experience throughout life. Each has its own trigger, and each has its own appeasement. Food won't fix any of these feelings. It may comfort for the short term, distract from the pain, or even numb you into a food hangover, but food won't solve the problem. If anything, eating for an emotional hunger will only make you feel worse in the long run. You'll ultimately have to deal with the source of the emotion, as well as the discomfort of overeating.

1. Ask yourself: "Am I biologically hungry?" If your answer is yes, honor your hunger and eat!

2. When you find yourself searching for food but know that you're not biologically hungry, take a time-out to ask yourself, "What am I feeling?"

- Are you scared, anxious, angry, bored, hurt, lonely, depressed? Or are you happy, excited, need a reward, or want to celebrate?
- To help identify your feelings, spend some quiet time writing in your journal or talking into a tape recorder. Or, if it's easier to get in touch with your feelings with another person, call a good friend or understanding relative. You might even need to call your psychotherapist or nutrition therapist. Use e-mail if that's an easier way to communicate.

3. Then ask yourself, "What do I need?"

- Do you actually need sleep, a hug, some intellectual stimulation, etc.? Food doesn't appropriately satisfy any of those needs.

4. In order to get your needs met, ask: "Would you please?" Sometimes, for needs to be fulfilled, you'll have to speak up and ask for help.

5. Meet your needs without using food in the following ways:

- Nurture yourself by taking bubble baths, listening to soothing music, getting a massage, taking a yoga class, buying yourself some flowers, etc.
- Deal with your feelings. Acknowledge what is troubling you. Allow your feelings to emerge. This will reduce your need to push them down with food.
- If necessary, provide yourself with a temporary distraction. It's okay to get away from the feelings from time to time, but you don't have to use food for this purpose. Try renting a movie, read-

ing an absorbing book, listening to music or an audio book, gardening, etc.

6. If you have an episode of using food to cope, see it as a red flag that something is going on in your life that needs attention. Whatever you do, don't beat yourself up for this behavior. Most people do it at times—just take it as a learning experience and go on.

STEP 8 — PRINCIPLE EIGHT: RESPECT YOUR BODY

Accept your genetic blueprint. Just as a person with a shoe size of eight would not expect to realistically squeeze into a size six, it is equally as futile (and uncomfortable) to have the same expectation with body size. But mostly, respect your body, so you can feel better about who you are. It's hard to reject the diet mentality if you are unrealistic and overly critical about your body shape.

1. Appreciate the parts of your body that you especially like—whether it's your hair, waist, feet, or nose.
2. Take bubble baths, and use lotions and creams that feel soothing as you rub them in.
3. Get massages and hugs and caresses that give your body the opportunity to be touched.
4. Get comfortable. Buy comfortable undergarments. Buy clothing that is flattering and fits you without being tight.
5. Don't hide your body in clothes that are too large.
6. Quit the body-check game. Stop comparing yourself to everyone else in the room. It blinds you from appreciating yourself and is a setup for more body dissatisfaction. It might even create a temptation to return to dieting.
7. Don't compromise for the "Big Event." Don't succumb to the pressure of "dieting down" to squeeze into that special outfit—it will only backfire.
8. Stop body bashing. Every time you focus on your imperfect body parts, it creates more self-consciousness and body worry. When you hear yourself making disparaging comments about your body, replace these comments with kind body statements.
9. Stop weighing yourself. It can only make you feel discontented with your body.

10. Respect body diversity, especially yours.

11. Be realistic about your genetic makeup. Accept your body type, and know that your body is likely to balance out at its natural weight when you're consistently listening to your intuitive signals and practicing self-care.

12. Be understanding of yourself. Respect the fact that you may be higher than your normal body weight if you are someone who has used food to cope when you knew no other way to handle your feelings, or because you've been a victim of the diet mentality. Be gentle with yourself and accept that your body is where it is because you had very little choice about these factors.

Step 9 — Principle Nine:
Exercise — Feel the Difference

Forget militant exercise. Just get active and feel the difference. Shift your focus to how it feels to move your body, rather than the calorie-burning effect of exercise. If you focus on how you feel from working out, such as energized, it can make the difference between rolling out of bed for a brisk morning walk or hitting the snooze alarm. If when you wake up, your only goal is to lose weight, it's usually not a motivating factor in that moment of time.

1. Break through exercise barriers:

  • Discover all the reasons behind any exercise resistance that you might have. It may be due to having been teased as a child, having rebelled against authority, feeling intimidated for not having a lean enough body, etc.
  • Focus on how it feels. Exercise is primarily for feeling good. It so happens that the better you feel, the less you'll need to use food as a way to cope. It can also give you increased energy, a general aura of well-being, a sense of empowerment, and sounder sleep.
  • Disassociate exercise from weight loss. Erase the tape of how exercise felt when you were dieting. You probably weren't getting enough calories or carbohydrates to give you the energy to exercise and feel good at the same time.
  • Focus on exercise as a way of taking care of yourself, feeling good now, and preventing health problems later in life.

- Don't get caught in exercise mind games such as:
- *The It's-Not-Worth It Trap*—i.e., feeling it's not worth it if it doesn't last a specified amount of time.
- *Couch-Potato Denial*—being busy is not the same as physical activity.
- *The No-Time-to-Spare Trap*—learn to prioritize.
- *The If-I-Don't-Sweat-It-Doesn't-Count Trap*—physical fitness doesn't have to mean rigorous workouts.

2. Get active in daily living. Make exercise convenient and fun:

- Park your car a few blocks from your destination so you can add some walking to your day.
- Walk up stairs instead of using the elevator.
- Ride your bike or walk to work if you live close enough.
- When you travel, take walking shoes or a jump rope. Consider choosing hotels that have workout facilities.

3. Make exercise fun.

- Consider playing a team sport such as volleyball (beach volleyball during the summer), softball, basketball, soccer, or tennis.
- Join a gym, if having others around you will motivate you.
- Buy a treadmill or other home exercise equipment and put a TV and DVR or DVD player in front of it so you can record and watch movies or interesting programs. Listening to music or an audio book might also make the exercise more fun.
- Find an exercise partner with whom you can take walks. Talking and walking can make the walk more enjoyable.

4. Make exercise a nonnegotiable priority.
5. Be comfortable while exercising.
6. Include strength training so you can rebuild muscle that was lost from dieting.
7. Include stretching as part of your exercise routine.
8. Remember rest. Make sure you give yourself days of rest within your exercise week. It will prevent burnout, as well as giving your muscles a chance to refresh and repair.

Step 10 — Principle Ten:
Honor Your Health with Gentle Nutrition

Make food choices that honor your health and taste buds while making you feel well. Remember that you don't have to eat a perfect diet to be healthy. You will not suddenly get a nutrient deficiency or gain weight from one snack, one meal, or one day of eating. It's what you eat consistently over time that matters. Progress, not perfection, is what counts.

1. Consider the tenets of food wisdom: variety, moderation, and balance. As with exercise, consider nutrition as your passport into feeling good.

2. Feed your metabolism. Be sure to stoke your metabolic fire by getting sufficient fuel throughout the day by eating whenever you're hungry.

3. Eat plenty of whole grains, fruits and vegetables, and beans for their fiber content, so your digestive tract works well. They're also a powerhouse of vitamins, minerals, and phytochemicals.

4. Eat sufficient protein, but not too much, for cellular repair and production of hormones, enzymes, hair, nails, etc.

5. Eat plenty of carbohydrates and sufficient calories so your protein can be used as a protein source and not be burned as an energy source.

6. Take in an adequate amount of dairy products to get enough calcium to keep your bones strong.

7. Drink plenty of water to aid digestion, prevent constipation, have sufficient blood volume, and cleanse your kidneys.

8. Eat an adequate amount of fat. We need fat in our diets for these reasons:

- to promote satiety,
- to help build cell walls, including brain cells,
- for absorption of fat soluble vitamins, and
- for production of hormones.
- Whenever possible, choose quality fats, such as avocado, olive oil, nuts, etc.

9. Allow for some *play foods* in order to balance your good health with pleasure and satisfaction. Let most of your food choices be made for physical health, while some of them are for simple pleasure.

10. Don't be duped by the *fat-free trap*. Fat free doesn't mean calorie free or nutrient dense. These foods tend to be limited in nutrients, while having an overabundance of sugar. Fat-free foods often are not as satisfying as low-fat foods. They also create an illusion of being low-calorie and lead to overconsumption before you know it.

11. Get off the food pedestal. You don't have to be perfect. Honor your health, your taste buds, and your humanness.

These guidelines summarize the chapters of this book. The order in which they're presented is not an absolute, just as nothing in this book is absolute, except for giving up the pursuit of dieting. Use them as your recipe card, as we suggested at the beginning of this appendix. But just as you might improvise in cooking your dish from the written recipe, be creative with these guidelines. Use what feels right for you, add to them if you like, and discard what doesn't fit. The bottom line is to trust your gut—use your intuitive talents to feel comfortable with eating and to release yourself from the prison of dieting.

References

Foreword and Introduction

Bacon, L., and Aphramor, L. Weight Science: Evaluating the Evidence for a Paradigm Shift. *Nutrition Journal* 10, 9 (January 2011), http://bit.ly/f4CKOK.

The Center for Mindful Eating's Web site: http://www.tcme.org/principles.htm. Accessed April 24, 2011.

Kristeller, J. L., and Hallett, B. Effects of a Meditation-Based Intervention in the Treatment of Binge Eating. *Journal of Health Psychology* 4, 3 (1999): 357–363.

Levine, P. A. *Waking the Tiger—Healing Trauma*. North Atlantic Press, 1997.

Chapter 1. Hitting Diet Bottom

Field, A. E., et al. Relation between Dieting and Weight Change Among Preadolescents and Adolescents. *Pediatrics* 112 (2003): 900–906.

Mann, T. Medicare's search for effective Obesity Treatments: Diets Are Not the Answer. *Am. Psychologist* 62, 3 (2007): 220–233.

Neumark-Sztainer, D., et al. Obesity, Disordered Eating, and Eating Disorders in a Longitudinal Study of Adolescents: How Do Dieters Fare Five Years Later? *J Am Diet Assoc.* 106, 4 (2006): 559–568.

Chapter 2. What Kind of Eater Are You?

Berg, F. *The Health Risks of Weight Loss*. Hettinger, ND: Healthy Living Institute, 1993.

Birch, L. L. Children's Eating: Are Manners Enough? *Journal of Gastronomy* 7, 1 (1993): 19–25.

Birch, L. L. The Role of Experience in Children's Food Acceptance Patterns. *Journal of the American Dietetic Association* 87 (1987): 9 supplement: S-36.

Birch, L. L. et al. The Variability of Young Children's Energy Intake. *New England Journal of Medicine* 324 (Jan. 24, 1991): 232.

Eating Guilt. *Obesity and Health* 6, 2 (1992): 43.

Forbes, G. B. Children and Food—Order Amid Chaos. *New England Journal of Medicine* 324 (Jan. 24, 1991): 262.

Gallup Organization. Gallup Survey of Public Opinion Regarding Diet and Health. Prepared for American Dietetic Association/International Food Information Council: Princeton, NJ: Gallup Organization, Inc. (January 1990).

Satter, E. Comments from a Practioner on Leann Birch's Research. *Journal of the American Dietetic Association* 87 (1987): 9 supplement: S-41.

Satter, E. *How to Get Your Child to Eat . . . But Not Too Much.* Palo Alto, CA: Bull Pub, 1987: 6.

Tylka, T. L. Development and Psychometric Evaluation of a Measure of Intuitive Eating. *J Counseling Psych* 53, 2 (April 2006): 226–240.

Tufts University Diet & Nutrition Letter. Warning: Keep Dieting Out of Reach of Children. 11, 10 (1993): 3.

Chapter 5. Principle 1: Reject the Diet Mentality

Associated Press (Washington). Vitamin Retailer to Pay Fine. *AP Online* (April 29, 1994).

Berdanier, C. D., and McIntosh, M. K. Weight Loss—Weight Regain: A Vicious Cyle. *Nutrition Today* 26, 5 (1991): 6.

Berg, F. M. *The Health Risks of Weight Loss.* Hettinger, ND: Healthy Living Institute, 1993.

Blackburn, G. L. et al. Why and How to Stop Weight Cycling in Overweight Adults. *Eating Disorders Review* 4, 1 (1993): 1.

Blackburn, G. L. et al. Weight Cycling: The Experience of Human Dieters. *American Journal Clinical Nutrition* 49 (1989): 1105.

Ciliska, D. *Beyond Dieting.* NY: Brunner/Mazel, 1990.

Field, A. E., et al. Relations Between Dieting and Weight Change Among Preadolescents and Adolescents. *Pediatrics*, 112 (2003): 900–906.

Foreyt, J. P. and Goodrick, G. K. Weight Management without Dieting. *Nutrition Today* (March/April 1993): 4.

Foreyt, J. P. and Goodrick, G. K. *Living without Dieting.* Houston, TX: Harrison Publ., 1992.

Gallup Organization. Women's Knowledge and Behavior Regarding Health and Fitness. Conducted for American Dietetic Association and Weight Watchers, June 1993.

Garrow, J. S. Treatment of Obesity. *The Lancet* 340 (1992): 409–413.

Goodrick, G. K. and Foreyt, J. P. Why Treatments for Obesity Don't Last. *Journal of the American Dietetic Association*. 91, 10 (1991): 1243.

Grodner, M. Forever Dieting: Chronic Dieting Syndrome. *Journal of Nutrition Education* 24, 4 (1992): 207–210.

Haines J., and Neumark-Sztainer, D. Prevention of Obesity and Eating Disorders: A Consideration of Shared Risk Factors. *Health Education Research,* 21(6) (2006): 770–782.

Hartmann, E. *Boundaries in the Mind. A New Psychology of Personality.* NY: Basic Books, 1991.

Hill, A. J. and Robinson, A. Dieting Concerns Have a Functional Effect on the Behaviour of Nine-Year-Old Girl. *British Journl of Clinical Psychology.* 30 (1991): 265–267.

Katherine, A. *Boundaries: Where you End and I Begin.* Park Ridge, IL: Parkside Publishing Company, 1991.

Kern, P. A., et al. The Effects of Weight Loss on the Activity and Expression of Adipose-Tissue Lipoprotein Lipase in Very Obese Human. *New England Journal of Medicine* 322, 15: 1053–1059.

Mann, T., et al. Medicare's Search for Effective Obesity Treatments: Diets Are Not the Answer. *American Psychologist,* 62(3) (2007): 220–233.

Neumark-Sztainer, D., et al. Obesity, Disordered Eating, and Eating Disorders in a Longitudinal Study of Adolescents: How Do Dieters Fare Five Years Later? *Journal of the American Dietetic Association,* 106(4) (2006): 559–568.

Patton, G. C., et al. Onset of Adolescent Eating Disorders: Population Based Cohort Study Over 3 Years. *British Medical Journal,* 318 (1999): 765–768.

Pietiläinen, K. H., et al. Does Dieting Make You Fat? A Twin Study. *International Journal of Obesity,* 36 (2012): 456–454.

Polivy, J. and Herman, C. P. Undieting: A Program to Help People Stop Dieting. *International Journal of Eating Disorders* 11, 3 (1992): 261–268.

Rodin, J. et al. Weight Cycling and Fat Distribution. *International Journal of Obesity* 14 (1990): 303–310.

Saarni, S. E., et al. Weight cycling of athletes and subsequent weight gain in middle-age. *International Journal of Obesity,* 30 (2006): 1639–1644.

Wilson, G. T. Short-Term Psychological Benefits and Adverse Effects of Weight Loss. *NIH Technology Assesssment Conference: Methods for Voluntary Weight Loss and Control,* March 30–April, 1992.

Wooley, S. C. and Garner, D. M. Obesity Treatment: The High Cost of False Hope. *Journal of the American Dietetic Association*. 91, 10 (1991): 1248.

Yanovski, S. Z. Are Anorectic Agents the Magic Bullet for Obesity (editorial). *Arch Family Medicine*. 2(Oct 1993):1025–1027.

Chapter 6. Principle 2: Honor Your Hunger

Birch, L. L., Johnson, S. L., Andresen, G., Peters, J. C. and Schulte, M. C. The Variability of Young Children's Energy Intake. *New England Journal of Medicine* 324(Jan. 24, 1991):232.

Boyle, M. A. and Zyla, G. *Personal Nutrition*, 2nd edition. pp 77, 217. St. Paul, MN: West Publishing, 1992.

[1] M. Ciampolini and R. Bianchi, "Training to estimate blood glucose and to form associations with initial hunger," Nutrition and Metabolism, vol. 3, article 42, 2006. [http://bit.ly/bXRdkD]

[2] M. Ciampolini, D. Lovell-Smith, R. Bianchi, et al., "Sustained Self-Regulation of Energy Intake: Initial Hunger Improves Insulin Sensitivity," Journal of Nutrition and Metabolism, vol. 2010, Article ID 286952, 7 pages, 2010. doi:10.1155/2010/286952 [Free full text. http://bit.ly/9OYSsw]

[3] M. Ciampolini, D. Lovell-Smith, and M. Sifone, "Sustained self-regulation of energy intake. Loss of weight in overweight subjects. Maintenance of weight in normal-weight subjects," Nutrition and Metabolism, vol. 7, article 4, 2010.

Drott, C. and Lundholm, K. Cardiac Effects of Caloric Restriction-mechanisms and Potential Hazards. *International Journal Obesity*, 16: (1992) 481–486.

Franchina, J. J. and Slank, K. L. Effects of Deprivation on Salivary Flow in the Apparent Absence of Food Stimuli. *Appetite*. 10: (1988) 143–147.

Garner, D. M. and Garfinkel, P. E. (eds). *Handbook of Psychotherapy for Anorexia and Bulimia*. (1985) NY: Guilford, chapter 21.

Polivy, J. and Herman, C. P. Diagnosis and Treatment of Normal Eating. *Journal of Consulting and Clinical Psychology* (1987). 55(5):635–644.

Leibowitz, S. , Brain Neuropeptide Y: An Integrator of Endocrine, Metabolic and Behavioral Processes. *Brain Research Bulletin*, Sept–Oct (1991):27 (3–4)33–7.

Marano, H. Chemistry and craving. *Psychology Today*. Jan/Feb (1993) 31.

Nicolaidis S. and Even, P. The Metabolic Signal of Hunger and Satiety, and Its Pharmacological Manipulation. *International Journal Obesity*, Dec (16 suppl 3) (1992):S31–41.

Polivy, J. and Herman, C. P. Dieting and Binging a Causal Analysis. *American Psychologist*. Feb (1985):193–201.

Scrimshaw, N. S. The Phenomenon of Famine. *Annual Review of Nutrition* (1987) 7:1–21.

Wolf, N. *The Beauty Myth*. NY: Anchor Books (1991) 179–217.

Chapter 7. Principle Three: Make Peace with Food

Baldwin, A. L. *Theories of Child Development, Second Edition*, (1980). John Wiley & Sons, Inc.: NY, NY.

Berk, L. E. *Child Development, Third Edition* (1994). Allyn and Bacon: Boston, MA.

Benton D. The plausibility of Sugar Addiction and Its Role in Obesity and Eating Disorders. Clinical Nutrition 29 (2010) 288–303.

Berridge K. C. & Kringelbach M. L. Affective Neuroscience of Pleasure: Reward in Humans and Animals. Psychopharmacology (Berl). 2008 (August) 199(3): 457–480.

Epstein L. H. Habituation as a Determinant of Human Food Intake. *Psychol Rev. 2009* April; 116(2): 384–407.

Epstein L. H. Long-term Habituation to Food in Obese and Nonobese Women. *Am J Clin Nutrition*. 2011; doi: 10.3945/ajcn.110.009035.

Erikson, Erik H. *The Life Cycle Completed. A Review.* W.W. Norton and Company: NY, NY., 1982

Ernst M. M. Habituation of Responding for Food in Humans. Appetite (2002) 38, 224–234 doi:10.1006/appe.2001.0484.

Gearhardt An et al. Preliminary Validation of the Yale Food Addiction Scale. *Appetite* 2009 (52):430-436.

Gilbert D. Stumbling on Happiness. Knopf. NY: NY, 2006, 130.

Herman, C. P. and Polivy, J. Restrained Eating. In Stunkard. A. *Obesity.* Philadelphia, PA.: WB Saunders, (1980), pp 208–225.

Kristeller J. L., & Wolever RQ (2011). Mindfulness-based Eating Awareness Training for Treating Binge Eating Disorder: The Conceptual Foundation. *Eating Disorders, 19* (1), 49–61 PMID: 21181579

Loro, A. D. and Orleans, C. S. (1981). Binge Eating in Obesity: Preliminary Findings and Guidelines for Behavioral Analysis and Treatment. *Addictive Behaviours.* 7, 155–166.

Miller, P. H. *Theories of Developmental Psychology.* (1993). W.H. Freeman and Company: NY, NY.

Mydans, S. 8 Bid Farewell to the Future: Musty Air, Roaches and Ants. *The New York Times*. Sept 27, 1993: p. A1.

Ogden, J. and Wardle, J. Cognitive and Emotional Responses to Food. *International Journal of Eating Disorders.* 10(3) (1991): 297–311.

Personal Communication. Ennette Larson, M.S., R.D. Research dietitian for NIH, Phoneix, AZ.

Salimpoor V. N. Anatomically Distinct Dopamine Release During Anticipation and Experience of Peak Emotion to Music. *Nature Neuroscience.* Feb (2011);14 (2):257–262.

Satter, E. *How to Get Your Kid to Eat . . . But Not Too Much.* (1987) Bull Publishing Company: Palo Alto, CA.

Seamon, J. G. and Kenrick, D. T. *Psychology,* Second Edition (1994). Prentice Hall: Englewood Cliffs, N.J.

Smitham, L. Evaluating an Intuitive Eating Program for Binge Eating Disorder: A Benchmarking Study. University of Notre Dame, November 26, 2008.

Snoek H. M. et al. Obese and Normal-weight Women. *Am J Clin Nutr* Vol. 80, No. 4, October 2004, 823–831.

Chapter 8. Principle 4: Challenge the Food Police

As the Chicken Turns. *Tufts University Diet and Nutrition Letter.* 11 (11) (1994):1.

Berne, Eric. *Games People Play.* Grove Press, Inc. New York, 1964.

Ellis, A. and Harper, R. A., *A New Guide to Rational Living.* 1975. Melvin Powers, Wilshire Book Company, 12015 Sherman Road, North Hollywood, CA, 91605.

Food Guilt. *Utne Reader.* Nov/Dec (1993):53.

Hiser, E. Butter paroled, margarine charged. *Eating Well.* Nov/Dec:104, 1993.

King, G. A., Herman, C. P., and Polivy, J. Food Perception in Dieters and Non-dieters. *Appetite,* 8 (1987):147–158.

Seid, R. P. *Never Too Thin.* NY, NY: Prentice Hall Press, 1989.

Chapter 9. Principle 5: Feel Your Fullness

Bray, G. A. The Nutrient Balance Approach to Obesity. *Nutrition Today.* (1993). 28(3):13–18.

De Castro, J. M. Weekly Rythms of Spontaneous Nutrient Intake and Meal Patterns of Humans. *Physiology & Behavior.* 50 (1991):729–738.

De Castro, J. M. Physiological, Environmental, and Subjective Determinants of Food Intake in Humans: A Meal Pattern Analysis. *Physiology & Behavior.* (1988), 44:651–659.

Chapter 10. Principle 6: Discover the Satisfaction Factor

Anderson, S. L. (1990). A look at the Japanese Dietary Guidelines. *Journal of the American Dietetic Association*, 90(11), 1527–1528.

Oldham-Cooper R. E., et al. Playing a Computer Game During Lunch Affects Fullness, Memory for Lunch, and Later Snack Intake. *Am J Clin Nutr* 93: February (2011) 308–313.

Epstein L. H. Habituation as a determinant of human food intake. *Psychol Rev.* 2009 April; 116(2): 384–407.

Visser, M. On having cake and eating it. *Journal of Gastronomy* 7(1):5–17, 1993.

Wisniewski, L., Epstein, L. H., and Caggiula, A. R. (1992). Effect of Food Change on Consumption, Hedonics, and Salivation. *Physiology and Behavior*, 92(52), 21–26.

Chapter 11. Principle 7: Cope with Your Emotions without Using Food

Arnow, B., Kenardy, J., and Agras, W. S. (1992). Binge Eating Among the Obese: A Descriptive Study. *Journal of Behavioral Medicine*, 15(2), 155–170.

Barnett, R. Appetite and the Meal. *The Journal of Gastronomy.* 7(1) (1993):59–72.

De Castro, J. M. (1990). Social Facilitation of Duration and Size but Not Rate of the Spontaneous Meal Intake of Humans. Physiology and Behavior, 47, 1129–1135.

De Castro, J. M. and Brewer, E. M. (1991). The Amount Eaten in Meals by Humans Is a Power Function of the Number of People Present. *Physiology and Behavior*, 51, 121–125.

De Castro, J. M. (1991). Weekly Rhythms of Spontaneous Nutrient Intake and Meal Pattern of Humans. *Physiology and Behavior.* 50, 729–738.

Goldman, S. J., Herman, C. P., and Polivy, J. (1991). Is the Effect of a Social Model on Eating Attenuated by Hunger? *Appetite.* 17, 129–140.

Heatherton, T. F., Herman, C. P. and Polivy, J. (1992). Effects of Distress on Eating: The Importance of Ego-involvement. *Journal of Personality and Social Psychology.* 62(5), 801–803.

Herman, C. P. and Polivy, J. Fat Is a Psychological Issue. *New Scientist.* Nov (1991):41–45.

Herman, C. P. and Polivy, J. (1988). Psychological Factors in the Control of Appetite. *Current Concepts in Nutrition*, 16, 41–51.

Herman, C. P., Polivy, J., Lank, C. N., and Heatherton, T. F. (1987). Anxiety, Hunger, and Eating Behavior. *Journal of Abnormal Psychology*, 96(3), 264–269.

Hill, A. J., Weaver, C. F. L., and Blundell, J. E. (1991). Food Craving, Dietary Restraint and Mood. *Appetite,* 17, 187–197.

Morton, C. J. Weight Loss Maintenance and Relapse Prevention. In: *Obesity and Weight Control* by Reva T. Frankle and Mei-Uih Yang. 1988. Aspen Publishers, Inc., Rockville, Maryland.

Ogden, J. and Wardle, J. (1991). Cognitive and Emotional Responses to Food. *International Journal of Eating Disorders*, 10(3), 297–311.

Polivy, J., Herman, C. P., Hackett, R., and Kuleshnyk, I. (1986). The Effects of Self-attention and Public Attention on Eating in Restrained and Unrestrained Subjects. *Journal of Personality and Social Psychology*. 50(6), 1253–1260.

Weissenburger, J., Rush, A. J., Giles, D. E., and Stunkard, A. J. (1986). Weight Change in Depression. *Psychiatry Research*, 17, 275–283.

Chapter 12. Principle 8: Respect Your Body

2011 Succeed Foundation Body Image Survey [http://www.responsesource.com/releases/rel_display.php?relid=63713&hilite=BOdy%20image *accessed June 6, 2011*]

Bacon L. and Aphramor L. Weight Science:Evaluating the Evidence for a Paradigm Shift. [2011]. *Nutrition Journal*, January. 10:9. [Free full text]. http://bit.ly/f4CKOK.

Brownell, K. The Debate to Nowhere. Posted Augst 23, 2006. http://bit.ly/je8eFU [*accessed June 12, 2011*].

Diet Winners and Sinners of the Year. *People Weekly*. January 10, 1994.

Dietary Guideline Advisory Committee. *Report of* Puhl R. M. The Stigma of Obesity: A Review and Update. *Obesity* (2009) doi:10.1038/oby.2008.636.

Rudd Report. Weight Bias a Social Justice Issue Policy Brief. 2009. Yale University.

Stice E. et al. An Effectiveness Trial of a Dissonance-Based Eating Disorder Prevention Program for High-Risk Adolescents Girls *J Consult Clin Psychol*. October (2009); 77(5):825–834. Free Full Text. [http://bit.ly/bw6gLV].

The Dietary Guidelines Advisory Committe on the Dietary Guidelines for Americans 1990. USDA.

Rodin, J. *Body Traps*. NY, NY: William Morrow, 1992.

Wiseman, et al. Cultural Expectations of Thinness in Women: An Update. *International Journal of Eating Disorders*. 11(1) (1992):85–89.

Chapter 13. Principle 9: Exercise—Feel the Difference

American College of Sports Medicine. Position Stand: The Recommended Quantity and Quality of Exercise for Developing and Maintaining Cardiorespiaratory and Muscular Fitness in Healthy Adults. *Med Scie Sports Exer*. 22 (1990):265–274.

American College of Sports Medicine. Position Stand: The Recommended Quantity and Quality of Exercise for Developing and Maintaining Cardiorespiratory and Muscular Fitness, and Flexibility in Healthy Adults. *Medicine & Science in Sports & Exercise.* 30(6):975–991, June 1998.

American College of Sports Medicine. Press Release: Experts Release New Recommendations to Fight America's Epidemic of Physical Inactivity. July 29, 1993.

American College of Sports Medicine. Two Minutes of Exercise a Day Can Keep the Pain Away. June 3, 2011. [http://bit.ly/mdFUog *accessed June 10, 2011*].

Calogero R. and Pedrotty K. (2007). Daily practices for Mindful Exercise. In L. L'Abate, D. Embry, & M. Baggett (Eds.), Handbook of Low-cost Preventive Interventions for Physical and Mental Health: Theory, Research, and Practice, Springer-Verlag, 141–160.

Chaput J. C. Physical Activity Plays an Important Role in Body Weight Regulation, *Journal of Obesity,* vol. 2011, Article ID 360257, 11 pages, 2011. doi:10.1155/2011 /360257.

Costill, D. L. Carbohydrates for Exercise: Dietary Demands for Optimal Performance. *International Journal of Sports Medicine,* 9:5, 1988.

Evans, B. and Rosenberg, I. *Biomarkers the 10 Determinants of Aging You Can Control.* Simon and Schuster: NY, NY. 1991.

Foreyt, J, et al. Response of Free-living Adults to Behavioral Treament of Obesity: Attrition and Compliance to Exercise. *Behavior Therapy* 24 (1993):659–669.

Gandey A. Exercise Reduces Silent Brain Infarcts. *Medscape News.* June 10, 2011.

Gavin, J. *The Exericse Habit.* Champaign, IL: Human Kinetics, 1992.

Lemon, P. W. R and Mullin, J. P. Effect of Initial Muscle Glycogen Levels on Protein Catabolism During Exercise. *Journal Applied Physiology: Respitr. Environ. Exercise Physiol.:*48(4) (1980): 624–629.

McGuire, K., & Ross, R. (2011). Incidental Physical Activity Is Positively Associated with Cardiorespiratory Fitness *Medicine & Science in Sports & Exercise* DOI: 10.1249/MSS.0b013e31821e4ff2

Miller, W. C. Exercise: Americans Don't Think It's Worth It. *Obesity & Health.* Mar/Apr:29, 1994.

Pollock, M. L., et al. Effect of Age and Training on Aerobic Capacity and Body Composition of Master Athletes. *J Appl Physiol* 62 (1987):725–731.

Tryon, W. W., Goldberg, J. L., and Morrison, D. F. Activity Decreases as Percentage Overweight Increases. *International Journal of Obesity.* 16 (1992):591–595.

Chapter 14. Principle 10: Honor Your Health with Gentle Nutrition

2010 Dietary Guidelines
http://www.cnpp.usda.gov/dietaryguidelines.htm [accessed May 30, 2011].

Calorie Control Commentary, 14(1):1–2, 1992.

Basdevant A. Prevalence of Binge Eating Disorder in Different Populations of French Women. *Int J Eat Disorders.* 1995;18(4):309-315.

Beardsley E. In Paris, Culinary Education Starts In Day Care. NPR. February 16, 2009.

Callaway, W. The Marriage of Taste and Health: A Union Whose Time Has Come. *Nutrition Today.* 27(3):37–42, 1992.

Calder P. The American Heart Association Advisory on n-6 Fatty Acids: Evidence Based or Biased Evidence? *British Journal of Nutrition,* 2010 /Volume 104(11):1575–1576.

CDC. Helicobacter pylori. Fact Sheet for Health Care Providers, http://www.cdc.gov /ulcer/files/hpfacts.PDF [accessed May 29, 2011].

Egolf, B., Lasker, J., Wolf, S., and Potvin, L. The Roseto Effect: A 50-year Comparison of Mortality Rates. *Am J Public Health* (1992) 82: 1089–1092

Evans, H. M. et al. A New Dietary Deficiency With Highly Purified Diets: The Beneficial Effect of Fat in the Diet. *Proceedings of the Society for Experimental Biology and Medicine* (1928); 25:390–397.

Getz L. Orthorexia: When Eating Healthy Becomes an Unhealthy Obsession. *Today's Dietitian.* 2009 (June): page 40.

Glore, S. R. et al. Soluble Fiber and Serum Lipids: A Literature Review. *Journal of the American Dietetic Association.* 94 (1994):425–436.

Guyenet S. Butter, Margarine and Heart Disease. *Whole Health Source.* December 27, 2008.
http://www.webmd.com/diet/news/20080813/the-olympic-diet-of-michael-phelps [*accessed May 23, 2011*].

Ledoux, S. Eating Disorders Among Adolescents in an Unselected French Population. *International Journal of Eating Disorder.* 10(1) (1991):81–89.

McCargar, L. J. et al. Physiological Effects of Weight Cycling in Female Lightweight Rowers. *Canadian Journal of Applied Physiology.* 18(3) (1993):291–303.

McEwen B. Central Effects of Stress Hormones in Health and Disease: Understanding the Protective and Damaging Effects of Stress and Stress Mediators. *Eur J Pharmacol.* 2008 April 7; 583(2-3): 174–185.

National Research Council. *Recommended Dietary Allowances.* National Academy of Sciences: Washington, D.C., (1989), 46–49.

OECD (2010), *OECD Factbook 2010: Economic, Environmental and Social Statistics*, OECD Publishing.

Ramsden C. E. et al. Omega 6 Fatty Acid-specific and Mixed Polyunsaturate Dietary Interventions Have Different Effects on CHD Risk: A Meta-analysis of Randomised Controlled Trials. *British Journal of Nutrition,* 104 (2010), 1586–1600.

Rozin, P. Food and Cuisine: Education, Risk and Pleasure. *Journal of Gastronomy.* 7(1) (1993):111–120.

Rozin, P. et al. Attitudes to Food and the Role of Food in the Life in the USA, Japan, Flemish Belgium & France: Possible Implications for the Diet-Health debate. *Appetite,* 1999 (33):163–180.

Rozin, P. et al. The Ecology of Eating: Smaller Portion Sizes in France Than in the United States Help Explain the French Paradox. *Psychological Science.* 2003;14(5): 450–454.

Rozin, P. Food Is fundamental, Fun, Frightening, and Far-reaching. *Social Research,* (1999). 66, 9–30.

Scrinis, G. On the Ideology of Nutritionism. *Gastronomica: The Journal Of Food And Culture.* 8, 1 (2008):39–48.

Schardt, D. Phytochemicals: Plants Against Cancer. *Nutrition Action Health Letter.* 21, 3 (1994).

Schneeman, B. et al. The Regulatory Process to Revise Nutrient Labeling Relative to the Dietary Reference Intakes *Am J Clin Nutr* (2006) 83: 5 1228S–1230S.

Stacey, M. *Consumed: Why Americans Love Hate And Fear Food.* Simon And Schuster: NY, NY 1994.

Stout, C., Morrow, J., Brandt, E. N., and Wolf, S. Unusually Low Incidence of Death From Myocardial Infarction: Study of an Italian American Community in Pennsylvania. *JAMA.* (1964); 188(10):845–849.

Thompson, J. L. et al. Effects of Diet and Diet-Plus-Exercise Programs on Resting Metabolic Rate: A Meta-analysis. *Intl. J Sport Nutrition* 1996 (6):41–61.

Urban, N. et al. Correlates of Maintenance of a Low-fat Diet Among Women in the Women's Health Trial. *Preventive Medicine* 21 (1992):279–291.

USDA. Human Nutrition Service. *USDA's Food Guide Pyramid.* Home and Garden bulletin, no. 249, April 1992.

USDHH. Healthy People 2000. *Nutrition Today.* 25(6):29–39, 1990.

Wolf, S. K. L. Grace, J. Bruhn, and C. Stout. Roseto Revisited: Further Data on the Incidence of Myocardial Infarction in Roseto and Neighboring Pennsylvania Communities. *Trans Am Clin Climatol Assoc.* 85 (1974): 100–108.

Chapter 15. Raising an Intuitive Eater: What Works with Kids and Teens

Birch L. L., Fisher J. O. and Davison K. K. Learning to Overeat: Maternal Use of Restrictive Feeding Practices Promotes Girls' Eating in the Absence of Hunger. *American Journal of Clinical Nutrition*. (2003) 78: 215–220.

Carper J. L., Fisher J. O., Birch L. L. Young Girls' Emerging Dietary Restraint and Disinhibition Are Related to Parental Control in Child Feeding. *Appetite*. (2000) 35:121–129.

Eneli, I. U., Crum, L. P. A, and Tylka, T. R. The Trust Model: A Different Feeding Paradigm for managing childhood obesity. *Obesity* 2008; 16: 2197–2204.

Field, A. E., et al. Relation Between Dieting and Weight Change Among Preadolescents and Adolescents. *Pediatrics*. (2003) 112:900–906.

Los Angeles Times, November 1, 2009, p. A1.

Neumark-Sztainer D., Wall, M., Jaiones, J., Story, M., Eisenberg, M. E. Why Does Dieting Predict Weight Gain in Adolescents? Findings from Project EAT-II: A 5-year Longitudinal Study. *Journal of the American Dietetic Association*. (2007) 107:448–455.

Rubenstein, T. B., McGinn, A. P., Wildman, R. P., Wylie-Rosett, J. Disordered Eating in Adulthood Is Associated with Reported Weight Loss Attempts in Childhood. *International Journal of Eating Disorders*. (2010) 43; 663–666.

Satter, E. M. *Child of Mine, Feeding with Love and Common Sense*. Bull Publishing Company: Boulder, CO, 2000.

Satter, E. M. *Your Child's Weight: Helping Without Harming*. Kelcy Press: Madison, WI, 2005.

Shunk, A. S., Birch, L. L. Girls at Risk for Overweight at Age 5 Are at Risk for Dietary Restraint, Disinhibited Overeating, Weight Concerns, and Greater Weight Gain from 5 to 9 Years. *Journal of the American Dietetic Association*. (2004) 104:1120–1126.

Stice, E., et al. Naturalistic Weight-reduction Efforts Prospectively Predict Growth in Relative Weight and Onset of Obesity Among Female Adolescents. *Journal of Consulting Clinical Psychology*. (1999) 67: 967–974.

Chapter 16. The Ultimate Path Toward Healing from Eating Disorders

American Psychiatric Association (APA). *Practice Guideline for the Treatment Of Patients with Eating Disorders*. 3rd ed. Washington (D.C.): American Psychiatric Association (APA); 2006.

Tribole, E. Intuitive Eating in the Treatment of Eating Disorders: The Journey of Attunement. *Perspectives*. Winter (2010):11–14.

Tribole, E. Intuitive Eating: Can You Be Healthy and Eat Anything? *Eating Disorders Recovery Today*, Winter 2009.

Tribole, E. Intuitive Eating in the Treatment of Disordered Eating. *SCAN's Pulse*. Summer 2006.

Chapter 17. The Science Behind Intuitive Eating

AED Guidelines for Childhood Obesity Prevention Programs. http://bit.ly/jypTHX [*accessed June 9, 2011*].

Augustus-Horvath, C. L. and Tylka, T. The Acceptance Model of Intuitive Eating: A Comparison of Women in Emerging Adulthood, Early Adulthood, and Middle Adulthood. *J Counseling Psychology* 2011 (Jan) 58:110–125.

Avalos, L.C., & Tylka, T.L. Exploring an Acceptance Model of Intuitive Eating With College Women. *Journal of Counseling Psychology*. (2006) 53, 486–497.

Bacon, L., et al. Size Acceptance and Intuitive Eating Improves Health for Obese, Female Chronic Dieters. *J Am Dietetic Assoc* (2005) 105:929–936.

Cole, R. E. & Horace, K. T. Effectiveness of the "My Body Knows When" Intuitive-eating Pilot Program. *Am J Health Behav*. (2010) 34(3):286–297.

Hahn, Wiseman, Hendrickson, Phillips & Hayden et al. Intuitive Eating and College Female Athletes (in press).

Hawks, S. R. Intuitive Eating and the Nutrition Transition in Asia. *Asia Pac J Clin Nutr*. (2004) 13(2):194–203.

Hawks, S. R. The Intuitive Eating Validation Scale: Preliminary Validation. *Am. J. Health Educ*. (2004) 35:26–35.

Hawks, S. R. Relationship Between Intuitive Eating and Health Indicators Among College Women. *Am. J. Health Educ* 2005; (Nov/Dec):331–336.

Heileson J. L. & R. Cole (2011). Assessing Motivation for Eating and Intuitive Eating in Military Service Members. *Journal of the American Dietetic Association*, 111 (9 Supplement), page A26.

Kristeller, J. L., & Wolever, R. Q. (2011). Mindfulness-based Eating Awareness Training for Treating Binge Eating Disorder: The Conceptual Foundation. *Eating Disorders, 19* (1), 49–61 PMID: 21181579.

Personal communication with J. L. Kristeller, May 20, 2011.

Kroon Van Diest, A. M. & Tylka, T. The Caregiver Eating Messages Scale: Development and Psychometric Investigation. *Body Image 7* (2010) 317–326.

MacDougall, E. C. An Examination of a Culturally Relevant Model of Intuitive Eating with African American College Women. University of Akron, 2010. Dissertation 218 pages.

Madanat, H. N., Hawks, S. R. Validation of the Arabic Version of the Intuitive Eating Scale. *Promot Educ.* 11(3)(2004):152–7.

Madden, C. E. Leong, S. L., Gray, A., and Horwath C. C. Eating in response to hunger and satiety signals is related to BMI in a nationwide sample of 1601 mid-age New Zealand women. *Public Health Nutrition*, (Mar 2012): 1–8.

Mensinger, J. Intuitive Eating: A Novel Health Promotion Strategy for Obese Women. Nov 2009.

Smith M. H. et al. Validation of Two Intuitive Eating Scales Among Females Receiving Inpatient Eating Disorder Treatment. [Abstract 2010 ICED conference]

Smith, T. and Hawks, S. Intuitive Eating, Diet Composition, and the Meaning of Food in Healthy Weight Promotion. *Am J Health Educ* (May/June 2006):130–134.

Smitham, L. Evaluating an Intuitive Eating Program for Binge Eating Disorder: A Benchmarking Study. University of Notre Dame, Dissertation. November 26, 2008.

Tylka, T. L. A Psychometric Evaluation of the Intuitive Eating Scale with College Men (in press).

Tylka, T. L., and Wei, M. Do Perceived Social Support and Self-esteem Mediate the Relationship Between Attachment and Intuitive Eating?

Tylka, T. L. and Wilcox, J. A. Are Intuitive Eating and Eating Disorder Symptomatology Opposite Poles of the Same Construct? *J of Counseling Psychology* 53(2006):474–485.

Tylka, T. L. Development and Psychometric Evaluation of a Measure of Intuitive Eating. *J Counseling Psychology* 53(2)(2006):226.

Vergakis B. DIET: Professor Loses Weight, Keeps It Off by Eating Whatever He Wants. Associated Press. Dec, 5, 2005. [accessed May 4, 2011]

Wei, M., and Tylka, T. L. Do Perceived Body Acceptance by Others and Body Appreciation Mediate the Relationship Between Attachment and Intuitive Eating? (in press).

Weigenberg, M. J. Intuitive Eating Is Associated with Decreased Adiposity (2009, Abstract). http://professional.diabetes.org/Abstracts_Display.aspx?TYP=1&CID=72812 [accessed May 13, 2010].

Young, S. Promoting Healthy Eating Among College Women: Effectiveness of an Intuitive Eating Intervention. Iowa State University, 2011, 147 pages; Dissertation. AAT 3418683.

Resources

Intuitive Eating audio CD, Sounds True, 2009

This is a set of four CDs, which is an excellent companion to our book. The CDs focus on the practical "how-to" aspects of Intuitive Eating. This is not a verbatim reading of the book, but a discussion format with guided practices for all of the ten principles of Intuitive Eating.

Intuitive Eating Official Web site

www.IntuitiveEating.org

Get the latest news from our blog and calendar of events. You will also find articles, research, interviews, and general information about Intuitive Eating.

Counseling and Support

Certified Intuitive Eating Counselor Directory

www.IntuitiveEatingCounselorDirectory.org

This is a listing of allied health professionals who are trained and certified in the Intuitive Eating process. We receive numerous requests for local Intuitive Eating health professionals. To help fill this gap, we offer certification for allied health professionals. These health professionals include dietitians, psychotherapists, physicians, physical therapists, nurses, chiropractors, dentists, occupational therapists, licensed massage therapists, licensed physical trainers, certified health education specialists, licensed health and life coaches, and others in the health profession who espouse the Intuitive Eating principles in their work.

Intuitive Eating Online Community
www.IntuitiveEatingCommunity.org
Get inspired, share your story, and partake of the many tools to empower your Intuitive Eating journey. This is your community—it's free, but you will need to sign up.

Professional Resources

How to Become a Certified Intuitive Eating Counselor
We are eager to spread the message of Intuitive Eating through allied health professionals who qualify to be certified and listed on our Intuitive Eating Counselor Directory. There are two main ways to become a certified Intuitive Eating counselor:

1. Self-study program administered by Helm Publishing, which is based on both on the Intuitive Eating book and a full-day workshop CD that Elyse and Evelyn facilitated for health professionals. Upon completion of the self-study program and passing an exam, you qualify as a Certified Intuitive Eating Counselor. This is an independent study on your own schedule. For more information see: http://bit.ly/k6CJDe.
2. Participate in training with either Elyse or Evelyn, in addition to passing a written exam.

For more details and information see these Web sites:

www.EvelynTribole.com
www.ElyseResch.com
www.IntuitiveEatingProTraining.com

Intuitive Eating Professionals on LinkedIn
http://linkd.in/mMrn2M
This is an international group of over nineteen hundred allied health professionals, where we share news, views, and resources. It's free to join.

Intuitive Eating Client Worksheets
www.Intuitive-Eating-Worksheets.com
Help your clients through the Intuitive Eating process by using this easy-to-use, reproducible set of twenty-one worksheets.

Index